COLLEGE LIBRARY
SUFFOLK UNIVERSITY
BOSTON, MASS. 02114

Hospital Organization and Management:
Text and Readings
Second Edition

Health Systems Management
Edited by **Samuel Levey, Ph.D.,** *City University of New York,* and **Alan Sheldon, M.D.,** *Harvard School of Public Health*

Volume 1:
Financial Management of Health Institutions
J.B. Silvers and C.K. Prahalad
ISBN 0-470-79173-X 1974

Volume 2:
Personnel Administration in the Health Services Industry: Theory & Practice
Norman Metzger
ISBN 0-470-59993-6 1974

Volume 3:
The National Labor Relations Act: A Guidebook for Health Care Facility Administrators
Dennis D. Pointer and Norman Metzger
ISBN 0-470-69146-8 1975

Volume 4:
Organizational Issues in Health Care Management
Alan Sheldon
ISBN 0-470-78275-7 1975

Volume 5:
Long Term Care: A Handbook for Researchers, Planners and Providers
Sylvia Sherwood, Editor
ISBN 0-470-78600-0 1975

Volume 6:
Analysis of Urban Health Problems: Case Studies from the Health Services Administration of the City of New York
Irving Leveson and Jeffrey H. Weiss, Editors
ISBN 0-470-14983-3 1976

Volume 7:
Health Maintenance Organizations: A Guide to Planning and Development
Roger W. Birnbaum
ISBN 0-470-14984-1 1976

Volume 8:
Labor Arbitration in Health Care
Earl R. Baderschneider and Paul F. Miller, Editors
ISBN 0-470-15037-8 1976

Volume 9:
The Consumer and the Health Care System: Social and Managerial Perspectives
Harry Rosen, Jonathan M. Metsch and Samuel Levey, Editors
ISBN 0-89335-005-2 1977

Volume 10:
Long-Term Care Administration: A Managerial Perspective, I & II
Samuel Levey and N. Paul Loomba, Editors
ISBN 0-89335-004-4 (I) 1977
ISBN 0-89335-015-X (II) 1977

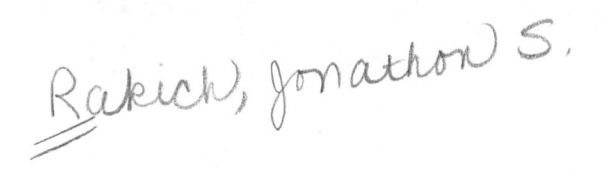

Hospital Organization and Management:

Text and Readings

Second Edition

Edited by

Jonathon S. Rakich, Ph.D.
Professor of Management
Director of Graduate Programs
College of Business Administration
University of Akron
Akron, Ohio

and

Kurt Darr, J.D., Sc.D.
Professor of Health Care Administration
Assistant Dean
School of Government and Business
The George Washington University
Washington, D.C.

SP

SP MEDICAL & SCIENTIFIC BOOKS
a division of Spectrum Publications, Inc.
New York • London

Distributed by Halsted Press
A Division of John Wiley & Sons

New York   Toronto   London   Sydney

Copyright © 1978 Spectrum Publications, Inc.

All rights reserved. No part of this book may be reproduced in any form, by photostat, microform, retrieval system, or any other means without prior written permission of the copyright holder or his licensee.

SPECTRUM PUBLICATIONS, INC.
175-20 Wexford Terrace, Jamaica New York 11432
Second Printing
Library of Congress Cataloging in Publication Data

Rakich, Jonathon S   comp.
   Hospital organization and management.

  (Health systems management ; 11)
  Includes bibliographies and index.
  1. Hospitals--Administration–Addresses, essays, lectures. I. Darr, Kurt II. Title.
[DNLM: I. Hospital administration--Collected works. W1 HE588F v. 11 / WX150 H83]
RA971.R25   1977   658'.91'3621108   77-24710
ISBN 0-89335-029-X

Distributed solely by the Halsted Press Division of John Wiley & Sons, Inc.
New York, New York
ISBN 0-470-99179-8

To the Hospital Manager

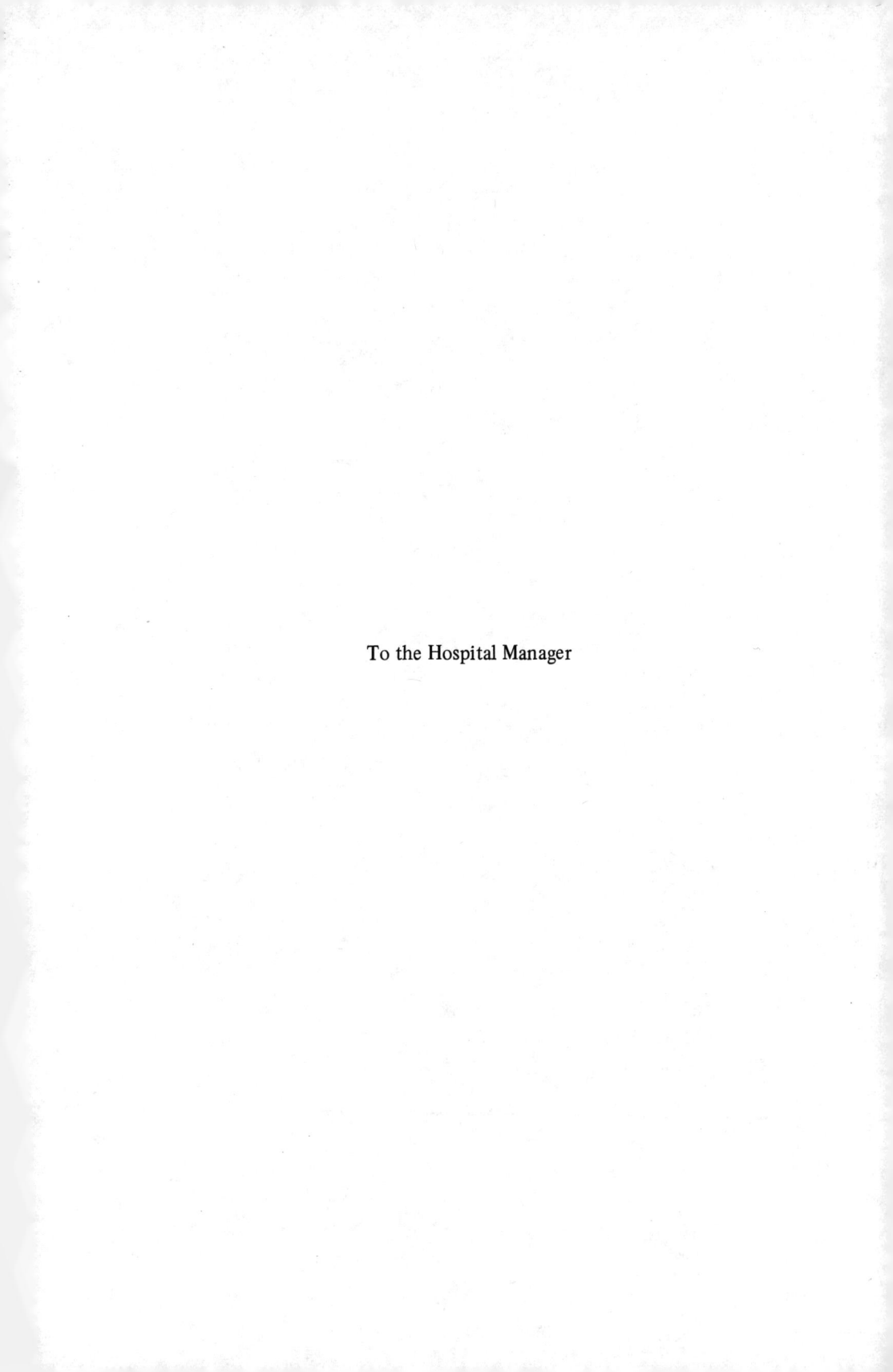

ACKNOWLEDGMENTS

We first acknowledge our wives, Tana Rakich and Anne Darr. Their cooperation and and encouragement made our work easier.

We would like to thank *Harvard Business Review, Hospital and Health Services Administration, Hospital Progress, Hospitals, Inquiry, Journal of Nursing Administration, The New England Journal of Medicine, Supervisor Nurse, Topics in Health Care Financing,* G.P. Putnam's Sons, and the Macmillan Company for permission to reprint articles and excerpts contained in this book. We thank the Catholic Hospital Association for releasing the first edition copyright.

Our warm appreciation is extended to those authors whose writing is contained in this book. To each we say, thank you. We acknowledge the editorial guidance given by Professor Samuel Levey, Director of the Graduate Program in Hospital and Health Administration at the University of Iowa, and the constructive reviews given by Professor Milton C. Devolites, Department of Health Care Administration, The George Washington University, Washington, D.C. We also thank our employers for providing the organizational support to assist us. Specifically, we acknowledge Professor Frank Simonetti, Professor Leon Gintzig, Dean James W. Dunlap, and Dean Peter B. Vaill.

Others provided research assistance and we thank them: David Hau, David Cox, Charles McKnight, and Suzanne Blumenthal. Those who helped in manuscript preparation are also owed our gratitude: Helen Scherrer and Syed Hossain. Finally, we thank Spectrum Publications' personnel for their cooperation and assistance; in particular, our editor, Leslie Tick.

CONTENTS

Acknowledgements
Preface
Foreword
Introduction

PART I. THE HOSPITAL AS AN ORGANIZATION   1

Introduction . . . 1
Complexity of Hospitals . . . 1
Historical Development of Hospitals . . . 2
    Hospitals and Early Christianity
    The Renaissance
    Period of Growth (1860-1920)
    Consolidation (1920-1950)
Hospital Organization (Triad) . . . 7
    New Models
The Governing Authority . . . 10
The Administrator . . . 11
The Medical Staff . . . 12
Bibliography . . . 13

SELECTIONS

    Organization

    1. The Hospital as an Organization, *Basil S. Georgopoulos and Floyd C. Mann*   19

    2. The Hospital as a Matrix Organization, *Duncan Neuhauser*   29

    3. Strictures and Structures, *Ray E. Brown*   43

    4. The Hospital as a Prototype Organization, *Alan D. Bauerschmidt*   46

    5. Hospital Administration and Systems Concepts, *Fremont E. Kast and James E. Rosenzweig*   53

    6. Corporate Models in Health Care Delivery, *Lynda Diane Baydin and Alan Sheldon*   64

Governing Authority

7. The Board of Trustees, *Temple Burling, Edith M. Lentz, and Robert N. Wilson*   75

8. Current Perspectives on Hospital Governance, *Lawrence D. Prybil and David B. Starkweather*   84

9. Should Doctors Be on Your Board? *C. Jerome Jorgensen*   91

10. Governing Boards, *Anthony R. Kovner*   97

The Administrator

11. What is Health Administration? *Charles J. Austin*   105

12. The Lessons of a Profession, *Everett A. Johnson*   117

The Medical Staff

13. Medical Staff Functions and Leadership, *William W. Jack*   125

14. The Hospital Medical Director: An Administrator's View, *James D. Harvey*   132

15. Hospital Medical Staff Organization: Structure, Process, and Outcome, *Stephen M. Shortell*   137

PART II. THE MANAGEMENT OF HOSPITAL PERSONNEL   **147**

Employee Motivation . . . **147**
Need Hierarchy . . . **147**
Job Satisfaction . . . **149**
Leadership and Supervision . . . **150**
    Leadership: Degree of Decision-making Authority
        Held by the Manager
    Leadership: Manner of Overseeing the Accomplishment
        of Work Activity
Linkage . . . **152**
Factors Affecting Styles . . . **152**

Managerial Approaches . . . 154
Theory X and Theory Y . . . 154
Participative Management . . . 156
Delegation . . . 157
Bibliography . . . 158

SELECTIONS

Employee Motivation

16. The Organization as a Social System, *Ted R. Brannen*	164
17. The Growing Need for Motivated Nurses, *Francis G. Edwards*	169

Leadership and Supervision

18. Effective Supervision Requires Leadership, *Thomas R. O'Donovan*	177
19. A Situational Approach to Supervision: Leadership Theory and the Supervising Nurse, *Paul Hersey, Kenneth H. Blanchard, and Elaine L. LaMonica*	184

Managerial Approaches

20. Participative Management: A Valid Alternative to Traditional Organizational Behavior, *Barbara Snyder Hill*	193
21. Mastering the Managerial Skill of Delegation, *Elena M. Volante*	199

PART III. HOSPITAL UNIONIZATION — 205

The Union Movement . . . 205
Wagner Act of 1935 and Employer Unfair Labor Practices . . . 207
Taft-Hartley Act of 1947 and Union Unfair Labor Practices . . . 207
Effect of the NLRA and Taft-Hartley Acts . . . 207
1974 Amendments to Taft-Hartley . . . 208
Unionization Issues and Procedures . . . 210
Why Employees Unionize . . . 211
Administrative Philosophy . . . 212

Strategy ... 214
Bibliography ... 215

SELECTIONS

The 1974 Taft-Hartley Amendments

22. Recognition and Negotiation Under Taft-Hartley, *Randyl D. Elkin*   221

23. Negotiating and Administering a Union Contract, *Randyl D. Elkin*   229

Unionization Issues and Procedures

24. The Effect of Unions on Hospital Management, *Leo B. Osterhaus*   240

25. The Nurse as a Professional and as a Unionist, *Richard L. Epstein and K. Bruce Stickler*   249

26. Solicitation Rules Will Need Revision, *William J. Emanuel and Alfred Klein*   260

27. Grievance Procedure: Outlet for Employees, Insight for Management, *Rod Clelland*   269

PART IV. QUANTITATIVE APPROACHES TO DECISION-MAKING   273

Resource Allocation ... 273 ✓
Objective Functions ... 274
Decision-Making ... 274
Quantitative Techniques ... 276
    Planning
    Control
    Evaluation of Alternatives
Bibliography ... 279

SELECTIONS

Decision-Making

28. Anatomy of a Decision, *Edward J. Spillane*   285

Quantitative Techniques

29. Operations Research in Health and Hospital Administration, *Ronald L. Gue* — 294

30. The Application of Linear Programming to Decision-Making in Hospitals, *William L. Dowling* — 308

31. Estimating Bed Needs By Means of Queuing Theory, *James K. Cooper and Timothy M. Corcoran* — 316

32. Capital Budgeting Decision-Making for Hospitals, *Richard F. Wacht* — 320 ✓

PART V. HEALTH CARE POLICY ISSUES AND TRENDS — 331

Government Involvement—Issues and Bases . . . 331
The Constitution . . . 331
Curative Medicine and Public Health . . . 333
Evolution of Federal Involvement . . . 334
    Pre-Medicare and Medicaid
    Post-Medicare and Medicaid
New Environment for Hospitals . . . 336
Regulation and National Health Insurance . . . 337
Accountability and Quality Assurance . . . 338
Bibliography . . . 340

SELECTIONS

Responsibility

33. A Trustee Views the Voluntary Hospital System, *Ray R. Eppert* — 345

34. The Social Responsibility of General Hospitals, *Bright M. Dornblaser* — 354

Planning and Programs

35. Effective Planning Committees for Hospitals, *James B. Webber and Martha A. Dula* — 363

36. Prospective Rate Setting: Concept and Practice,
    William L. Dowling — **377**

37. Institutional Providers and the Professional Standards Review
    Organization, *Kurt Darr* — **411**

   Health Care Policy Issues

38. The Crisis in the Health Care System: A Contrary Opinion,
    S. David Pomrinse — **423**

39. What Can Be Learned from Regulation of Other Industries?
    David B. Starkweather — **438**

40. Policy Considerations in National Health Insurance, *Kurt Darr* — **444**

41. Health and Public Policy, *Herman M. Somers* — **456**

SUBJECT INDEX — **469**

PREFACE

The first edition of this book was published in 1972. Its purpose was to offer a compilation of readings on hospital organization and management from a managerial perspective. The second edition has the same purpose and the five part categorization of subject matter is similar: I. THE HOSPITAL AS AN ORGANIZATION: II. THE MANAGEMENT OF HOSPITAL PERSONNEL; III. HOSPITAL UNIONIZATION; IV. QUANTITATIVE APPROACHES TO DECISION-MAKING; and V. HEALTH CARE POLICY ISSUES AND TRENDS. Of the 41 selections in the second edition, 24 are new. The 17 retained from the first edition are among classics in the field.

In this edition, the manner of presentation has changed. Each of the five parts contains editor's textual material which introduces the articles selected. This textual material serves to 1. orient the reader to the subject matter under consideration, 2. link the specific selections in each part to the general subject, thereby amplifying the text material, and 3. tie all the parts together. In addition, this edition includes a new and useful feature—a bibliography at the end of each text portion. It will assist those readers who wish to pursue a subject in greater depth. When certain bibliographic entries are in point, they are cited, by author, in the textual material. The topic index will be useful as a ready means of reference. J.S. Rakich authored the introductory material for Parts II, III, and IV; K. Darr authored the introductory material for Parts I and V.

We believe various professionals will be interested in the material this book presents. Students enrolled in graduate programs in health services administration will find this a useful source. Those pursuing baccalaureate education in the allied health professions, particularly nursing, may have coursework which addresses issues and problems contained in this book. It can serve as a reference text for instructor lecture and/or class discussion. Finally, we anticipate that busy managers employed by hospitals and other health services institutions will find this book a practical tool.

We are hopeful that this work will be a constructive contribution to the hospital and health services administration field. The focus and orientation of this book reflects our attempt to isolate one segment.

Jonathon S. Rakich
Akron, Ohio

Kurt Darr
Washington, D.C.

FOREWORD

As one astute observer has already pointed out, many of the modern disciplines possess a long history, but a short past. Health care management is very much a member of that family.

Twenty years ago the total body of literature on hospital administration was fully within a single individual's capacity to review, and even perhaps to own. Today, that body reflects an explosive and relentless expansion similar in magnitude to that which began among the professional medical specialties much earlier. If one thing becomes necessary in the face of this avalanche of material—both good and bad—it is the exercise of selectivity.

In this volume two young authors offer—above all—an expertly selected range of material. As with the initial edition in 1972, selectivity marks each element of all of its parts.

Those of us engaged in management of modern health care institutions owe our compliments to Jonathon Rakich and Kurt Darr, as well as to the contributors of the selected, original articles. Taken as a whole, this volume instructs, enlightens, and provokes. It will prove inspiring to some, and useful to all.

L.R. Jordan
President
Alton Ochsner Medical Foundation
New Orleans, Louisiana

INTRODUCTION

The contemporary hospital in the United States bears little resemblance to the hospital of the latter half of the 19th century. Today's hospital is the major institution in the health care delivery system. Advances in technology and medicine have increased its importance and continue to enlarge its role. The hospital is the organizational entity in which sophisticated equipment, technology, and paraprofessional and professional personnel are gathered to provide health care services. Since 1950 the hospital has rapidly expanded its use of our nation's resources for health care and is taking an increasingly disproportionate share. The concept of "health care as a right" has emerged and will be a factor in the enactment of some form of national health insurance. Consequently, increased governmental involvement and intervention, consumer scrutiny, and demands for accountability and efficiency are forces confronting today's hospital administrator.

COSTS

The dramatic rise in health care and hospital expenditures since 1950 is shown in Figure 1. In 1950 total health care expenditures were $12 billion, representing 4.6 percent of the nation's gross national product (GNP). By 1975 they had risen tenfold to almost $120 billion and represented 8.3 percent of GNP. Expenditures for hospital services have had a similar growth rate and currently approximate 40 percent of all health care expenditures. In total, health care is one of the largest industries in our nation's economy.

NUMBER OF HOSPITAL ADMISSIONS AND OTHER DATA

Table 1 and Figure 2 provide data from which several conclusions can be drawn. Although the number of hospitals and beds has not increased appreciably since 1950, Table 1 indicates that employed personnel has more than tripled, from 1.0 million

Hospital Organization and Management

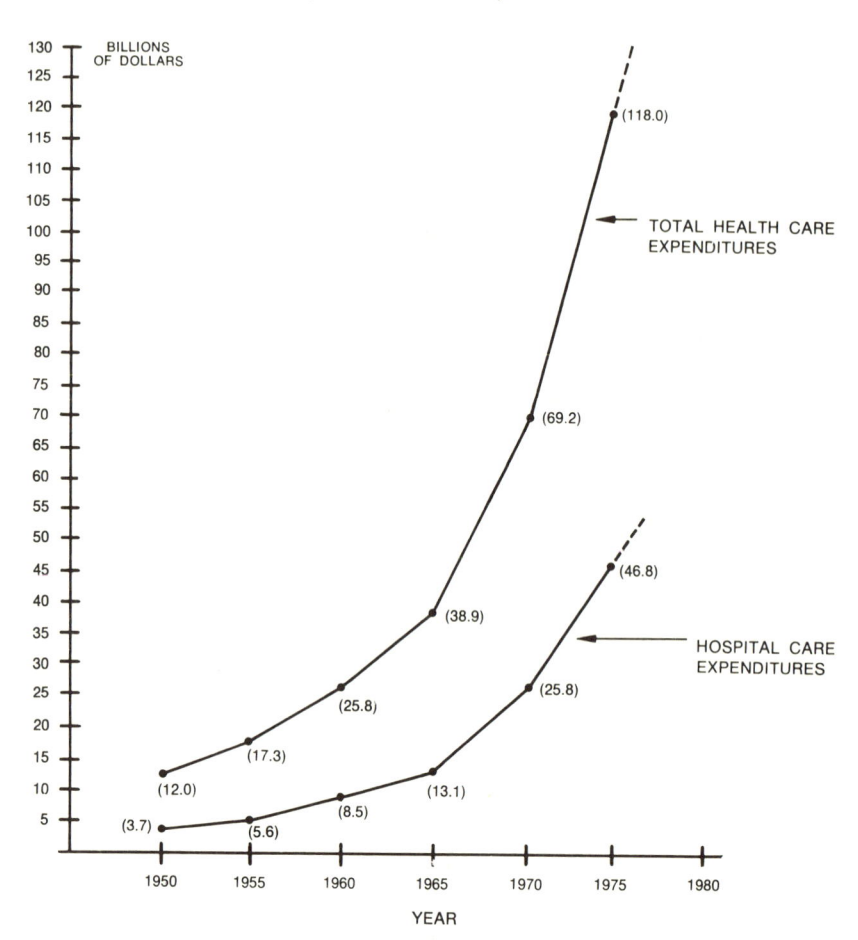

Figure 1. Total United States Health Care and Hospital Care Expenditures, Selected Years (in billions of dollars)

Source: "National Health Care Expenditures, Fiscal 1975," *Social Security Bulletin,* Vol. 39, (February, 1976) and "National Health Care Expenditures, 1929-73," *Social Security Bulletin,* Vol. 37, (February, 1974).

to 3.0 million (84 to 269 per 100 beds). Initially, this appears inconsistent. However, the data on annual hospital admissions and outpatient visits presented in Figure 2 indicate that more people are being served by roughly the same facility base (5 percent increase in the number of hospitals with no significant increase in the number of beds), partly because of the utilization of more personnel, but primarily because of decreased length of inpatient stays and more emphasis on outpatient services.

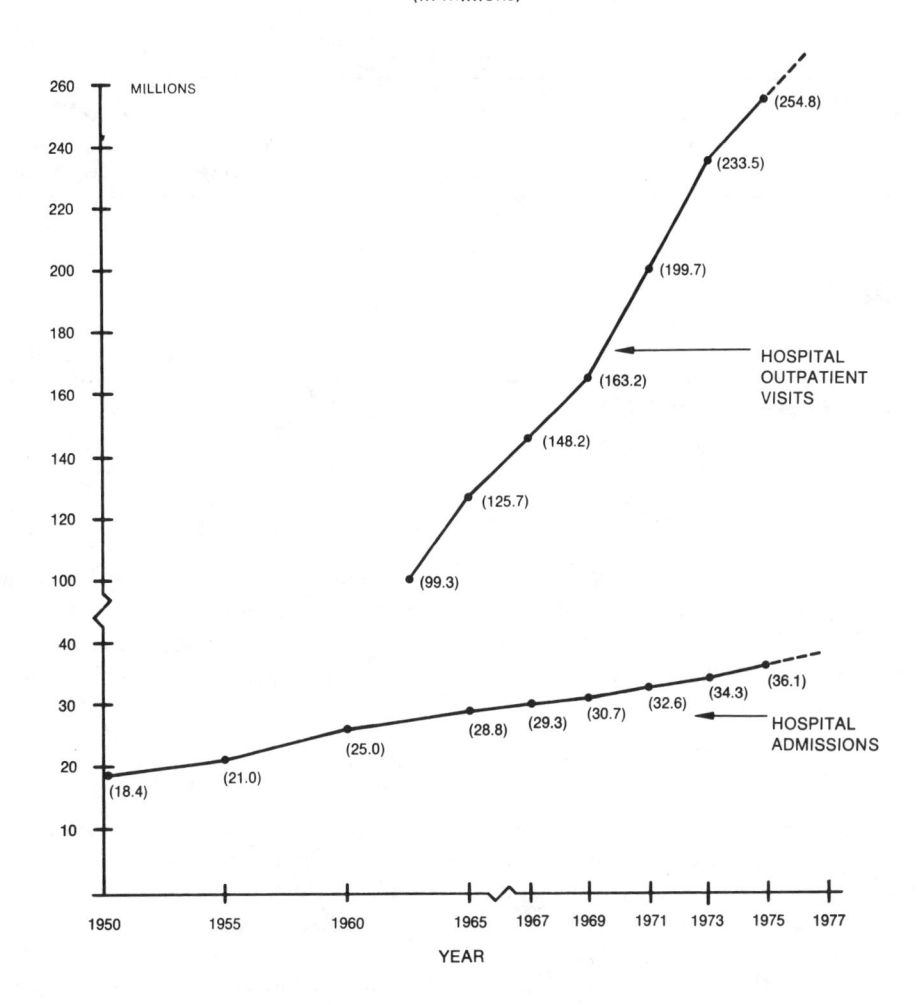

Figure 2. Hospital Admissions and Outpatient Visits, Selected Years
(in millions)

Source: Hospital Statistics, 1976. Chicago: American Hospital Association (1976), p. 3.

Hospitals can be classified in several different categories: length of stay (short-term or long-term), type of service, and type of control. The length of stay category is based on whether patients stay fewer than 30 days (short-term or acute), or 30 days or more (long-term). Approximately 90 percent of our nation's hospitals are short-term. "Type of service" denotes whether the hospital primarily provides general medical and surgical services, rehabilitative, maternity, psychiatric, or pediatric ser-

TABLE 1

NUMBER OF AHA REGISTERED HOSPITALS AND PERSONNEL, SELECTED YEARS

Year	Number of AHA registered Hospitals	Number of beds (in thousands)	Personnel (in thousands)	Personnel per 100 bed census
1950	6,788	1,456	1,058	84
1955	6,956	1,604	1,301	95
1960	6,876	1,653	1,598	114
1965	7,123	1,704	1,952	139
1970	7,123	1,616	2,537	196
1975	7,156	1,466	3,023	269

Source: *Hospital Statistics, 1976.* Chicago: American Hospital Association (August, 1976), Table 2.

vices. The third category classifies hospitals by type of control, or ownership; not-for-profit, profit (investor-owned), and government (federal, state, local). Approximately 50 percent of hospitals are not-for-profit, 12 percent are investor-owned, and 38 percent are government-controlled with two-thirds of them controlled by local government.

A SYSTEMS FRAME OF REFERENCE

There are many problems and challenges facing today's hospital administrator. Among them are rising health care costs which are expected to exceed $200 billion by 1980, greater consumer expectations, demands for increased accountability and cost containment, greater federal control, and structural changes in the delivery of health care.

To demonstrate the importance of these challenges, portraying hospitals from a systems perspective is helpful. The hospital is unique. To its patients, it is a place to receive care. To physicians and employees, it is a place to work. To the administrator, it is a multi-faceted organization embracing patient care, facility maintenance, financial, custodial, and food service activities. This complex organization functions within a larger set of institutions providing health care and requires the coordination of people and activities.

When viewed from a systems model (Figure 3) the hospital consists of a set of subsystems, each interrelated and interdependent.[1] All of them must be managed, coordinated, and directed so that the institution's purposes can be accomplished. In terms

Figure 3

The Hospital as a System

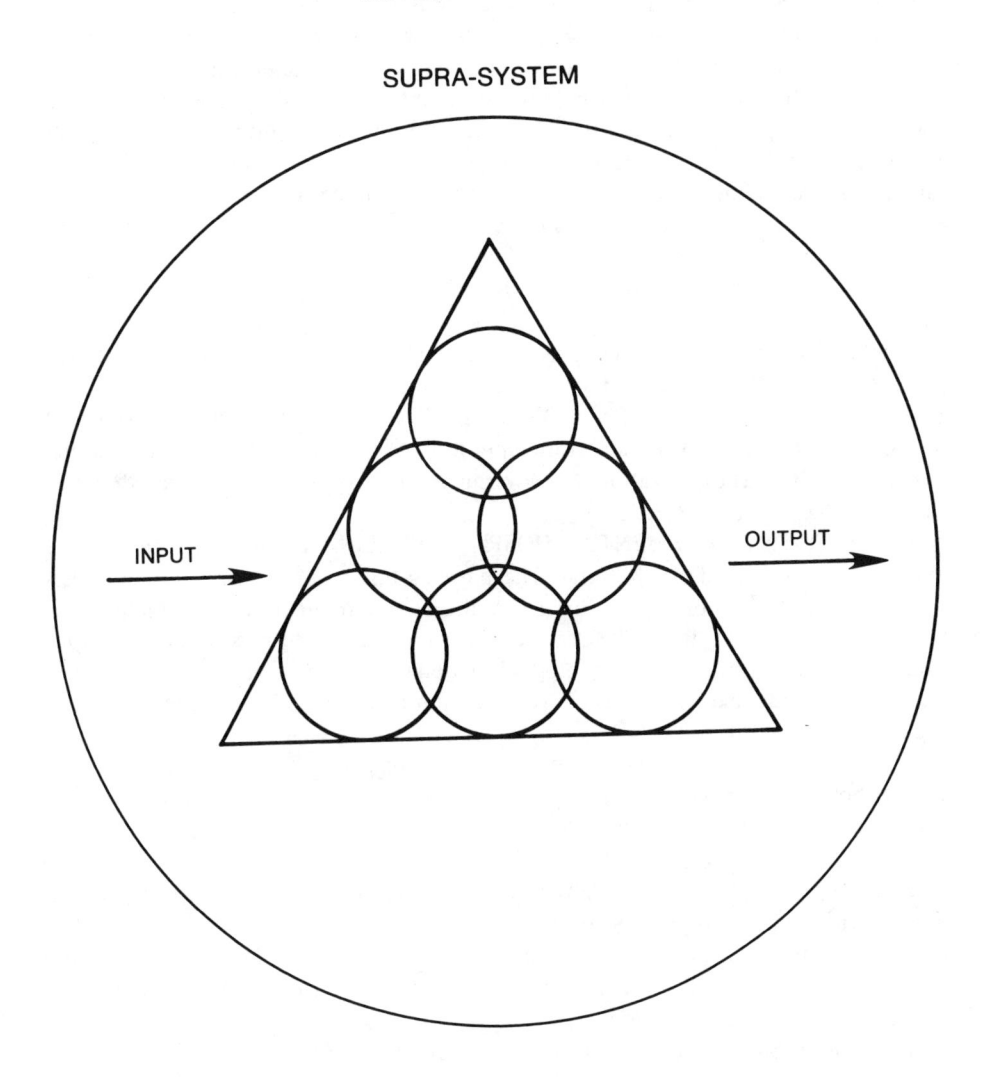

SUPRA-SYSTEM

INPUT →

OUTPUT →

of management, "the administrator must understand the hospital, not as a number of isolated parts, but as a system; he must have knowledge of the relationships between the parts and be aware of their interaction."[2]

Portrayed as a system, the hospital resides within a "supra-system," which is its external environment. When viewing the larger supra-system (health care delivery), the individual hospital with its own subsystems becomes a subsystem within itself. The hospital does not exist in isolation, but in a dynamic environment. It must react to the environment and cope with it. At the same time the hospital must be aware of its impact on the environment. The 1960s and 1970s brought changes in that environment which have and will continue to have a major impact on hospitals in terms of responsibilities, resource utilization, and costs, to name only a few.

Extending the systems model permits an examination of input and output. The hospital as an organizational entity utilizes input resources to generate output. Austin views hospital administration as the process of converting input composed of organization resources (men, money, material, and technology) into output which is identified as patient care, education, and/or research.[3]

LINKAGE

This book is divided into five parts. Each part introduces the broad subject area and contains carefully selected articles which address specific issues.

Part I, THE HOSPITAL AS AN ORGANIZATION, focuses on the organizational design of the hospital. In this structure input is converted into output. Sections which describe hospital (a) organization, (b) governing authority, (c) the administrator, and (d) the medical staff are included.

Part II, THE MANAGEMENT OF HOSPITAL PERSONNEL, is concerned with the manpower resources of the hospital. The nation's hospitals employ 3.0 million persons. Two-thirds of hospital annual expenditures, approximately $47 billion, comprises employee costs. It can be argued that manpower is the most important input utilized by the hospital. The technological, material, and financial resources are inert and only when people serve as a catalyst can input be converted to the final output of the organization.

If one acknowledges manpower to be a major ingredient (input) for the provision of the hospital's service, it is also possible to view manpower as an organizational asset. Part II contains selections which discuss the motivation of hospital employees and their leadership and supervision.

Part III is HOSPITAL UNIONIZATION. Passage of the not-for-profit hospital amendments to the Taft-Hartley Act in 1974 was an event which has and will continue to have an impact on the "supra" health care delivery system and on individual hospitals. The first section in Part III is concerned with the 1974 Taft-Hartley Amendments; the second presents unionization issues and procedures.

Decisions regarding hospital management consider output (objectives) and input (resources). Particularly important are decisions which involve organizational change, planning, directing, and controlling. The decision-making process and quantitative techniques are examined in Part IV, QUANTITATIVE APPROACHES TO DECISION-MAKING.

The final part, HEALTH CARE POLICY ISSUES AND TRENDS, focuses on the "supra-system," the hospital's external environment. Sections in this part review the societal responsibility of the hospital, internally and externally imposed plans and programs, and health care policy issues of importance in governance and management of the contemporary hospital.

FOOTNOTES

[1] See: Samuel Levey and N. Paul Loomba, *Health Care Administration: A Managerial Perspective,* (Philadelphia: J.B. Lippincott Company, 1973), Chapter 2.

[2] See selection 5. , p. 62.

[3] See selection 11, p. 110.

Hospital Organization and Management:
Text and Readings
Second Edition

Part I
THE HOSPITAL AS AN ORGANIZATION

INTRODUCTION

Persons representing a variety of disciplines have turned their attention to health care. Operations researchers, engineers, accountants, attorneys, political scientists, and politicians are participating in health care administration. Hospitals are the major recipient of this increased attention. In addition to being highly visible, bricks-and-mortar organizations, hospitals are suggested as the focal point of health care delivery. It follows that concern about the ever increasing rise in the cost of health care services has also focused on hospitals (Prims and Delesie).

For hospitals and their personnel, from governing authority on down, this is future shock. Hospitals are faced with new environments and confronted with new rules. Many of the old assumptions regarding hospitals and their philosophies are being challenged. Those in leadership positions, both within and outside the health care field, have asserted that there is a health care crisis. Although it is a crisis with many facets, it is not a crisis to cause the system to collapse or disintegrate. Questions are raised about the costs and the efficacy of medical care, the desirability of receiving it, the fallibility of the physician, and the ability of the health care system to save people from imprudent lifestyles, unhealthy environment, and individual genetic makeup. Best stated, it is a crisis of confidence.

COMPLEXITY OF HOSPITALS

The hospital has been and continues to be one of the most complex organizations in existence. This complexity requires organizational arrangements which have been termed by some authors as prototypical, e.g., task teams composed of a wide variety of skilled professionals are commonplace in hospitals. Some theorists who have conducted studies about hospitals are surprised that such institutions function at all.

The complexity of the modern hospital results from a number of attributes:

1. *Within the institution, there is a wide diversity of objectives and goals for different personnel and subsystems.* Various segments of the hospital will be responsible for, or involved in, patient care, education, research, hotel-type accommodations and problems, and carrying out complex and sophisticated medical and surgical procedures. These various activities are sometimes contradictory and often in conflict.

2. *The diversity of personnel ranges from the most highly skilled and educated physicians and administrators to unskilled and uneducated employees.* Enabling them to work together is a major responsibility of the hospital manager.
3. *The hospital is in continuous operation.* This requires high standby costs and involves substantial personnel and scheduling problems.
4. *In many areas of hospital operations there are dual lines of authority.* Administrators are responsible for solving a wide variety of management problems, and physicians are responsible for patient care, education, and research. Often these two seemingly distinct areas of activity overlap, and, in fact, some employees may have two or more persons to whom they are responsible.
5. *Hospitals deal with problems of life and death.* This puts a special psychological and physical stress on personnel at all levels of the organization—it is not the usual service organization. Often the setting and results cause consumers to be hypercritical.
6. *There is a problem in measuring the major product.* The patient care rendered in the hospital has eluded precise measurement. Although there has been some progress in determining the quality of care, many questions remain unanswered and substantial disagreement exists among the experts as to how and what should be measured.

These attributes are unlikely to change. In fact, increasingly the technology used by hospitals is more expensive and complicated; therefore, managing the institution is likely to become more difficult (Schulz and Johnson).

HISTORICAL DEVELOPMENT OF HOSPITALS

Historically, the earliest evidence of institutionalized care for the ill can be found about 1200 B.C. in Greek temples. Hippocrates (460?-370? B.C.), the most prominent Greek physician, was instrumental in separating medicine from religion and philosophy. He is credited with addressing medicine from a rational standpoint and the foundations of modern medicine are built upon his work. Medical training gained importance in this era, as did recognition of environmental influences on health and disease. Religion, however, undoubtedly continued to play a fundamental role in the development of hospitals.

Greek medicine reached its zenith during the Golden Age of Greece, about 400 B.C., when the temples of Aesculapius emerged.[1] Considered among the earliest hospitals in Greek and Roman civilizations, the temples were used both as houses of worship and as shelters for the diseased. The patients were often ambulatory. The care in Aesculapia was non-brutal, emphasizing patient exposure to the open air and sunshine as well as a regimen of rest, relaxation, baths, exercise, and proper diet. Such temples were similar in nature to modern day spas—the individual and his body were given the support for recuperation and restoration to health. Limited medication was prescribed to patients at the Aesculapia; the records show that many did regain their health as a result of these simple regimens.

The first hospitals evidencing modern features were found in ancient Egypt and India.[2] In Egypt, at approximately 600 B.C., medical care was often rendered in healing temples. Egyptian priest-physicians were among the first to prescribe practical drugs, and they performed limited surgery and set fractures. Between 273-232 B.C., hospitals called Cikista were built in India. Hindu physicians were adept surgeons and medications were administered. Such institutions were noted for their high state of cleanliness and sanitation. Patients remained overnight and were cared for by attendants.

Hospitals and Early Christianity

The Christian era stressed humanitarianism. During that period ecclesiastic hostels were built adjacent to churches so that priests could conveniently care for and offer solace to patients. By the year 500 A.D., almost every city throughout the old Roman empire had established church-related hospitals. Religious beliefs superseded scientific, Hippocratic knowledge in treatment of patients. Christianity prevailed in the provision of medical care, emphasizing above all else the importance of compassion and care for each patient, often at the expense of scientific knowledge.

After the fall of Rome, and especially during the Middle Ages (A.D. 500-1450), hospitals were marked by increasingly strong religious influence. Medical advances used in India, Egypt, and the Roman empire were lost as these civilizations disintegrated. During the Middle Ages, a very bleak period for hospitals, medical knowledge which had been developed went unused, primarily because of social and religious pressures. Renewed emphasis on supernatural influences in health and disease occurred as the Christian church gained a prominent role in dictating the processes of medical treatment.

The Middle East did not have the decline in the quality of medicine which occurred in western Europe during the Middle Ages. Mohammedan physicians were acquainted with use of inhalation anesthesia and they originated the use of a vast number of new drugs. Moslem countries had asylums for the mentally ill a thousand years before such institutions appeared in Europe.[3] Built in Cairo in the 13th century, Al-Mansur Hospital was equipped with separate wards for more serious diseases, had outpatient clinics, and operated homes for the convalescent.[4]

The Renaissance

The value of scientific medical knowledge was not rediscovered until the Renaissance, beginning in the 14th century. Ironically, though Christianity was a major inhibiting force in the use of such medical knowledge, much of it was recorded in books prepared and preserved by monasteries during the Middle Ages. As the writings of early Greeks were revived, 16th century scholars applied their knowledge in the development of new scientific theories. This rebirth of interest in scientific medicine encouraged physicians to attempt procedures which exceeded their knowledge of science and their ability to prevent or understand the consequences of their actions. The hospital's reputation was not enhanced by these increasingly daring surgeons. During the late 18th and early 19th centuries, wound infection was ubiquitous and puss drainage was considered a sign of healing. Brutal medical treatment such as bleeding, purging, violent emetics, and cathartics were commonly used. A good surgeon was one who could operate quickly—the lack of anesthesia made the patient's pain unbearable and he was rather difficult to control.

The hospital* had shifted from religious orientation to medical orientation. The Renaissance succeeded in substantially separating science from religion, establishing clearly the scientific approach to medical matters. Although religious conflicts were to emerge occasionally, scientific inquiry finally became the dominant influence in medical care delivery.

The oldest existing hospital in western Europe is the Hotel-Dieu, Paris, France, founded in A.D. 550 and rebuilt in the 13th century. Malcolm T. MacEachern,[5] hospital historian, writer, and theorist, describes it as a hospital not unlike today's facility. In its construction the importance of separating individuals in different disease states and various stages of recovery was emphasized and the hospital was divided into wards. For instance, there were sections for convalescent and maternity patients. Departments with specialized functions were directed by a department head, and others were assigned to specialty tasks such as food, drugs, laundry, and dressings. A kind of governing authority, the board of provisors, inspected the institution twice a year.

Period of Growth (1860-1920)

The first hospital in the United States, the Pennsylvania Hospital, was founded in 1751. In 1798 Congress passed legislation establishing the Marine Hospital Service for merchant seamen. However, in the United States, 1860 to 1920 was the period of explosive hospital growth. Hospitals increased from several hundred in the 1870s to a peak of 7,370 in 1924.[6] During these years medicine evolved from an age of ignorance to an age of basic technology and science. Advances during this period laid the foundation for 20th century medicine and the modern hospital. The discovery of anesthesia in the late 1840s was the first of many events which led to changes in medical philosophy and treatment modes. The homeopaths and eclectic medical sects reached a peak of influence, but declined as allopathic medicine matured after the turn of the century. The heroic and vigorous therapy treatment modes gave way to those based on scientific knowledge. Use of antiseptic surgery in the 1860s yielded to aseptic surgery based on the germ theory of disease after the bacteriologists discovered the link between micro-organisms and disease. Koch's study of anthrax and tubercu-

---

*The English word hospital is derived from the Latin "hospitalis" and "hospes," meaning a host or guest.

losis, and Pasteur's work with rabies and cholera in the 1880s were part of these break-throughs.[7]

Diagnostic techniques also contributed to the emerging role of the hospital. Roentgen's discovery of the X-ray in 1895,[8] blood typing in 1900 (safer transfusions), development of the electrocardiograph in 1902, and the Curies' experimentation with radium were only a few of the era's scientific advances.

These developments permitted surgeons to increase their intervention in disease processes and to do so with decreasing mortality and greater efficacy. A place for the focus of this technology had to be found. Hospitals, already established, offered surgeons a physical facility, equipment, personnel, and perhaps most importantly, an organizational framework within which modern surgery could be performed. Primarily, the development of the 20th century hospital is a history of the growth of efficacious surgery.

Also during this period medical education evolved from a state of "nonenlightenment" to one which began to utilize the growing scientific base. Before 1900 most medical schools were proprietary. Their entrance requirements were minimal and exit requirements were not much higher. Most did not have laboratory facilities or clinical training for their students. In 1893 the Johns Hopkins medical school was formed. Modeled after German universities, it soon became the premier American institution for medical education. It was the first to require an undergraduate degree as part of its admission requirements, and the first to have four years of study, as compared with two years in most of the other 131 schools.[9]

In 1910, Abraham Flexner was commissioned by the Carnegie Foundation to evaluate all medical schools in the United States and Canada. Some major deficiencies reported were: low or nonexistent admission standards; poor facilities; inadequate staff; and lack of basic science and clinical instruction.[10] The issuance of the Flexner report was a turning point in medical education, and it was to have a major impact on hospitals.

Concurrent developments helped to shape the modern hospital's role: emergence of nursing as a profession, and changes in society's attitudes toward hospitals. Preceding the Crimean War, nursing was often performed by religious orders. Sectarian nursing had low status and standards, and attracted persons who sometimes abused and robbed their patients. However, the period 1860-1920 witnessed advances in nursing, expansion of the nurse's role in health care delivery, and establishment of professional schools of nursing. Florence Nightingale, a pioneer in English nursing, and Dorothea Dix, a pioneer in American nursing, were instrumental in fostering these changes. The first three schools of nursing in the United States were established in 1873. In 1890 there were 35 schools of nursing; by 1910 there were 1,129.[11] The role of these new professionals began evolving to a partnership with physicians in the delivery of health care.

The change in society's attitude toward the role of hospitals in delivering health care did not occur quickly. Crowded and unsanitary conditions, high mortality rates, and meager medical care deterred people from entering hospitals voluntarily. These conditions and attitudes were changing; the industrialization of the United States during the 1860-1920 period and the urbanization of our society assisted the growth of hospitals. As society became more urbanized sanitation worsened, and slum conditions and the spread of diseases became more prevalent. In many instances hospitals became the place for care of those individuals migrating to the cities. Finally, a shift in attitude occurred; the hospital was seen less as a charitable institution and it was respectable for a paying patient to be admitted. The 1947 Commission on Hospital Care indicated that the "lack of public interest, because of ignorance and prejudice, resulted in slow hospital growth and a low quality of service during early periods."[12] Once prejudice was eliminated then illness rather than economic status was recognized as the basis for hospital admission. The pay-patient system assisted the expansion of hospitals by disassociating "Hospital" from the connotation of charity.

Consolidation (1920-1950)

By 1920 the foundation had been laid. In the following thirty years refinements were made and consolidation occurred. In 1924 there were 7,370 hospitals in the United States, the highest number ever. By 1950 there were 6,788 hospitals; however, the total number of beds increased from 813,000 (an average of 110 per hospital) in 1924 to 1,456,000 (an average of 214 beds per hospital).[13] At the end of the period more beds (113%) were located in fewer facilities and the quality of care provided improved dramatically. Two significant events which had a major impact on hospitals during this period were accreditation and the beginning of private health insurance.

In 1913, the American College of Surgeons was formed. Criteria for physicians seeking fellowship included submission of one hundred case histories of patients on whom the surgeon had operated. Discovering that many could not do so because hospitals had inadequate patient records, the College outlined a set of requirements including: medical staff, patient records, and diagnostic and therapeutic equipment requirements. These had to be met before a hospital was placed on its approved list.[14] This process was carried out by the college until 1951 when its activities were transferred to the Joint Commission on Accreditation of Hospitals.

The impact of approval by the American College of Surgeons was to force the closing of many substandard hospitals. In addition, the College's standards hastened acquisition and use of therapeutic and diagnostic equipment in hospitals and the establishment of laboratories. Consequently, it was an important force in reshaping the hospital, altering its role in developing as the major element in the delivery of health care.

The second major event affecting hospitals in this period was the emergence of private hospitalization insurance plans. One of the earliest, that between the Baylor University Hospital (Texas) and 1500 local teachers, was signed in 1929. For a fixed fee the hospital agreed to provide, if necessary, up to 21 days of hospitalization to each subscriber.[15] By the mid 1940s there were 87 private hospitalization plans covering over 20 million people.[16] The effect was substantial. First, they kept a number of hospitals from going bankrupt during the Depression. Second, they enabled enrollees to prevent the financial disaster of a major illness by spreading risk over a larger enrolled population. Third, they permitted the fee-for-service health care delivery system to become further entrenched. Finally, they helped consolidate hospitals as the major institution in the health care delivery system.

Unlike its European contemporaries, the American hospital system was largely developed and built without government involvement. The vast general acute hospital network which emerged in the United States from 1900 through the end of World War II was predominantly the product of voluntary initiative on the part of the American people and of certain religious groups. Government participation in health care at the federal level was limited to special groups: servicemen, veterans, American Indians, and merchant mariners; and psychiatric hospitals at the state level. A large number of city and county government hospitals were built.

HOSPITAL ORGANIZATION (TRIAD)

Voluntary not-for-profit hospitals evolved some unique aspects. The most important of these was the sharing of power in a triad, which includes the governing authority (board of trustees), chief executive officer (administrator), and medical staff. Theoretically, this arrangement permits a sharing of power among the three participants, but can best be characterized as an accommodation. The triad results from: the independent contractor status of staff physicians who care for their patients in the hospital (K. Taylor) and the need for governing authorities to delegate responsibility for day-to-day operation of the facility to an administrator. Despite its many shortcomings and the increasing number of attacks on its efficiency and desirability, the triad has continued to be the dominant form of organization for voluntary, not-for-profit hospitals (see Figure I-1).

New Models

Recently, a new title has been proposed for the largest category of hospitals. It is suggested that "public general" hospital is a more meaningful generic grouping for all hospitals which offer a broad range of medical and surgical services to the public at large. This title includes hospitals of all types of ownership which serve more than a select group of beneficiaries or specific disease entities and recognizes the quasi-public utility status which hospitals have.

A new organizational model proposed for voluntary not-for-profit hospitals is the corporate structure (see Figure I-2). In this form the governing authority delegates power to a chief executive officer (CEO) who is responsible for all activities within the facility, including medical care. While this may be desirable from an administrative standpoint, it ignores the power and influence of medical staffs generally, and is likely to gain acceptance slowly, if at all.

Closer links between the chief executive officer and the governing authority may tend to minimize the CEO's independence. However, only in hospitals where physicians are employed (such as veterans administration, military, and some in university

Figure I-1
Hospital organization. Typical voluntary not-for-profit

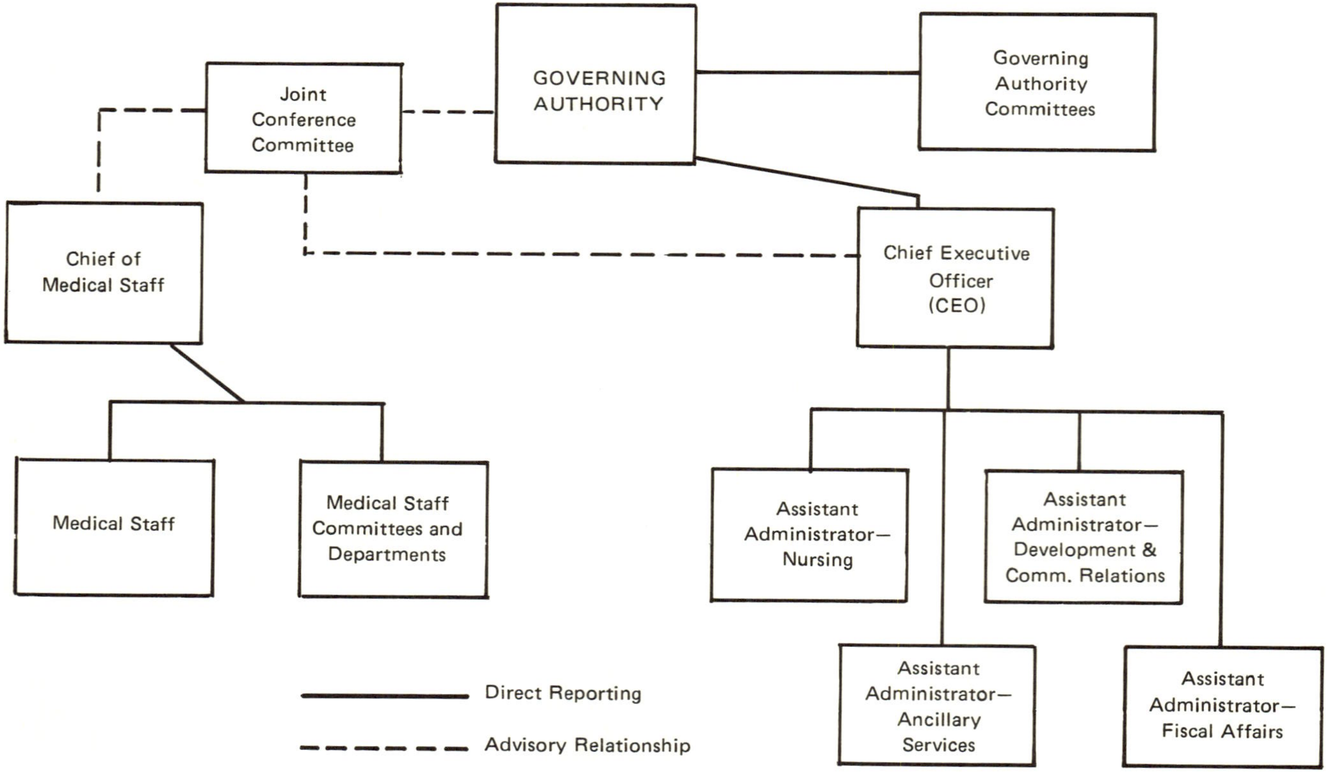

Figure I-2
Hospital organization. Evolving corporate structure.

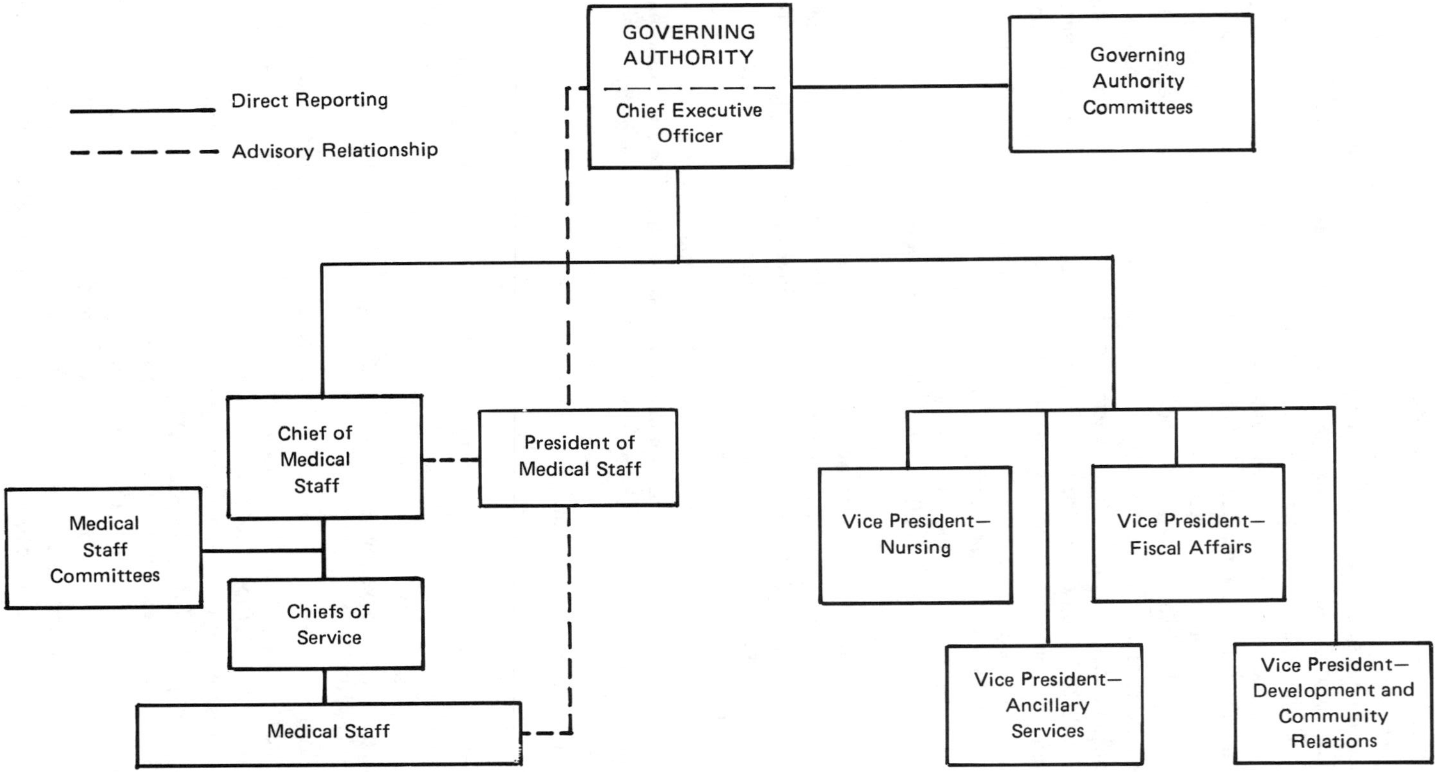

teaching) has there been established a greater degree of line authority over physicians—at least over the administrative aspects of hospital medical practice. By the very nature of the physician's education and professional activity, however, functional independence is a necessary and desirable element. In investor-owned, not-for-profit, and other community hospitals, medical staffs retain a high degree of independence and in most situations hospitals have relied on moral suasion to gain physician cooperation. Increasingly, however, this may not be adequate. The courts have declared that despite the lack of an employment relationship, the hospital, through its governing authority, is accountable for the medical practice rendered (Mountz). The inevitable result of this will be increased control of what physicians do and a greater willingness to use sanctions such as limitation or suspension of hospital privileges. Attenuating or removing privileges is the most direct control point which hospitals have over physicians; however, this happens only rarely (Springer).

THE GOVERNING AUTHORITY

As the result of diverse pressures the hospital board of trustees or as it is increasingly called, the governing authority, has come under close scrutiny (Johnson and Johnson). These pressures include community interest, governmental regulation, third party payor involvement, and malpractice decisions (Pfeffer). Boards are often asked pointed questions about community responsibility and involvement (F. Taylor). Court decisions on malpractice have sharpened the accountability of governing authorities for medical staff activities (Prybil, Sommer). Increasing economic difficulties have made a thorough understanding of financial matters imperative. To remedy these problems, various proposals have been made to increase competence of governing authority members, especially in technical areas. (Berger and Donelson; Schechter). These proposals include seminars, continuing education, and outside resources such as consultants (Howard; Tower).

Based on previous experience, these suggestions for developing internal competence of a voluntary board must be questioned. To do so in no way belittles or besmirches the conscientious efforts of thousands of participants nationwide. The demands being placed on them have changed dramatically, primarily because the hospital's environment is so different.

Trustees of voluntary hospital governing authorities have traditionally come from the educated and upper socioeconomic groups. Board membership for the hospital chief executive officer and/or hospital physician was roundly debated for many years. Its undesirability is infrequently mentioned today and increasing numbers of hospitals include both (McMahon; Rosenkrantz).

The increasing accountability of governing authority members is likely to result in a natural selection process. The ramifications of membership will cull those individuals who have neither the time nor the expertise to be truly effective. Nonchalant or superficial involvement is likely to become a thing of the past. It is doubtful that even the most effective education program can do more than partially offset the chronic shortage of time which most members experience. It has been suggested that the hospital administrative staff should provide the expertise to assist governing authority members. Consultants have also been used as means to offset this deficit. Of the two, more highly qualified administrative staff is probably a better solution. However, neither approach is adequate. Policy decisions of acceptable quality by the governing authority can only result when the membership has virtually as much expertise as do CEOs and their staffs or consultants especially in terms of the external forces (Kovner). One is led, therefore, to the conclusion that evolution will be toward paid governing authority members who devote a specific amount of time to governance of a facility and are paid for that time—a pattern long since adopted by business boards.

For those governing authority members who are defined as trustees (usually in voluntary not-for-profit hospitals) there are additional burdens of serving. In the eyes of the law, trustees are similar to fiduciaries (Davis). They are held to a very high standard of conduct (Mace). They are charged with safeguarding the assets of the organization, protecting the patient from harm, and not getting any secret personal gain from their relationship. Conflict of interest—or more precisely stated, differing interests—on the parts of trustees has increasingly been the subject of journalistic and legal inquiries. Recent court decisions have identified nonfeasance as an important a shortcoming as malfeasance. This increasing emphasis on ethical conduct for governing authority members will make even honest candidates less likely to want to serve.

THE ADMINISTRATOR

MacEachern identified Florence Nightingale, an Englishwoman, as the first hospital administrator.[17] Since Nightingale did her work during the mid-19th century, his conclusion makes emergence of the hospital executive a relatively recent phenomenon. Hospital administration was identified as having a distinct body of knowledge when the University of Chicago established the first U.S. graduate program in hospital administration in 1934. The number of programs increased slowly during the years that followed, until the mid-1960s when a period of rapid growth occurred. In 1976 there were 35 graduate education programs (31 in the United States, 4 in Canada) accredited by the Accrediting Commission on Education for Health Services Administration. There are numerous graduate and undergraduate programs not accredited, but the growth of undergraduate education has been most explosive—it is estimated there are well over 100 nationwide.

Hospital managers are educated in a variety of institutional settings: schools of business, public health, economics, and medicine (Wren, 1967). Similarly the content within these settings is different, but one requirement for accreditation is that certain types of subject matter be taught. This is consistent with the development of a distinct body of knowledge in the field—albeit eclectic. The Master's degree is usually awarded after two years of study, divided into didactic (one academic year minimum) and residency portions of varying lengths. Most programs contend they are educating generalist managers for top leadership positions.

Among hospital managers there is a continuing discourse about whether the field of hospital administration has achieved professional stature (Boissoneau). There is little doubt that it has been professionalized through use of education, income, titles, and other accouterments of office. Furthermore, hospital personnel—including physicians— and the public generally recognize the role and importance of hospital managers. However, hospital managers have not joined the ranks of the historic learned professions, e.g., law, medicine, and the clergy. In addition, there continues to be evidence that many physicians do not consider administrators to be their peers (Bellin; Sheinbach).

As the hospital administrator became a usual entity in the hospital hierarchy a primary task was to implement policy developed by the governing authority (Cathcart). Depending on the relative strengths and weaknesses of the board vis-a-vis the administrator, the scopes of their roles have been quite varied. Within the past ten years, however, the importance of external forces on hospitals has grown dramatically (Elder; Griest). We have reached the point where hospitals are so influenced by external forces, that two individuals are commonly responsible for hospital activities. One is charged with managing the internal functioning of the facility; the second, usually the superior, interacts in and evaluates the external environment of the hospital and makes this knowledge and information available to the governing authority and the internal management. Regardless of the specific approach used, there is no doubt that the hospital executive will have to be increasingly well-educated and sophisticated to function effectively in the health care environment; above all, leadership and management skills are required (Longest, Mecklin).

THE MEDICAL STAFF

The medical staff is an indispensable element of hospital operation (Martin, Perkins). Society has recognized the physician as having unique knowledge and ability in dealing with the ill (Balint). Through the licensing process it verifies that this individual has, in fact, achieved basic abilities. By virtue of the license, then, the physician is permitted to exercise a number of powers which are not given to others, e.g., control of prescription drugs. This power is found in hospitals—the whole treatment of hospital in- and out-patients is dependent on the physician personally carrying out medical treatment and/or directing and supervising others in performing certain tasks (Fuchs). This importance, in addition to professional independence and social status, has necessitated a relationship in the hospital hierarchy in which physicians have substantial power (Riddle; Roemer). This unique relationship has added immensely to the complexity of hospital management and organization (Fischer).

The hospital-based specialists, e.g., anesthesiologists and pathologists, are often employees; increasingly fulltime chiefs-of-staff and chiefs-of-service are being hired (Norville and Halonen). This has occurred because proper management by physicians of medical activities can no longer be done on a part-time or voluntary basis. This change is not only consistent with good management practice, but is necessitated by increasing emphasis on scrutinizing hospitals and holding them accountable for the quality of medical care.

Often, persons unfamiliar with the American hospital system and hospital organization are surprised to learn that the physicians pay nothing for the privilege of treating patients in the facility. At the time when hospitals had charity wards, and physicians contributed their time and effort to treating those patients, there was a true exchange between the facility and the physician. The physician assisted the hospital in meeting a prime social responsibility—caring for indigent patients. At present there are few patients for whom no payment is received by either hospital or physician. The question of what it is that the physician contributes to the hospital has been asked in some quarters. Is it a symbiotic relationship from which society benefits, and is this fact alone adequate? Or does the hospital provide an indispensable workshop, which, if not provided by the hospital, would have to be furnished by the physician? Neither can function without the other, yet the relationship is probably more beneficial to the physician than it is to the facility.

The long-term trend will likely result in greater control by hospitals over physicians. Increased demands for accountability from government, consumer, and third-party payor will bring this about. It may well be that the end result is hospital-based specialists—specialist physicians attached to hospitals without office practices.

The hospital is today and likely will remain one of the most complex and fascinating organizational entities in existence. Hospitals have been thrust into a milieu where those who lead them will have many opportunities to demonstrate their skills, or shortcomings. Regardless of future developments of regulation and control, as long as there are hospitals, means to effectively and efficiently manage them must and will be found. For those who will take up the gauntlet, the challenge is momentous.

BIBLIOGRAPHY

American Hospital Association. *The Hospital Trustee Reader.* Chicago: American Hospital Association, 1975.
American Medical Association. *Physician-Hospital Relations/1974.* Chicago: American Medical Association, 1974.
Arnold, Mary F.; Blankenship, L. Vaughn; and Hess, John M., eds. *Administering Health Systems.* Chicago: Aldine-Atherton, 1971.
Balint, Michael. *The Doctor, His Patient and the Illness.* London: Pitman Medical, 1964.

Beaudry, Sister M. Laurice. "Broadening the Institution's Health Care Base." *Hospital Progress* 56(March): 66-69, 1975.

Bellin, Lowell Eliezer. "The Health Administrator as a Status Seeker." *Journal of Medical Education* 48(October): 896-904, 1973.

Bennett, Adison C. *Methods Improvement in Hospitals*. Philadelphia: J.B. Lippincott Co., 1964.

Berger, Robert O. Jr., and Donelson, J. Garfield. "What Directors Need to Know . . . And How to Get It to Them." *Financial Executive* 42(September): 22-27, 1974.

Blain, Gilbert. "The Hospital as a 'Professional' Bureaucracy." *Trustee* 28(October): 13-16, 1975.

──────. "The Professional in a Bureaucratic Structure." *Hospital Medical Staff* 4(October): 1-6, 1975.

Boissoneau, Robert. "A Matter of Degree: Education in Health Care Administration." *Hospital Administration* 20(Summer): 22-32, 1975.

Cathcart, H. Robert. "Governance and Administration: A Joint Venture." *Trustee* 28(October): 19-21, 1975.

Chandler, Marvin. "It's Time to Clean Up the Boardroom." *Harvard Business Review* 53(September-October): 73-82, 1975.

Checker, Armand, and Knapp, Richard M. "A Profile of Teaching Hospital Governing Boards." *Trustee* 28(August): 20-22, 1975.

Creason, Robert D. "Administrators Waste Time, Don't We?" *Osteopathic Hospitals* 19(May): 12-14, 1975.

Davis, C. Dean. "Fiduciary Responsibilities of Hospital Trustees." *Texas Hospital* 31(March): 26-29, 1976.

Elder, Max Q. "Hospital/Community Relations." *Hospitals* 50(1 April): 109-17, 1976.

Ewell, Charles M. Jr.; Johnson, Alton C.; and Von Ehren, Warren R. "Management: Administrators Identify the Problems." *Hospitals* 48(16 December): 52-55, 1974.

Fischer, Donald C. "Physician-Directors: A Logical Next Step." *Hospital Progress* 56(March): 29, 1975.

──────. "Relationship of Physician-Director to Chief Executive Officer and Medical Staff." *Hospital Progress* 56(June): 46, 1975.

Freeman, Sister Roberta. "Management of People—What is Your Philosophy?" *Hospital Administration in Canada* 16 (June): 46, 1974.

Fuchs, Victor. *Who Shall Live?* New York: Basic Books, 1974.

Garrett, Raymon D. *Hospitals: A Systems Approach*. Philadelphia: Petrocelli Books, 1973.

Georgopoulos, Basil S., ed. *Organization Research on Health Institutions*. Ann Arbor: The University of Michigan Institute for Social Research, 1972.

Glover, G.I., and Laycock, Eric P. "Participative Management and Its Impact on the Organizational Structure of the Enterprise." *Hospital Administration in Canada* 16(March): 27-30, 1974.

Griest, Dorothy. "There's More to Public Relations Than Press Releases." *Hospital Financial Management* (May): 32-40, 1975.

Guzwell, G.A. "The Hospital Ombudsman." *Hospital Administration in Canada* 16(August): 15-18, 1974.

Hancock, Walton M. "Dynamics of Hospital Operational Control Systems." *Hospital and Health Services Administration* 21(Summer): 23-42, 1976.

Heydebrand, Wolf. *Hospital Bureaucracy: A Comparative Study of Organizations*. New York: Dunellen, 1973.

Hicks, Allen M. "Governance: Annual Administrative Review." *Hospitals* 49(1 April): 41-43, 1975.

Hofmann, Paul B. "Establishing Standards of Institutional Performance." *Hospital Progress* 57 (February): 50-53, 1976.

Howard, Godfrey G. "Anatomy of a Hospital Trustee." *Harvard Business Review* 51(May-June): 65-71, 1973.

Jacobs, Donald J. "Care Ensured for Unassigned Patients." *Hospitals* 49(1 January): 79-82, 1975.
Johnson, Everett A., and Johnson, Richard L. *Contemporary Hospital Trusteeship.* Chicago: Teach-'em, 1976.
Kernaghan, Salvinija G. "A Slow Move to the Front of the Class." *Trustee* 28(February): 22-25, 1975.
Kovner, Anthony R. "Hospital Board Members as Policymakers: Role, Priorities, and Qualifications." *Medical Care* 12(December): 971-82, 1974.
Leader, Alan H., and Payne, Michael H. "An Analysis of Health Care Production in Hospitals: A View of Sub-System Outcomes." *Hospital Topics* 54(Jan.-Feb.): 35, 1976.
Levey, Samuel, and Loomba, N. Paul, eds. *Health Care Administration: A Managerial Perspective.* Philadelphia: J.B. Lippincott Co., 1973.
Longest, Beaufort B., Jr. *Management Practices for the Health Professional.* Reston, Va.: Reston Publications, 1976.
Lyon, Herbert L., and Ivancevich, John M. "An Exploratory Investigation of Organizational Climate and Job Satisfaction in a Hospital." *Academy of Management Journal* 17(December): 635-48, 1974.
McKnight, John L. "Hospitals Must Work to Change Image." *Hospitals* 49(16 May): 72-74, 1975.
McMahon, John A. "Hospital-Physician Relations: Where Do We Go From Here?" *Trustee* 28 (March): 25-26, 1975.
Mace, M.L. "Standards of Care For Trustees of Nonprofit Organizations." *Harvard Business Review* 54(January-February): 14, 1976.
Makowski, Robert J. "Mandate, Maintain, Monitor: A Model for Hospital Governance." *Trustee* 29(January): 34-36, 1976.
Martin, Jack D. "Doctors vs. Hospitals: A New Deal for Medical Staffs." *Medical Economics* 52(3 March): 35, 1975.
Mecklin, John M. "Hospitals Need Management Even More Than Money." *Fortune* 81(January): 96, 1970.
Moore, Terence F., and Lorimer, Bernard E. "The Matrix Organization in Business and Health Care Institutions." *Hospital and Health Services Administration* 21(Fall): 26-34, 1976.
Morse, George, and Morse, Robert. *Protecting the Health Care Facility.* Baltimore: Williams and Wilkins, 1973.
Mountz, Wade. "The Malpractice Impact on Hospitals." *Investor-Owned Hospital Review* 8(June-July): 11, 1975.
Mueller, Robert K. *Board Life: Realities of Being a Corporate Director.* New York: American Management, 1974.
Murray, Ralph T.; Donnelly, Paul R.; and Threadgould, Margaret. "How Administrators Spend Their Time." *Hospital Progress* 49(September): 49-58, 1968.
Nash, Al. "Hospital Values, Conflicts and Supervisory Practices." *Personnel Journal* 52(December): 1056-60, 1973.
Norville, Jerry, and Halonen, Robert J. "Negotiating and Administering Contracts with Hospital-Based Physicians." *Hospital Progress* 56(June): 61-67, 1975.
Perkins, Roy F. "The Physician's View of the Hospital: A Love-Hate Relationship." Part 1 *Hospital Medical Staff* 4(April): 1-7; and Part 2 *Hospital Medical Staff* 4(May): 10-14, 1975.
Pfeffer, Jeffrey. "Size, Composition, and Function of Hospital Boards of Directors: A Study of Organization-Environment Linkage." *Administrative Science Quarterly* 18(September): 349-64, 1973.
Prims, A.V., and Delesie, L.B. "Economic Efficiency of Hospitals and Their Ancillary Services." *Hospital Administration* 20(Spring): 30-46, 1975.
Prybil, Lawrence D. "Governance Accountability Vested in Trustees." *Hospitals* 50(1 April): 48-50, 1976.
Riddle, Hasty W. "The Interrelationship of Physicians and Hospitals." *Journal of the Kentucky Medical Association* 73(March): 163-64, 1975.

Roemer, Milton I., and Friedman, Jay W. *Doctors in Hospitals: Medical Staff Organization and Hospital Performance.* Baltimore, Maryland: Johns Hopkins Press, 1971.

Roos, Noralou P.; Roos, Leslie L.; and Schermerhorn, John R. "Hospital Performance: Analyzing Power and Goals." *Journal of Health and Social Behavior* 15(June): 78-92, 1974.

Rosen, Daniel. "The Profitable Nonprofit Field." *Dun's Review* 100 (October): 97-99, 1972.

Rosenkrantz, J.A. "Should Administrators Serve on Hospital Boards?" *Hospitals* 41(1 August): 63, 1967.

Schechter, Daniel S. "Trustees: Educational Have-Nots." *Trustee* 28(February): 18-21, 1975.

Schulz, Rockwell, and Johnson, Alton. *Management of Hospitals.* New York: McGraw-Hill Book Co., 1976.

Sheinbach, Jerry. "Prestige of the Health Administrator." *Journal of Medical Education* 49(March): 314, 1974.

Sommer, A.A. Jr. "Directors' Liability-Preventive Measures." *Financial Executive* 42(September): 18-21, 1974.

Springer, Eric W. "Changing Hospital-Physician Relations: Power of Board to Deny Privileges." *Hospital Topics* 51(July): 21-23, 1973.

Szilagyi, Andrew D., and Sims, Henry P. Jr. "An Exploration of the Path-Goal Theory of Leadership in a Health Care Environment." *Academy of Management Journal* 17(December): 622-34, 1974.

Taylor, Frank. "Do Trustees Meet Today's Community Needs?" *Trustee* 27(January): 26-32, 1974.

Taylor, Keith. "Formal Liaison Between Governing Board and Medical Staff." *Hospital Forum* 17(January): 9, 1975.

Thompson, David W. *The Manager: Understanding and Influencing Behavioral Change.* Chicago: Bradford Press, 1974.

Tower, Robert. "Orienting the Hospital Governing Board." *Osteopathic Hospitals* 20(January): 10-12, 1976.

Whiting, Roger N. "Suggested Organizational Changes for the Hospital Industry." *Health Services Reports* 88(October): 743-49, 1973.

Witt, John A. "Managerial Titles Creating Identity Crisis." *Hospital Progress* 56(June): 60, 1975.

Wren, George. "Graduate Education for Hospital Administration: A Comparison of the Public Health and Business School Programs." *Hospital Administration* 12(Fall): 33-64, 1967.

Wren, George R., and Hilgers, Sharon M. "Titles of Hospital Administrators." *Hospital Administration* 19(Spring): 68-82, 1974.

FOOTNOTES

[1] Mary Risley, *House of Healing,* (Garden City, N.Y.: Doubleday & Co., 1961), pp. 53-66

[2] *Ibid.,* pp. 29-52.

[3] Malcolm T. MacEachern, *Hospital Organization and Management,* 3rd ed. (Berwyn, Illinois: Physicians Record Company, 1962), pp. 8-10.

[4] *Ibid.,* p. 10.

[5] *Ibid.,* pp. 8-10.

[6] United States Department of Commerce, *Historical Statistics of the United States: Colonial Times to 1957,* (Washington, D.C.: U.S. Government Printing Office, 1960), p. 35.

[7] H.S. Hartzog, Jr., *Triumphs in Medicine,* (New York: Doubleday, Page, and Company, 1927), pp. 161-163, 144-148.

[8] Fielding H. Garrison, *History of Medicine,* (Philadelphia: W. B. Saunders Co., 1929, 4th edition), p. 721.

[9] For data on the number of United States medical schools by sect (regular, homeopathic, and eclectic) for the years 1850-1920 see: "Medical Education in the United States," *Journal of the American Medical Association,* Vol. 79, No. 8 (August 19, 1922), pp. 629-659.

[10] A review of the Flexner report is strongly recommended. See: Abraham Flexner, *Medical Education in The United States and Canada,* (New York: The Carnegie Foundation, 1910).

[11] United States Department of Commerce, *Op. cit.,* p. 34.

[12] Commission on Hospital Care, *Hospital Care in the United States,* (New York: The Commonwealth Fund, 1947), p. 49.

[13] United States Department of Commerce, *Historical Statistics of the United States: Colonial Times to 1970* (Washington, D.C.: Government Printing Office, 1975), pp. 78-79. When examining the number of beds relative to the total United States population the following results are obtained: (1) extrapolating between the 1920 and 1930 censuses, the 1924 population was 112 million people which results in 7.3 beds per thousand population; the 1950 population was 151 million people which results in 9.6 beds per thousand population. Stated another way, the population increased 35 percent between 1924 and 1950 while the number of hospital beds increased 79 percent. Census data were obtained from the previously cited source, page 9.

[14] Laura G. Jackson, *Hospital and Community,* (New York: Macmillan, 1964), p. 357.

[15] C. Rufus Rorem, *Non-Profit Hospital Service Plans,* (Chicago: American Hospital Association, 1940), p. 9.

[16] Nathan Sinai, Odin W. Anderson, and Melvin L. Dollar, *Health Insurance in The United States,* (New York: The Commonwealth Fund, 1946), p. 44.

[17] MacEachern, *Hospital Organization,* p. 17.

Organization

Selection 1, "THE HOSPITAL AS AN ORGANIZATION" by Basil S. Georgopoulos and Floyd C. Mann, despite its date, 1962, provides an excellent review of the hospital and its distinguishing characteristics. The complexities and interactions are highlighted. Duncan Neuhauser discusses management theory and the vertical and horizontal coordination necessary for hospitals in *Selection 2*, "THE HOSPITAL AS A MATRIX ORGANIZATION." He describes the theoretical basis for use of matrix theory in hospitals and concludes it is appropriate.

The late Ray E. Brown in *Selection 3*, "STRICTURES AND STRUCTURES," describes some of the philosophical problems associated with hospital organization and management. While a number of management writers have criticized hospitals for failing to meet the traditional patterns, Alan D. Bauerschmidt has a different perspective. In *Selection 4*, "THE HOSPITAL AS A PROTOTYPE ORGANIZATION," he argues that other industries can and will have to learn from organizational and managerial arrangements already used by hospitals.

Fremont E. Kast and James E. Rosenzweig introduce general systems theory in *Selection 5*, "HOSPITAL ADMINISTRATION AND SYSTEM CONCEPTS," and describe how it is useful in understanding the complexities of hospital administration. As part of this effort they review general systems theory and show how these concepts are applied outside hospitals.

Finally, *Selection 6*, "CORPORATE MODELS IN HEALTH CARE DELIVERY" by Lynda Diane Baydin and Alan Sheldon, is especially useful in understanding how new forms of organization and interrelationships can assist hospitals in performing their functions more efficiently and effectively. The authors discuss their advantages, disadvantages, and why some of these efforts do not succeed.

1.
The Hospital as an Organization

BASIL S. GEORGOPOULOS, PH.D. AND FLOYD C. MANN, PH.D. *

Basil S. Georgopoulos, Ph.D., is Program Director of the Survey Research Center and Professor of Psychology at the University of Michigan. Floyd C. Mann, Ph.D., is the director of the Center for Research on Utilization of Scientific Knowledge at the University of Michigan.

The community general hospital is an organization that mobilizes the skills and efforts of a number of widely divergent groups of professional, semiprofessional, and nonprofessional personnel to provide a highly personalized service to individual patients. Like other large-scale organizations, it is established and designed to pursue certain objectives through collaborative activity. The chief objective of the hospital is, of course, to provide adequate care and treatment to its patients (within the limits of present-day technical-medical knowledge, and knowledge of organizing human activity effectively, as well as within limits that may be imposed by the relative scarcity of appropriate organizational resources or by extraorganizational forces). Its principal product is medical, surgical, and nursing service to the patient, and its central concern is the life and health of the patient. A hospital may, of course, have additional objectives, including its own maintenance and survival, organizational stability and growth, financial solvency, medical and nursing education and research, and various employee-related objectives. But, all these are subsidiary to the key objective of service to the patient, which constitutes the basic organizing principle that underlies all activities in the community general hospital.

There is little ambiguity, if any, about the main organizational objective of the community general hospital. Unlike many organizations, the hospital is able to make the role it performs in the larger community psychologically meaningful to its members. And most of its members try to give unstintingly of their energies to perform the tasks assigned to them. Many doctors and nurses look upon their profession as a sacred calling. Others find working in the hospital deeply satisfying of needs that they cannot easily express in words. They see the hospital as a nonprofit institution dedicated to works of mercy, and they sense their mission in life to give of themselves in order to help others. Immediate personal comfort and satisfactions, and even material rewards, are defined by most members as less important than giving good

*Current address for Floyd C. Mann: University of Colorado, Boulder.

Reprinted with permission of Macmillan Publishing Co., Inc., from *The Community General Hospital* by Basil S. Georgopoulos and Floyd C. Mann, pp. 5-15. Copyright 1962 by Macmillan Publishing Co., Inc.

care to the patient and meeting a higher order of obligation to mankind. Serious conflicts regarding material rewards, such as those found in organizations where profit is the chief motive, are virtually nonexistent in the hospital. For all these reasons, motivating organizational members toward the objectives of the organization is much less of a problem in the hospital by comparison to other large-scale organizations. The goals of individual members and the objectives of the organization are considerably more congruent in the case of the hospital.

EXTENSIVE DIVISION OF LABOR

To do its work, the hospital relies upon an extensive division of labor among its members, upon a complex organizational structure which encompasses many different departments, staffs, offices, and positions, and upon an elaborate system of coordination of tasks, functions, and social interaction.

Work in the hospital is greatly differentiated and specialized, and of a highly interactional character. It is carried out by a large number of cooperating people whose backgrounds, education, training, skills, and functions are as diverse and heterogeneous as can be found in any of the most complex organizations in existence. And much of the work is not only specialized but also performed by highly trained professionals—the doctors—who require the collaboration, assistance, and services of many other professional and nonprofessional personnel. In addition to the medical staff, which itself is highly specialized and departmentalized, there is the nursing staff, which includes graduate professional nurses in various supervisory and nonsupervisory positions, practical nurses, and untrained nurses' aides. In addition to the nursing staff and the medical staff, which are the two largest groups in the community general hospital, there are the hospital administrator and a number of administrative-supervisory personnel who head various departments or services (e.g., nursing, dietary, admissions, maintenance, pharmacy, medical records, housekeeping, laundry) and are in charge of the employees in these departments. There are also a number of medical technologists and technicians who work in the laboratory and X-ray departments of the hospital, as well as a number of miscellaneous clerical and secretarial personnel. And apart from all these staffs and professional-occupational groups, there is a board of trustees which has the overall formal responsibility for the organization, and which consists of a number of prominent people from the outside community. The trustees offer their services to the hospital without remuneration and are not employees of the organization. In short, professionalization and specialization are two of the hallmarks of the hospital.

HIGH INTERDEPENDENCE OF SERVICES

Because of this extensive division of labor and accompanying specialization of work, practically every person working in the hospital depends upon some other person or persons for the performance of his own organizational role. Specialists and professionals can perform their functions only when a considerable array of supportive personnel and auxiliary services is put at their disposal at all times. Doctors, nurses, and others in the hospital do not, and cannot, function separately or independently of one another. Their work is mutually supplementary, interlocking, and interdependent.

In turn, such a high interdependence requires that the various specialized functions and activities of the many departments, groups, and individual members of the organization be sufficiently coordinated, if the organization is to function effectively and attain its objectives. Consequently, the hospital has developed a rather intricate and elaborate system of internal coordination. Without coordination, concerted effort on the part of its different members and continuity in organizational operations could not be ensured.

It is also interesting and important to note here that, unlike industrial and other large-scale organizations, the hospital relies very heavily on the skills, motivations, and behaviors of its members for the attainment and maintenance of adequate coordination. The flow of work is too variable and irregular to permit coordination through mechanical standardization. And the product of the organization—patient care—is itself individualized rather than uniform or invariant. Because the work is neither mechanized nor uniform or standardized, and because it cannot be planned in advance with the automatic precision of an assembly line, the organization must depend a good deal upon its various members to make the day-to-day adjustments which the situation may demand, but which cannot possibly be completely detailed or prescribed by formal organizational rules and regulations. This is all the more essential, moreover, if one takes into account the fact that the patient, who is the center of all activity in the hospital, is a transient rather than a stable element in the system—in the short-stay hospital, he comes and goes very rapidly.

HOSPITALS: AUTHORITARIAN-DEMOCRATIC?

Fundamentally, then, the hospital is a human rather than a machine system. And even though it may possess elaborate and impressive-looking equipment, or a great variety of physical and material facilities, it has no integrated mechanical-physical systems for the handling and processing of its work. The patient is not a chunk of raw material that passively goes through an ordered progression of machines and assembly-line operators. At every stage of his short stay in the hospital, he is mainly dependent upon his interaction with the people who are entrusted with his care, and upon the skills, actions, and interactions of these different people. All of these factors necessitate heavy reliance upon the members of the organization to coordinate their activities on a voluntary, informal, and expedient basis.

Paradoxical as it may seem, however, the hospital is also a highly formal, quasi-bureaucratic organization which, like all task-oriented organizations, relies a great deal upon formal policies, formal written rules and regulations, and formal authority for controlling much of the behavior and work relationships of its members. The emphasis on formal organizational mechanisms and procedures and on directive rather than "democratic" controls, along with a number of other factors, gives the hospital its much talked about "authoritarian" character, which manifests itself in relatively sharp patterns of superordination-subordination, in expectations of strict discipline and obedience, and in distinct status differences among organizational members.

MAINTAINING AUTHORITARIANISM

The authoritarian character of the hospital is partly the result of historical forces having their origins at a time when professionalization and specialization were at a primordial stage, and when nursing, medicine, and the hospital were all closely associated with the work of religious orders and military institutions. The absence of substantial professionalization and specialization characteristic of hospital personnel at those times, along with the emphasis of religious and military institutions on social arrangements in which the occupant of every position in the organization presumably knew "his place," and kept to his place by strictly adhering to specified rights, duties, and obligations, had much to do with the hospital's adopting a strict hierarchical and authoritarian system of work arrangements. But, the advent of professionalization and specialization, the gradual independence of hospitals from religious and military institutions, and the impact of an increasingly secular culture have greatly reduced the authoritarian character of the hospital. As Lentz has noted, within the last 50 years the hospital has undergone marked changes, dropping some of its authoritarian and paternalistic characteristics and taking on those of a bureaucratic, functionally rational organization.

Today's community general hospital, however, still has some of its traditional authoritarian characteristics along with its emphasis on rational organization. Moreover, it is unlikely that it will rid itself of all authoritarianism in the near future. There are several major counterforces at work, in this connection. First, there is the fact that the hospital constantly deals with critical matters of life and death—matters which place a heavy burden of both secular and moral responsibility on the organization and its members. When human life is at stake, there is little tolerance for error or negligence. And, if error and negligence can be prevented by adherence to strict formal rules and quasi-authoritarian discipline, such rules are important to have and obedience cannot very well be questioned (although blind obedience is mitigated because the hospital increasingly relies on the expertness, judgment, and ethics of professionals who, while abhorring regimentation, are presumably capable of a good deal of self-discipline). Second, there is the great concern of the hospital for maximum efficiency and predictability of performance. In the absence of mechanically regulated workflows, this concern virtually forces the organization to use many quasi-authoritarian means of control (including rigid rules and procedures, directive supervision, rigorous discipline, etc.), in the hope of: (1) attaining some uniformity in the behavior of its members, (2) regulating their interaction and checking deviance within known limits of accountability, and (3) appraising their performance. Third, there is the temptation to adhere to traditional, familiar ways of doing things which, coupled with the lack of apparently equivalent or superior alternatives that could be employed to ensure clarity of responsibility and efficiency and predictability of performance, also serves to perpetuate organizational reliance upon customary directive means of control.[1]

HISTORY OF REGIMENTED BEHAVIOR

In brief, while historical forces might account for the origins of the authoritarian characteristics of the hospital, it is not likely that some of these characteristics would continue to persist (especially within the context of a highly secular culture) unless

---

[1] Incidentally, the apparent unavailability of equivalent or superior organizational alternatives is partly the result of our inadequate knowledge about how best to organize and manage human activity in a situation such as that of the community general hospital, and partly the result of the inability of hospitals to utilize the findings of modern research to best advantage.

they were more functional than not. And this clearly appears to be the case. In the first place, as in any organization designed to mobilize resources quickly in order to meet crises and emergencies successfully, a good deal of regimented behavior is required in the hospital. Lines of authority and responsibility have to be clearly drawn, basic acceptance of authority has to be assured, and discipline has to be maintained. In the second place, the hospital is expected to be able to provide adequate care to its patients at all times, with the precision of a machine system and with minimum error, even though it is a human rather than a machine system. It is expected to perform well continuously and to produce a machinelike response toward the patient, regardless of such things as turnover, absenteeism, and feelings of friendship or hostility among its personnel, or other organizational problems that it may be experiencing. It is also expected to be responsive to the health-related needs and demands of its community, and to meet a variety of medicolegal requirements. Because of these expectations, the hospital places high premium on being able to count upon and predict the outcome of the performances of its members. And predictability of performance can be partly attained through directive, quasi-authoritarian controls which, in the absence of apparently superior alternatives, are rather tempting to the organization.

PUBLIC DEMANDS EFFICIENCY

Coupled with this great concern for predictability of performance, moreover, there is an increasing concern that the hospital operate as efficiently and economically as possible. As the hospital has become a resource for all members of the community, and not just the indigent and the impoverished, the public has come to expect of it the best medical and nursing services that can be offered. These services, however, are quite costly, as are the facilities, equipment, supplies, and medicines that are required. And while the public may be willing (though not necessarily able to afford) to pay for these essential costs of hospital care, it also expects the best care possible at reasonable cost or even at least cost. At the same time, it is neither willing to tolerate nor prepared to pay any costs that may result from inefficient operations, poor administration, duplication of services, waste, negligence, and the like. It expects its hospitals to reduce to a minimum or eliminate altogether costs of this latter type and to operate with maximum economy. The hospitals themselves are quite aware of these and other pressures for efficiency, and have come to place very high emphasis on greater efficiency. Great emphasis on economic efficiency, however, is not entirely compatible with the hospital's traditional humanitarian orientation and objective of best service to the patient; the "best" service is not always or necessarily the most economical. Furthermore, this concern for efficiency is resulting both in progressive rationalization of hospital operations and in the institution of more rigid controls within the organization. Such controls, incidentally, serve to maintain the remaining authoritarian characteristics of the community general hospital.

NEEDED: ORGANIZATIONAL COORDINATION

But, efficiency of operations and predictability of performance in the hospital could not possibly be attained only through directive and quasi-authoritarian controls. In fact, if carried to extremes, such controls would in the long run be inimical both to efficiency and to predictability. Efficiency and predictability of performance are also, and perhaps primarily, attained through a number of other factors, which are essential to effective organizational functioning. Probably the most prominent of these factors in the case of the community general hospital are organizational coordination and professionalization.

Because of the high degrees of specialization and functional interdependence found in the hospital, coordination of skills, tasks, and activities is indispensable to effective organizational performance and its predictability. The different specialized, but interacting and interdependent, parts of the organization must fit well together; they must not work at cross purposes or in their own separate directions. If the organization is to attain its objectives, its different parts and members must function according to each other's needs and expectations of the total organization. In short, they must be well coordinated. But, as we have already pointed out, the hospital is dependent very greatly upon the motivations and voluntary, informal adjustments of its members for the attainment and maintenance of good coordination. Formal organizational plans, rules, regulations, and controls may ensure some minimum coordination, but of themselves are incapable of producing adequate coordination, for only a fraction of all the coordinative activities required in this organization can be programed in advance.

THE SUBJECT OF PROFESSIONALIZATION

The other relevant factor that we wish to consider here, in addition to coordination, is that of professionalization—professionalization being one of the major distinctive features of the community general hospital. The majority of those who hold the principal therapeutic and nontherapeutic positions in the hospital are trained as professionals. The doctors, through their training, have been schooled in certain professional obligations, ethics, and standards of appropriate behavior, and have acquired a number of common attitudes, shared values, and mutual understandings about their work and work relations with others. The same is true about the registered nurses. Other groups in the organization are also on the road to professionalization: the administrators, the medical librarians, the medical technologists, the dietitians, and others in paramedical positions.

COMPLEMENTARY EXPECTATIONS

This high degree of professionalization among those entrusted with the care of the patient has developed along lines of rational, functional specialization, and has had the effect of inculcating many complementary expectations and common norms and values in the members of the principal groups of the hospital—values, expectations, and norms that are essential to the integration of the organization. These include the norms of giving good care, devotion to duty, loyalty, selflessness and altruism, discipline, and hard work. This normative structure underpins the formal rational structure of the organization, and enables the hospital to attain a level of coordination and integration that could never be accomplished through administrative edict, through hierarchical directives, or through explicitly formulated and carefully specified organizational plans and impersonal rules, regulations, and procedures. However, increased professionalization and specialization have also had the effect of sharpening some of the status differences among the people working in the hospital—and sharp status distinctions bespeak of some authoritarianism.

Among other things, increased professionalization in the hospital has helped guarantee that certain minimum levels of competence and skill would exist in the organization, thus having a direct impact upon performance and organizational effectiveness. Similarly, professionalization and specialization have contributed to greater public confidence in the hospital, and to a wider acceptance of the hospital as a resource for the health needs of all people, for high professionalization and specialization imply expertness and knowledge. Increased professionalization has undoubtedly resulted in improved patient care and, in so doing, it has also raised the expectations of the public for both high-quality care and high efficiency in hospital operations. More and more of us go to the hospital for our various health needs nowadays but, because of improved service, we stay there for a shorter and shorter period of time. In the last 30 years, the average length of stay for adult patients in general hospitals has decreased by about a third, from 12.6 to 8.6 days—making it increasingly appropriate to refer to the community general hospital as the short-stay hospital.

NO SINGLE LINE OF AUTHORITY

Another of the distinctive characteristics of the community general hospital, closely related to professionalization and specialization, is the absence of a single line of authority in the organization. This feature has already been the subject of considerable discussion by Smith and others, but is important enough to warrant some brief observations here. Essentially, authority in the hospital is shared (not equally) by the board of trustees, the doctors, and the administrator—the three centers of power in the organization—and, to some extent, also by the director of nursing. In the hospital, authority does not emanate from a single source and does not flow along a single line of command as it does in most formal organizations.

A formal organizational chart of the hospital shows the board of trustees as having ultimate authority and overall responsibility for the institution. The board delegates the day-to-day management of the organization to the hospital administrator. In turn, the administrator delegates authority to the heads of the various nonmedical departments (including the director of nursing, who also wields a different kind of authority that originates in her professional expertness). The heads of these departments, in turn, have varying degrees of authority over the affairs of their respective departments and personnel. In the formal organizational chart, the medical staff, its officers, and its members are not shown as having any direct-line responsibility; they are outside of the lay-administrative line of authority. Yet, as is well known both within and outside the hospital, the doctors exercise substantial influence throughout the hospital structure at nearly all organizational levels, enjoy very high autonomy in their work, and have a good deal of professional authority over others in the organization. Over the nursing staff and over the patients, their professional authority is dominant. And although the board of trustees is in theory shown as the ultimate source of authority, the board actually has very limited *de facto* authority over the medical staff. Partly because the doctors are not employees of the hospital (they are "guests" who are granted practice privileges), partly because they enjoy high status and great prestige, partly because they have almost supreme authority in professional-medical matters, and partly for other reasons, they are subject to very little lay-organizational authority.

THE DIFFICULTIES THAT ARISE

Professionals in staff capacities in business corporations—lawyers, doctors, accountants, and others—have little or no authority to be involved in the activities of the line; they mainly serve as consultants and advisors. But this is not so in the case of the hospital. The absence of a single line of authority in the hospital, of course, creates various administrative and operational problems, as well as psychological problems having to do with the relative power and influence on organizational functioning on the part of doctors, trustees, administrators, and others. For one thing, it makes formal organizational coordination rather difficult. For another thing, it allows for instances in which it is not clear where authority, responsibility, and accountability reside. Similarly, it allows for a situation wherein a large number of organizational members, particularly members of the nursing staff, must be responsible to and take orders not only from their supervisors but also from the doctors. The lay authority and the professional authority to which nurses are subject, of course, are not always consistent. The absence of a single line of authority also makes for difficulties in communication, difficulties in the area of discipline, and difficulties in resolving problems that must be resolved through cooperative efforts on the part of both the lay-administrative and medical-professional sides. Frequently, the administrator, feeling that the responsibility for the overall management of the organization is his, and feeling that doctors through their power and pressures interfere in the discharge of his responsibilities, is motivated or actively attempts to circumvent the medical staff on various matters, and this, too, is apt to lead to problems. (The doctors, in turn, are likely to try to circumvent the administrator.) For the same reasons, the administrator is likely to be prone toward more and more bureaucratization in the hospital. And increased bureaucratization of organizational operations is likely to be fought and resented by the doctors, for it eventually means a reduction in their influence.

DELICATE BALANCE OF POWER

In general, multiple lines of authority require the maintenance of a very delicate balance of power in the organization—a balance of power that is rather precarious. On the positive side, multiple lines of authority may serve as a system of "checks and balances," which may prevent other kinds of possible problems, such as organizational inflexibility and authoritarianism, or may serve to lighten the burden of responsibility in situations where responsibility may be too great for any single group or individual to shoulder. Regardless of the advantages and disadvantages of a system of multiple lines of authority, such a system is an integral part of the community general hospital. Not only is it an integral part, moreover, but also a part that is virtually inevitable for an organization such as this. This is because much of the work in the hospital is performed by influential professionals and not by low-status workers, and because of the high degrees of both professionalization and specialization characteristic of the organization. As Parsons has aptly observed, "The multiplication of technical fields, and their differentiation from each other ... leads to an essential element of decentralization in the organizations which must employ them." For this reason, he goes on to explain that, unlike business and military organizations, "A university can not be organized mainly on a 'line' principle...." In this respect, the community general hospital is very similar to a university. (Hospitals and universities have a number of other interesting characteristics in common, but here we are interested only in hospitals.)

In summary, the community general hospital is an extremely complex social organization that differs from business and other large-scale organizations on a number of important characteristics. Among its main distinguishing characteristics, the following are worth reemphasizing:

MAIN DISTINGUISHING CHARACTERISTICS

1. The main objective of the organization is to render personalized service—care and treatment—to individual patients, rather than the manufacture of some uniform material object. And the economic value of the organization's products and objectives is secondary to their social and humanitarian value.

2. By comparison to industrial organizations, the hospital is much more directly dependent upon, and responsive to, its surrounding community, and its work is much more closely integrated with the needs and demands of its consumers and potential customers. To the hospital and its members, the patients' needs are always of supreme and paramount importance. Moreover, there is high agreement about the principal objective of the hospital among the members of the organization, and the personal needs and goals of the different members conflict little with the objectives of the organization.

3. The demands of much of the work at the hospital are of an emergency nature and nondeferrable. They place a heavy burden of both secular-functional and moral responsibility upon the organization and its members. Correspondingly, the organization shows great concern for clarity of responsibility and accountability among its different members, and very little tolerance for either ambiguity or error.

4. The nature and volume of work are variable and diverse, and subject to relatively little standardization. The hospital cannot lend itself to mass production techniques, to assembly-line operations, or to automated functioning. It is a human rather than a machine system, with all the attributes this entails. Both the raw materials and end products of the organization are human. And, being human, they participate actively in the production process, thus having a good deal of control over it.

5. The principal workers in the hospital—doctors and nurses—are professionals, and this entails various administrative and operational problems for the organization.

6. By comparison to industrial organizations, the hospital has relatively little control over its workload and over many of its key members. In particular, it has little direct control over the doctors and over the patients—two of its most essential components. In the short-stay hospital, the patients are not only a very heterogeneous

and very transient group, but are also, mainly and ultimately, in the hands of their doctors, who are not employees of the organization.

7. The administrator has much less authority, power, and discretion than his managerial counterparts in industry because the hospital is not and cannot very well be organized on the basis of a single line of authority. The simultaneous presence of lay, professional, and mixed lay-professional lines of authority in the hospital creates a number of administrative and other problems, which business organizations are largely spared.

8. The hospital is a formal, quasi-bureaucratic, and quasi-authoritarian organization which, like most organizations of this kind, relies greatly on conventional hierarchical work arrangements and on rather rigid impersonal rules, regulations, and procedures. But, more importantly, it is a highly departmentalized, highly professionalized, and highly specialized organization that could not possibly function effectively without relying heavily for its internal coordination on the motivations, actions, self-discipline, and voluntary, informal adjustments of its many members. Coordination of efforts and activities in the hospital is indispensable to organizational functioning, because the work is of a highly interactional character—the activities of organizational members are highly interlocking and interdependent, and the various members can perform their role only by working in close association with each other.

9. The hospital shows a very great concern for efficiency and predictability of performance among its members and for overall organizational effectiveness.

10. Finally, the community general hospital is an organization which is important to us all, and which is becoming increasingly important. Several basic social trends tend to ensure this: the accelerating accumulation of new medical knowledge, new medical, surgical, and nursing procedures, and new drugs and medicines; rising levels of family income in the nation; increased use of the general hospital for numerous different diseases and health needs; and a growing demand by the general public for the best possible quality of medical-surgical and nursing care.

It has been the purpose of this section to introduce the reader to some of the key characteristics and organizational problems of the community general hospital. (Many of these will be examined in detail in subsequent chapters.) The characteristics and problems discussed above, along with many others to be dealt with throughout the book, show how complicated an organization the hospital is, and lead one to suspect that increased understanding of such problems and characteristics might help ease some of the management difficulties and perhaps also improve the organizational effectiveness of our hospitals.

2.
The Hospital as a Matrix Organization

DUNCAN NEUHAUSER

Duncan Neuhauser, Ph.D. is Associate Professor of Health Services Administration and Associate Director of the yearly six-week Program for Health Systems Management - School of Public Health, Harvard University.

It does not take much reading in organization theory to discover a major divergence of opinion among those writers who praise the efficiency of large formal organizations and the centralized hierarchical authority structure associated with it. (Max Weber, Henri Fayol and Georgopoulos and Mann for hospitals come to mind.)[1] In contrast, the human relations writers have focused on the human problems apparently inherent in such organizations, including Likert, Katz and Kahn, and Argyris for hospitals,[2] and have recommended more participation in decision-making by workers. They are in fundamental disagreement as to the degree to which procedures should be specified hierarchically and imposed on organizational members. Both schools of thought believe they have found the best way to run an organization.

THE NEW RELATIVISM IN ORGANIZATIONS

More recently a number of writers have come up with a different approach saying that the appropriate management style, more or less hierarchical or conversely more or less participatory, will vary depending on the circumstances, principally, the complexity of the tasks being performed.[3] In doing so, they have made a significant contribution to our understanding of organizations by reconciling these apparently divergent points of view. The relativism of this approach makes it appropriately called The Contingency or Situational Theory of Management.[4] Some of these studies are described briefly below.[5]

Reprinted by permission from *Hospital Administration* (currently *Hospital and Health Services Administration*): *Quarterly Journal of the American College of Hospital Administrators*, Chicago, Vol. 17 (Fall, 1972), pp. 8-25. © 1972 by the American College of Hospital Administrators. All rights reserved.

CONTINGENCY THEORY

Morris Janowitz[6] observed in 1959 that increasing technological complexity in the armed forces called for a more highly skilled personnel which, in turn, has led away from the traditional hierarchical authoritarian military discipline and toward more decentralized decision making by skilled personnel.

Joan Woodward[7] in England and Robert Blauner[8] in the United States have studied different types of industrial settings, such as unit production (craft), mass production (the assembly line), and process production (oil refineries), and observed differences in management structure and employee attitudes that seem to result from differences in technology. Blauner describes the alienation among workers which comes from the simple repetitive tasks that are associated with the assembly line and the lack of both employee discretion and potential for initiative.

Harold Leavitt[9] in laboratory studies of small groups observed differences in communication patterns. For simple tasks having the *workers* report to one *boss* was efficient but boring for the workers and inflexible in adapting to changes. For difficult tasks a more participatory approach where everyone talked with everyone else on a more equal basis was more efficient. The members were happier, and they produced more new ideas.

PARTICIPATORY DECISION-MAKING

Aaron Lowin,[10] in his review of the literature on participatory decision-making, proposes that there are some persons who prefer to work in more hierarchical settings where they are told what to do and perform simple tasks, while others prefer freedom to make their own decisions. He says those people with a preference will gravitate toward the appropriate organizations or careers which satisfy this preference.

Burns and Stalker[11] in their study of twenty British industrial firms distinguish between organic and mechanistic organizational structures. Mechanistic organizations are hierarchical and centralized, performing routinized production activities in stable markets with unskilled workers. Organic organizations are more loosely structured and participatory. They have complex tasks, a skilled workforce, and face rapidly changing technologies and markets.

WORKING WITH DIFFERENT ORGANIZATIONAL STRUCTURES

While Burns and Stalker distinguished between organizations as a whole, Lawrence and Lorsch[12] looked at differences in task complexity (they call it environment) within organizations and differences in management styles associated with them. Departments performing routinized activities (production) had more task-oriented workers and more formalized structure than research departments which were informally structured, had a longer time horizon and were more interpersonally rather than task-

TABLE 1

GERALD BELL'S PERCEIVED DISCRETION SCORE FOR HOSPITAL OCCUPATIONS IN ONE 180-BED HOSPITAL. THE HIGHER THE SCORE THE MORE DISCRETION BASED ON QUESTIONNAIRE RESPONSE BY HOSPITAL EMPLOYEES

1. Housekeeping, laundry	1.3
2. Dietary helpers	1.4
3. Cooks	2.0
4. Nurse's aides	2.2
5. X-ray technicians	2.3
6. Orderlies	3.0
7. Lab technicians	3.0
8. Pharmacists	3.0
9. Secretaries	3.1
10. Plumbers, carpenters (semi-skilled worker)	3.2
11. Dietary supervisors	3.7
12. Nurses (staff)	4.5
13. Assistant department head (nursing)	4.9
14. Assistant department head (other)	5.0
15. Department head (nursing)	5.4
16. Department head (other)	5.4
17. Doctors	5.6
18. Administrators	5.7

oriented. The efficient organizations were those which clearly differentiated management styles in conjunction with different levels of task complexity. They pointed out the paradox that organizations facing different levels of task complexity not only have to be differentiated but also need a high degree of coordination (integration) between their differentiated departments.

THE HOSPITAL AS A DIFFERENTIATED ORGANIZATION

Gordon and Becker (1964)[13] and Durbin and Springall (1969)[14] have theorized along similar lines for hospitals. They propose that complex tasks and highly skilled professionalized workers call for a colleagial participatory decision-making structure while the repetitive tasks performed by unskilled workers call for a hierarchical formalized structure. At the extreme ends in a hospital are the physicians with their loose organic structure and the relatively unskilled workers of housekeeping, dietary, and laundry with more hierarchical centralized supervision. Nurses and skilled technicians fall in between. Gerald Bell developed an index of discretion in one hospital he studied for various different types of hospital workers.[15] See Table 1. His discretion score is based on whether these workers decided to perform tasks, and how and in what order to perform them. As one can see, there is a relationship between the complexity of tasks these workers perform, the amount of education or experience required (professionalism) and the amount of discretion they have. The converse of discretion presumably is hierarchical control and supervision.

Eugene Baldwin repeated Lawrence and Lorsch's study in 14 hospitals.[16] He observed a substantial difference in organizational structure (formalization, task orientation, time orientation) between doctors, paraprofessional, nonprofessional staff, fiscal staff, and administration. He found that a differentiated structure is significantly related to high performance. He further found that those hospitals, where these different groups were perceived to be well coordinated (integrated), had significantly higher performance.

In the author's study of 30 Chicago community hospitals, the hospital was conceptually divided into physician and non-physician components.[17] The relatively high complexity-physician component had higher quality of care if there was a high level of participation by physicians. The relatively low complexity non-physician component (dietary, housekeeping, laundry, lab, and X-ray workers) was more efficient if it was more hierarchically organized.[18]

The findings from these studies are summarized in Table 2.

As Table 2 indicates, there is no way to avoid problems. The high degree of centralized coordination, routinized tasks, division of labor into simplified jobs and automation come at the price of alienation and boredom on the part of unskilled workers. The participatory approach that may lead to high self fulfillment on the part of skilled workers can lead to a lack of centralized coordination and high labor costs.

Table 2 implies that sometimes even with highly complex tasks management would prefer to substitute less skilled for more skilled workers. For example, when professionals become too scarce there may be no choice (e.g., the development of physician assistants) or when there is so little goal congruence between professionals and organization, participation may be disasterous. Conversely, when the alienation is engendered by simple tasks and intelligent workers, a program of job enlargement may be appropriate. Just as management, to some extent, can vary the skill mix of the workforce, they can vary the complexity of tasks: for example, the housekeeping personnel can clean with mop and bucket or they can use more complicated automatic floor washers. In recent decades, the U.S. workforce has become more highly educated, more professionalized and the tasks generally more complex. This would suggest the general trend toward more flexible, participatory, organic, structures throughout the economy.

There is, in theory, an alternative to high goal congruence for professionals who specify their own procedures (means). This is when the quality of the end results of professional activities is clearly visible to the organization's managers, and they are in a position to replace low performing professionals. Neither is the case for hospitals where quality of care is not believed to be easy to measure and where it is difficult to expel a poorly performing physician from the medical staff.

TABLE 2

ADVANTAGES AND DISADVANTAGES ASSOCIATED WITH
DIFFERENT MANAGEMENT STYLES[1,9]

	Participatory Decision-Making (low specialization of procedures)	Hierarchical Decision-Making (high specialization of procedures)
Complexity	Appropriate for highly complex tasks	Appropriate for simple repetitive tasks
Type of worker	Highly skilled professionalized work force	Unskilled workers
Labor costs	Highly paid workers	Low paid workers
Worker alienation	Employee participation allows for more satisfying working conditions	Worker alienation
Goal congruence	Usually calls for a high degree of commitment to the goals of the organization (high goal congruence) often obtained as part of professional training	Goal congruence not as important and may be difficult to obtain from alienated workers
Employee compensation	Tasks too complex, rapidly changing and interdependent to allow for piece rate payment to be closely linked to performance	Artificial goal congruence obtained by piece rate for simple repetitive tasks
Control and coordination	Loss of centralized control and coordination	Maintains centralized control over the organization and obtains the benefits of coordination

GOAL CONGRUENCE

Participation calls for increased goal congruence.[20] To grant autonomy and discretion to a professional is appropriate to the extent that he will act in accordance with the best interests of the organization. Thus, much professional education and continuing education can be viewed as instilling and reinforcing in students an ideology consistent with the industry in which they will work. Researchers are instilled with the value of the scientific method, lawyers the value of the law, and doctors and nurses the value of health.

Etzioni distinguishes between three types of organizations depending on the degree of compliance.[21] In coercive organizations like jails, the inmates are hostile to organizational goals. In utilitarian organizations like business, members are comparatively indifferent to organizational goals. In normative organizations like universities or religious groups, there is a high degree of goal congruence. Consistent with their differentiated structure, hospitals are partly utilitarian and partly normative organizations, depending on the degree of professionalization of the personnel.

It is this necessity for high goal congruence on the part of professionals that apparently explains why hospitals, universities, and research institutes are not-for-profit corporations.[22] They adhere to altruistic goals which can be more readily subscribed to by professional membership performing the highly complex and unpredictable tasks carried out within their walls.

BEYOND DIFFERENTIATION

The contingency theory of management not only resolves some fundamental dilemmas in the literature on organizations, but it also explains the otherwise peculiar organizational structure of the general hospital with its administrative hierarchy on one hand and its loosely structured medical staff on the other. Contingency theory would suggest, and the empirical evidence supports the idea, that this is fundamentally a rational way to organize a hospital given the current technology and tasks involved. It also explains the persistence of this organizational form in thousands of independent hospitals.

Differentiation is necessary but not sufficient for an efficient hospital. The hierarchically differentiated departments also must coordinate their efforts (integration). This can be done in a variety of different ways,[23] some of which are listed in Table 3.

TABLE 3

TECHNIQUES FOR MAINTAINING COORDINATION[24]

Technique	Example
I. *Hierarchical Coordination*	
(a) Traditional scalar hierarchy	The classical organization chart, hierarchically imposed rules and regulations.
	When the organization's tasks become too complex and too rapidly changing the traditional hierarchy is inadequate and other coordination mechanisms are brought into play.
(b) Staff personnel and departments	"Assistants-to" who back up the hierarchy, staff, planning, clerical personnel.
(c) Automation	Information processing and decision making by computers.
II. *Lateral Coordination*	
(a) Management committees, task forces	Used to coordinate activities between hierarchically separate departments and people.
(b) Direct contact by individuals from different departments to solve problems	Individual contacts, face to face, telephone, or in writing.

(c) Work teams made up of members from different departments at the production level	The patient care team using the patient's medical record as a coordinating device.
(d) Integrators, integrating departments	Unit managers, scheduling departments, expeditors.
III. *Structural Characteristics Effecting Need for Coordination*	
(a) Self containment	Decentralization through independent autonomous subunits (product departmentalization) needing less interunit coordination.
(b) Less specialization	Specialists require coordination while generalists perform a larger range of tasks.
(c) Duplication	Duplication of service departments to coordinate with decentralized production departments; for example, having inpatient and outpatient pharmacy, x-ray, etc.
(d) Decentralization and professionalization (appropriate for complexity not coordination)	Push decisions down to lower levels and increase worker goal congruence. Professional education may lead to ability to coordinate one's work without close supervision.
IV. *Environmental Relationships*	
(a) Buffer departments	Admissions office, discharge planning, purchasing, personnel, public relations.
V. *Resource Characteristics Related to Coordination*	
(a) Input inventories	"Floor stocks" provide surplus production inputs and lessen the need for close interdepartmental coordination, but at the price of higher inventory costs.
(b) Queues	As a way of minimizing coordination or as a result of lack of coordination, e.g., waiting lines at cafeteria or x-ray
(c) Delays	If more coordination is required then the task can be carried out over a longer period of time.
(d) Stabilizing the production process	Advanced scheduling and booking avoids the problems associated with peak loads.

The traditional hierarchy is the principal source of coordination. The problem sets in when the amount of coordination required produces information overload in the hierarchy, and it fails to keep up with the need for rapid and complex decisions. The hierarchy can then be strengthened by the use of staff personnel, planning departments, assistants-to, clerical personnel, etc. If this is not sufficient, lateral coordinating mechanisms come into play such as management committees, work teams (e.g., the patient care team), special integrators (e.g., unit managers) or most frequently direct contact between people in different departments. Also there are structural changes which can be undertaken. Decentralization and professionalization can push complex decisions down the hierarchy, however at the price of coordination between decentralized divisions or between independent professionals. One way of minimizing the need for coordination is through self-contained sub-units (product differentiation) where ancillary services are duplicated in each subunit in order to make them independent. If specialization compels coordination between specialists, reverting to generalists minimizes this.

Either as a failure to coordinate or as specific policy, delay, queues, and input inventories develop. If there is not adequate coordination between nursing and X-ray, patients may queue up at X-ray. If department "B" uses or works on products made by department "A," having a buffer inventory between the two will minimize the need to coordinate closely their production. Of course, there are costs to the organization of these delays, queues, and inventories.

Of these lateral coordinating devices, the most prominent in hospitals are management committees, the medical staff organization, unit managers, and the patient care team. The patient care team, consisting of the physician in charge of the patient and those consultants and paraprofessionals who aid and assist him, is of great importance when one considers that physicians initiate most hospital activities and expenditures.

THE MEDICAL STAFF ORGANIZATION (MSO)

This consists primarily of staff committees, elected officers and department heads. Basically there are three possible options to MSO:

1. Decisions and structure can be imposed in a hierarchical authoritarian manner by the board and administrator on the medical staff without their participation. Contingency theory suggests that this approach with its lack of participation by professionals is non-optimal.

2. Physicians can act independently with minimal MSO, each going his own way. The study by Roemer and Friedman suggests that this is not conducive to high quality of care.[25]

3. The third approach is to combine a high degree of participation by professionals with a highly structured MSO. This form of self-structuring would seem to be the best arrangement for the hospital medical staff.

The traditional task structure of physicians, each with independent responsibility for his own patients, has not called for extensive, rapid coordination between doctors outside of the patient care team. This is not the case for aircraft designers, for example, who are all working on the same aircraft, where decisions about weight, size and shapes of parts are all interdependent.

There are at least two functions to colleagial organization: (1) to provide coordination (e.g., house staff training) and (2) to maintain and reinforce standards of professional excellence which might otherwise deteriorate if the professionals functioned in an isolated manner. *The Patient Care Team* is perhaps the most important form of coordination in the hospital. It is headed by the physician and may include a variety of consultants, nurses, technicians and other paraprofessional workers. A patient care team forms around each patient and dissolves as the patient leaves. Thus, teams are constantly forming, dissolving and forming again, perhaps rarely with the same membership. Traditionally this team has been quite hierarchical in nature with the physician in charge specifying orders to be followed precisely by nurses and technicians. The increasing skill levels of non-physician members of this team would lead one to predict via contingency theory that this hierarchical approach is increasingly inappropriate. It may have perpetrated itself longer than it might, because most of the paraprofessional team members are women who may possibly have tolerated dependence better than men. The existence of a Women's Liberation Movement suggests that this is no longer as true as it was a century ago when the doctor-nurse relationship was cast into its present mold.

When a physician admits a patient for, say, a herniorrhaphy, he specifies exactly what the patient care team is to do: chest X-ray, barium enema, urinalysis, pulmonary exercise, or what have you. Contingency theory would suggest that such detailed specification of procedures is inappropriate to the extent that the other patient team members are skilled professionals. Instead of giving detailed orders, perhaps the admitting physician should say, "Work this patient up for a hernia," leaving it to the rest of the team to decide what that work-up should consist of and how it should be scheduled. To some extent, this latter approach is taken between an attending doctor and an intern or resident who presumably is more skilled and professionalized than a nurse and who demands more participation in patient care decision making.

Realization of the importance of the patient care team as a form of lateral coordination highlights the role of the medical record as a coordinating device both between team members and over time as nursing shifts change.

THE HOSPITAL AS A MATRIX ORGANIZATION

The existence of both hierarchical (vertical) coordination through departmentalization and the formal chain of command and simultaneously lateral (horizontal) coordination across departments (the patient care team) is called a Matrix Organization. One can schematically represent the hospital as a matrix organization as shown in Figure 1. on the following page.

It is this form of diagram that leads to the use of the word matrix.[26] By way of contrast and comparison it is interesting to look at an example of a university as a matrix organization.

UNIVERSITIES AS MATRIX ORGANIZATIONS

Unlike hospitals, universities customarily have felt little need to coordinate activities of their various academic departments. Sociologists never need talk to economists, and neither need talk to professors of divinity. This is beginning to change as an increasing demand emerges for universities to bring their experts to focus on particular social problems.

While hierarchical functional departmentalization without coordination was sufficient in the past, it is inadequate to meet these new demands. The result has been the development of interdisciplinary research or study centers focused on a particular problem and bringing together different academic disciplines in doing so. For example, a Center for Population Studies may include biologists, physiologists, sociologists, and ethical philosophers. The biologist will be both a member of the center and of the academic department of biology (see Figure 2).

Figure 1

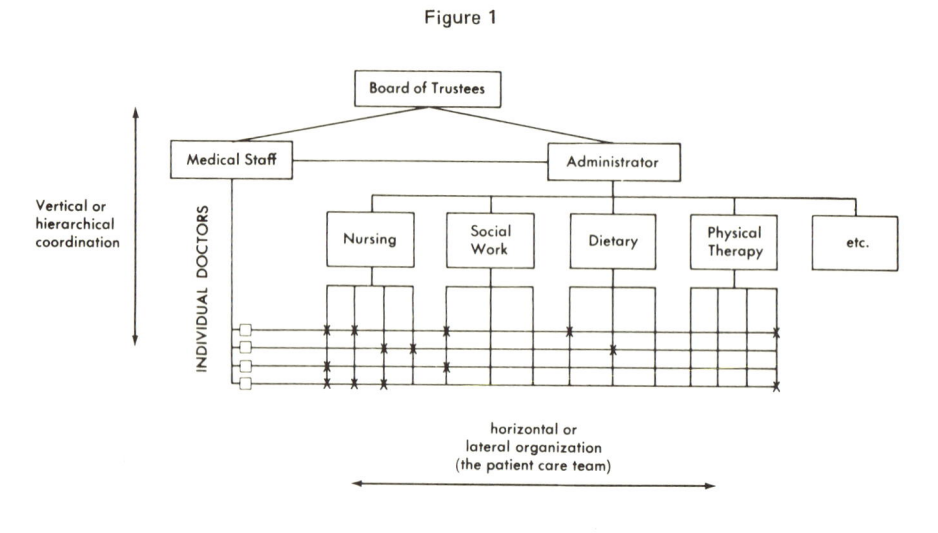

[Figure 1: Organizational chart showing Board of Trustees at top, with Medical Staff and Administrator below. Administrator oversees Nursing, Social Work, Dietary, Physical Therapy, etc. Individual doctors shown on left side. Vertical or hierarchical coordination indicated on left; horizontal or lateral organization (the patient care team) indicated at bottom.]

(x) Indicates both a member of a department and a patient care team.

DIFFERENCES BETWEEN THE ORGANIZATIONAL STRUCTURES

In this way, the new university has become similar in structure to hospitals, since both are matrix organizations. However, there the similarity ends. Unlike the hospital's patient care team, the university center's membership is stable over time and probably more colleagial or democratic in its organization—to name only two obvious differences.

This is not to say that hierarchical organization should be always functionally divided and that lateral organization should be product organized as in hospitals and universities. For example, the army functions in the opposite way. It is hierarchically divided into divisions or armies, which are approximately complete fighting units (hierarchical product organization), and staff specialists, such as the division's chief medical officer who reports both hierarchically to the division (or base) commander and also laterally to the surgeon general's office (lateral functional organization). It is interesting to speculate how such an arrangement might work in hospitals. In fact, it does approximately occur in some of the extremely large hospitals like the Massachussetts General Hospital in Boston or the Karolinska Sjukhuset in Stockholm. Such hospitals may be subdivided along product lines: surgical divisions, pediatric divisions, and psychiatric divisions, each headed by a chief physician and having its own nursing departments, laboratories, dietary departments, etc.

In turn, each of the product divisions has its own matrix organizations. In addition,

Figure 2

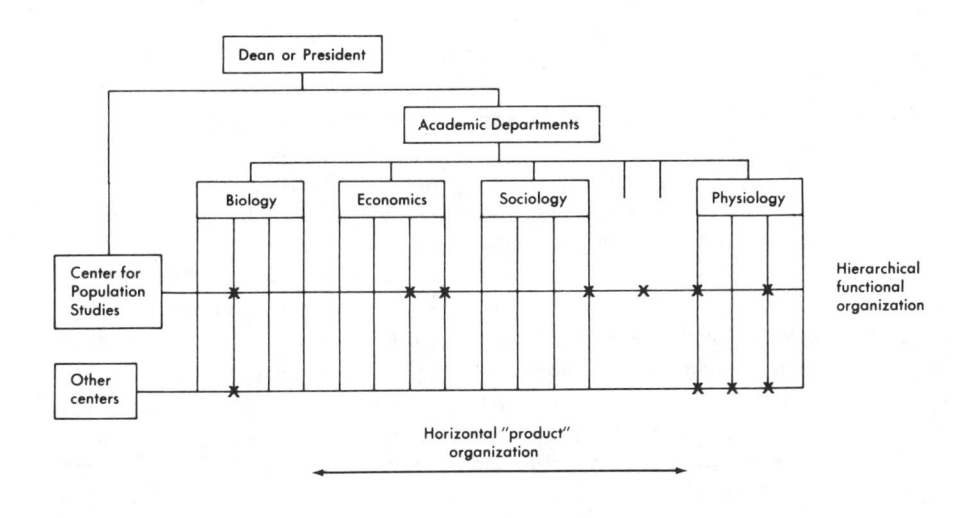

```
                    Dean or President
                           │
              ┌────────────┴────────────┐
              │                  Academic Departments
              │           ┌───────┬────────┬───────┬───────┐
              │        Biology Economics Sociology      Physiology
 Center for     │  │  │     │  │      │  │         │  │  │       Hierarchical
 Population     ─┼──┼──┼─────┼──┼──────┼──┼─────────┼──┼──┼─     functional
 Studies        │  │  │     │  │      │  │         │  │  │       organization
                │  │  │     │  │      │  │         │  │  │
 Other          ─┼──┼──┼─────┼──┼──────┼──┼─────────┼──┼──┼─
 centers
         ←──────── Horizontal "product" organization ────────→
```

Figure 3

```
                    General Director
                           │
         ┌─────────────┬───┴───┬─────────────┐
      Surgical      Pediatric  Psychiatric   Support
      Hospital                               departments
      Chief            │          │          serving
                     Matrix     Matrix       all
                                             divisions
    ┌─────┬─────┬─────┐
  Nursing Labs  etc.
P ──*─────*─────*──
H
Y
S
I
C
I
A
N
S
```

there are a large number of specialized ancillary departments serving all the product divisions. However, for most of the world's hospitals, which are smaller, the proportionately large number and size of ancillary departments serving all parts of the hospital apparently compel hierarchical functional organization.

Another interesting question is whether matrix organizations should have two separate cost reporting systems: one using the functional departments as cost centers and the other using patient care teams or nursing floors as cost centers. In the latter case, housekeeping, nursing, X-ray, etc., costs would all be allocated to patient groups.

UNITY OF COMMAND

The matrix organization leads to the view that a worker can have more than one boss. For example, the nurse is answerable hierarchically to her supervisor and laterally follows the orders of the doctor(s) in charge of her patient care teams. Unity of command was considered one of the basic assumptions of the classical approach to management. The even more basic assumption here is that the alienated worker would play one boss against the other, which could be done when the superiors disagreed. If workers are alienated and/or supervisors disagree, there is a problem. On the other hand, if workers are committed to the goals of the organization and the supervisors are largely in agreement, then unity of command is no longer necessary. For example, in the Russian factory the union, the party, and management all have some control over the workers. Management's message is to produce to meet the quota; the labor union head's message is to produce to meet the quota; and the party chairman says the same thing. The same is true for the family where mother and father both supervise the children. The studies of leadership development in small groups suggest that two leaders (task and socio-emotional) usually emerge. In short, multiple bosses are probably more the rule than the exception in this world.

CONCLUSION

H. L. Smith in a widely cited article states that for hospitals two lines of authority are one too many.[27] This implies that centralized bureaucratic authority over physicians would be much more efficient. Other writers have viewed the typical hospital organization as an anomaly.[28]

In contrast, Contingency Theory argues that the colleagially structured medical staff, coupled with the hierarchically controlled nonprofessional areas and with the paraprofessional departments falling in between, is fundamentally the appropriate form of organization. In addition, the Matrix Organization approach implies that hierarchical departmentalization around functional specialties and lateral coordination by patient care teams is also an appropriate way to coordinate the departmentalized specialists. In short, the hospital is rationally and appropriately organized given the tasks it is faced with. This is not to say that hospitals all run at 100 percent efficiency. Some hospitals are better organized than others. The complexity of the tasks and the degree of coordination required mean that there must be a significant amount of unproductive friction and perhaps considerably more than in organizations coping only with simple tasks in a stable environment where means-ends relationships are well-known.

From this point of view, it may come as some relief to hospital administrators that they have been doing the right thing all along, and recently organization theorists have come to realize it.

IMPLICATIONS FOR HOSPITAL MANAGEMENT

Hospital administrators are attempting to manage one of the most complex organizational forms in existence. They must be skilled in different management styles, both participatory and hierarchical. They must maintain a high degree of differentiation along departmental lines and integrate them simultaneously. They must do so in an industry where performance is exceedingly difficult to measure. Not only is the state of the hospital as a matrix organization complex, it is constantly changing. Technologies are changing, levels of professional competence are increasing, and once-difficult tasks are being routinized and taken over by less skilled people. The hospital, with its participation by professional employees, its difficulty in measuring performance and its potential for abuse of multiple authority, calls for maintenance of a high degree of goal congruence on the part of professional and paraprofessional workers.

The concept of the matrix organization brings into focus the importance of the patient care team for lateral coordination and the need for promoting good team management. Contingency theory suggests that the tradition of the attending doctor, specifying in detail the tasks of other team members, is an inappropriate management technique to the extent that these other team members are truly professionalized.

FOOTNOTES

[1] Max Weber, *The Theory of Social and Economic Organization* (Glencoe, Illinois: The Free Press, 1947); Henri Fayol, "General Principles of Management," *Classics in Management* (New York: American Management Association, 1960), p. 217; and Basil S. Georgopoulos and F.C. Mann, *The Community General Hospital* (New York: The Macmillan Co., 1967).

[2] Rensis Likert, *New Patterns of Management* (New York: McGraw-Hill, 1961), pp. 9-21; Daniel Katz and R. Kahn, *The Social Psychology of Organizations* (New York: John Wiley & Sons, 1966), pp. 332-334; and Chris Argyris, *Diagnosing Human Relations in Organizations*, A Case Study of Hospital Studies in Organizational Behavior, no. 2 (New Haven, Conn.: Labor and Management Center, Yale University, 1956).

[3] Or programmed (low complexity) versus unprogrammed (high complexity) tasks of James March and Herbert Simon, *Organizations* (New York: John Wiley & Sons, 1958).

[4] George F. Lombard, "Relativism in Organizations," *Harvard Business Review*, March/April 1971, p. 55; and Robert J. Mockler, "Situational Theory of Management," *Harvard Business Review*, May/June 1971, p. 146.

[5] Any brief summary is an injustice to the original. The only answer is for the interested reader to refer to them.

[6] Morris Janowitz, "Changing Patterns of Organizational Authority: The Military Establishment," *Administrative Science Quarterly* 3 (March 1959): 473-493.

[7] Joan Woodward, *Industrial Organization: Theory and Practice* (Oxford University Press, 1965).

[8] Robert Blauner, *Alienation and Freedom* (Chicago: University of Chicago Press, 1964).
[9] Harold J. Leavitt, *Managerial Psychology,* 2nd Edition (Chicago: University of Chicago Press, 1964).
[10] Aaron Lowin, "Participative Decision Making: A Model, Literature Critique and Prescriptions for Research," *Organizational Behavior and Human Performance* 3 (1968): 68-106.
[11] Tom Burns and G. M. Stalker, *Management of Innovation* (London: Tavistock, 1961).
[12] Paul R. Lawrence and Jay W. Lorsch. *Organization and Environment* (Cambridge, Mass.: Division of Research, Graduate School of Business Administration, Harvard University, 1967).
[13] Gerald Gordon and Selwyn W. Becker, "Changes in Medical Practice Bring Shifts in the Patterns of Power," *The Modern Hospital,* February 1964, pp. 89-91; S.W. Becker and G. Gordon, "An Entrepreneurial Theory of Formal Organizations, Part I," *Administrative Science Quarterly* 2, no. 3 (December 1966): pp. 315-344; and G. Gordon, "Greater Institutionalization," in *The Impact of Changing Medical Practice on Hospital Administration,* Proceedings of the 6th Annual Symposium on Hospital Affairs, Chicago Graduate Program in Hospital Administration, University of Chicago, Dec., 1963.
[14] Richard L. Durbin and W. Herbert Springall, *Organizations and Administration of Health Care* (St. Louis: C. V. Mosby Co., 1969); and John C. Aird, "Professions Within an Organization: Conflict and Adaptation," (masters thesis, University of California, June, 1967), Chapter 4.
[15] Gerald D. Bell, "Formalism Versus Flexibility in Complex Organizations, A Comparative Investigation within a Hospital." (Ph.D. dissertation, Yale University, 1965), p. 51.
[16] L. Eugene Baldwin, "Differentiation and Integration in Hospital Organization," unpublished (Pensacola: University of West Florida, Nov. 13, 1970).
[17] Duncan Neuhauser, *Administrative Activities and Hospital Performance* (Research #28, Center for Health Administration Studies, University of Chicago, 1971).
[18] Those hospitals where department heads and administrators specified a higher proportion of procedures had lower standardized costs and staffing ratios.
[19] Also see Daniel Katz and Robert L. Kahn, *The Social Psychology of Organizations* (New York: John Wiley & Sons, 1966), pp. 212-214; and R. Tannenbaum and W. H. Schmidt, "How to Choose a Leadership Pattern," *Harvard Business Review* 36 (1959): 95-101.
[20] This is similar to the "loyalty" of Durban and Springall loc. Cit. and the "commitment" of Milton Roemer and Jay W. Friedman, *Doctors in Hospitals* (Baltimore: Johns Hopkins Press, 1971).
[21] Amitai Etzioni, *A Comparative Analysis of Complex Organizations* (New York: Free Press, 1961).
[22] Bruce Steinwald and D. Neuhauser, "The Role of the Proprietary Hospital," *Journal of Law and Contemporary Problems,* Autumn 1970, pp. 817-838.
[23] Jay Lorsch, *Product Innovation and Organization* (New York: Macmillan Co., 1965).
[24] Modified from Jay R. Galbraith, "Organization Design: An Information Processing View," mimeographed (Cambridge Mass.: M.I.T., Sloan School of Management, October, 1969).
[25] M. I. Roemer and J. Friedman, *op. cit., Doctors in Hospitals* (Baltimore: The Johns Hopkins Press, 1971).
[26] Many hospital departments do not actively participate on the patient care team (e.g., maintenance and plant), and others participate indirectly (business office, admissions). To the extent that they don't need to coordinate their work with the patient care team, these departments fall outside the matrix type of organization.
[27] H. L. Smith, "Two lines of authority are one too many," *Modern Hospital* 84 (March 1955): 59-64.
[28] Charles Perrow, "Hospitals: Technology, Structure and Goals," in *Handbook of Organizations,* ed. James March, (Chicago: Rand McNally, 1965); and Hans O. Mauksch, "It Defies All Logic–But a Hospital Does Function," *Modern Hospital,* October 1960, pp. 67-70, reprinted in James K. Skipper and Robert C. Leonard, *Social Interaction and Patient Care* (Philadelphia: J. B. Lippincott Co., 1965), pp. 251-265.

3.
Strictures and Structures

RAY E. BROWN

The late Ray E. Brown was Executive Vice President of the McGaw Medical Center of Northwestern University.

The governance of the American hospital has always been elusive, amorphous, and confusing. Bewildered students of management have been able to find no theories to fit the apparently headless enterprise and have dismissed the situation as an enigma in much the same manner as aerodynamics engineers have treated the notion of the bumblebee flying. Hospitals had to coordinate too many diverse parts and divergent interests to remain organizationally inexplicable, however, and so they invented their own explanation. Because hospitals weren't anxious to admit to the organizational anomaly of a headless enterprise—and even less anxious to face up to the confrontation of the interests at contest by establishing a clear-cut hierarchical structure—they retreated to the other end of the anatomical scale and created the concept of the multilegged organization. Thus was born the presently existing organizational model with no avowed head but three proclaimed legs—trustees, administrator, and medical staff. This organizational arrangement has served the same purpose as the Soviet troika by ensuring an uneasy standoff between the three principal contenders for organizational authority. But it provided capabilities more for legwork than headwork. It also was magnificently designed to ensure that the hospital could move in three different ways without going in any direction.

The awkward and fragmented governance arrangement of the hospital is an inheritance from its past. The hospital was originally conceived as an agency dedicated to doing good rather than well. It was little more than a home away from home for the sick poor. The physicians didn't need the hospital in the beginning and the hospital didn't need management. Money was almost the sole problem of the early hospital and it was not a serious one. The persons who put up the needed sums of money thereby solved the major problem. These persons were the trustees, and they sat alone in the governance saddle because they were responsible for the saddlebags. That arrangement was natural and appropriate and it still persists in many welfare agencies whose

---

From *Hospitals, J.A.H.A.:* Reprinted, with permission, from *Hospitals, Journal of the American Hospital Association,* (Vol. 44, No. 16, August 16, 1970, pp. 79-81). Copyright 1970 by the American Hospital Association. All rights reserved.

purpose is assistance rather than operations. Sitting on top was neither too difficult nor too threatening to others as long as hospital trustees were sitting largely on their own funds.

SOME CHANGES MADE

Scientific medicine changed the seat on which hospital trustees were sitting, however. Scientific medicine changed the nature and the traditions of hospitals and brought both the doctor and his private patients into the hospital. The hospital became the depository of the community's medical resources and, with that change, the hospital trustee began sitting on the doctor's professional and economic prerequisites. At the same time, the hospital trustee started sitting on the hospital patients' funds rather than his own. He also began sitting on top of a complex, expensive, and multipurpose operating enterprise. All this produced a need for management in large doses. It also spelled dependency for a very independent medical profession and it necessitated operational disengagement by deeply engaged hospital trustees.

The present model of fragmented, divergent, and indecisive governance of the hospital represents a stalemate between the aspirations, the fears, and the needs of the three principal participants in that governance. It is more a result of compromise than of organizational logic. In a real way it can be described as a product of organizational treaty rather than organizational treatise.

NOT TOO DAMAGING

The accommodation arrangement under which hospitals have been governed for the past half century was not too damaging to hospital effectiveness. In some ways it was highly effective. If one discounts the frustration experienced by the participants, and the occasional abortive upheaval that has occurred in a few hospitals, the individual hospital has fared well. Reviewing this apparent paradox, one sees several reasons for it. Foremost is the rapid growth in utilization and support that hospitals have experienced. It is hard to go wrong when everything is going right. Also, the momentum of growth helps an enterprise run away from its deficiencies and run over its problems. In another vein, the very rapidity of change along all environmental fronts has served to both lay the dust over hospital miscues and lay the path for them to follow. Perhaps most importantly, the expertness in brinkmanship developed by all three components of the hospital governance triad enabled the hospital to hold together and to maintain a course. Perceptivity regarding how far one can go in bucking the crew or the tide preserves sufficient order to keep things moving. In the case of the hospital, this has meant a large unity of effort, instead of large dissension, despite the diffusion of authority.

CHANGING CIRCUMSTANCES

The governance by sufferance that has characterized the hospital to date is not being challenged by changing circumstances and by other claimants to a piece of the governance. Running hospitals to suit the compromised notions of trustees, administrators, and doctors is being attacked on both organizational grounds and on public policy grounds. There is mounting concern and criticism from various groups and organizations that hospitals are not running well nor running in the right direction.

The concerns and criticisms reflect in part the changing circumstances in which hospitals find themselves. Inflation, medical advances, and increasing utilization have caused hospital costs to rise precipitously and have raised questions regarding the operating efficiency and quality of hospital management. Third-party payers are now picking up most of the tab for the hospital, meaning that hospital costs and hospital programs are concerns of the paying public—whether through private sector or governmental third parties. Social policy, now committed to adequate medical and hospital care for all members of the population, denotes governmental responsibility to redeem this commitment. At the same time, those to whom the commitment was made are asserting a right to help determine how the commitment will be met. So, the long-standing obscurity in the governance of the hospital is further clouded by the strong claims of third parties, government, and organized community groups to have an input in that governance.

It is not simply a question of adding the new claimants as legs to a three-legged entity. The present three legs have themselves become restive because of the criticism and the threats of the new claimants. Each entity is asking for a clearer definition of its role and a better structured mode of role expression. A multitude of court decisions and a host of private and governmental approval and regulatory agencies are making similar demands.

As hospitals become more expensive, involved, and committed, the need for restructuring of their governance becomes imperative. The demand for this will grow increasingly loud and incessant by all parties at interest. The organizational model that is developed must provide strength in both program determination and in operations. It also must afford a proper amount and mode of input into the governance process from each of the interest groups. Most of all, the governance must be designed to coalesce rather than to checkmate the diverse interests represented. The present governance arrangement provides an easy means for everyone to say "no" and very little means for the hospital to say "yes." The central position hospitals now have in the total medical care program of the community requires positive leadership on the part of the hospital. This does not mean that it is supposed to be easy prey for all claims made on its program or resources. It does mean that if it is to program effectively, and operate efficiently, it must have an effective governance arrangement for making up its mind and carrying out its decisions.

4.

The Hospital as a Prototype Organization

ALAN D. BAUERSCHMIDT

Alan D. Bauerschmidt, Ph.D., is Associate Professor of Management - College of Business Administration - The University of South Carolina.

The administrator who has been exposed to traditional management theory in the process of his formal or continuing education has experienced a distinct disadvantage in the application of these concepts to his working situation. If he is astute, he has recognized that the principles involved will not work in his organization. If he has a blind bent for accepting the conventional wisdom of the authorities, he has failed himself and his organization in one way or another. This is one type of administrator. The more critical administrator can be further classified into one of two categories: the administrator who knows that the principles of management won't work in his organization, and who, therefore, makes no attempt to exercise any recognizable form of management, following instead a course of day-to-day accommodation of events over which he has little, if any, control; the second critical administrator, while recognizing the inappropriateness of traditional management concepts, accepts the challenge of his unique situation and performs his coordinative tasks through a personally developed theory of organization and management.

While the first two administrators would provide interesting case studies of faulty response, the last administrator is of much more interest to the student of management practice. In fact, because of certain modifications which are occurring in our society, the administrator who has accepted the managerial challenge may provide a model of administrative response to a prototype organization. There is reason to believe that traditional forms of organization which have been managed within the context of time-honored principles may be passing from the scene, with the strong sug-

---

This paper is based on an address delivered at the forty-eighth annual meeting of the South Carolina Hospital Association, at Columbia, South Carolina, on January 24, 1969. The argument presented here is amplified in the author's unpublished dissertation, *The Anomalies of Hospital Organization,* University of Florida, Gainesville, Florida, August, 1968.

Reprinted by permission from *Hospital Administration* (currently *Hospital and Health Services Administration):* Quarterly Journal of the American College of Hospital Administrators, Chicago, Vol. 15 (Spring, 1970), pp. 6-14. Copyright 1970 by the American College of Hospital Administrators. All rights reserved.

gestion that they will be replaced by managerial situations much like that of the hospital administrator. The period of isolation of the hospital administrator may well be replaced by a phase within which a variety of students and theorists from the business world will be peering over the shoulder of the hospital administrator to observe both his form of organization and his methods of management.

Before an attempt is made to explore the prototype characteristics of the hospital situation, it would be appropriate to review briefly the traditional structure of organization which the hospital administrator has found wanting or unacceptable in his own situation. In a very broad brush treatment, the foundation of accepted management principles rests upon a structure which includes a requirement for the rigid breakdown of functional specialization. Each element of organizational accomplishment can be identified and linked with an occupational or functional identity. In effect, it is postulated that the various functions which are identified can be rationalized. That is, the tasks can not only be identified, but can also be defined as the specific duties of definite individuals, with overlaps and gaps in the accomplishment of activities avoided. Finally, the various task elements which have been identified and rationalized can be linked together in a systematized manner through a well-developed command hierarchy which performs the coordinative functions called management. This feature of the traditional concepts approach is basically predicated upon the overriding principle of unity of command.

What this arrangement nets is a basic element of good management: a neat, orderly structure of enterprise within which management can go about its work. This structure, in its traditional format, might well be called the workbench of management. In common with other skilled artisans, all proficient managers realize that one cannot go about the tasks at hand without a sturdy bench upon which to operate. However, this form of structure serves another useful purpose—it provides a framework within which the techniques of management can be transferred from one form of enterprise to another, the theory being that management effectively applied in any form of enterprise can be as effectively applied elsewhere, if the structure of organization is similarly arranged. Undoubtedly, many hospital administrators have been faced with the supposition that if they are to employ the suggestions for improved operations advanced by the management scientist, the decision-theorist, the operations researcher, the industrial engineer, or the systems analyst, they must rationalize their organizational structure to conform with that employed by the business organization where the techniques of these specialists were developed. Through a deeper understanding of his own organizational situation, the astute hospital administrator will not feel remiss in rejecting such a suggestion even though he may be in agreement with the logic involved.

WHERE HOSPITAL STRUCTURE DIFFERS

The problem the hospital administrator faces in considering the adaptability of his organizational structure to the more familiar business model is well documented. The discussions in the literature describing the dichotomy between hospitals and the modal organizations of our society are undoubtedly quite familiar to the hospital administrator.[1] While these arguments may provide valuable ammunition to the administrator in his contests with a business-oriented board of trustees, they afford little opportunity to the dedicated hospital manager who wishes to seize upon the advantages provided by the management disciplines which have been mentioned. What the hospital administrator needs is a bridge between the structures of business and hospital organization upon which the techniques of management can be transferred to the gain of the hospital enterprise. Important new management research indicates that in two significant areas of organizational identity such a bridge is rapidly becoming available, and that, in fact, the hospital does lie on a continuum of universal enterprise, although it departs from the modal organizations of our society in these two aspects at the present time.

The first basis for affinity between the hospital and certain business enterprises is the form of production technique employed. There are a variety of production processes used in typical hospital situations, but the predominant form, the one which directly serves the primary objective of the operation is that which effects the care and treatment of the patient. Under analysis, this process is revealed as being directed toward a unique output. Each patient is a singular personality with a malady uncommon in its manifestation in the individual. There is also a particular physician who prescribes a course of care and treatment rare in its appreciation of the individual patient and his disease within a framework of the physician's personal experience and education. While it is impossible to enumerate completely the variables involved, one might guess that the probability would be of low order that the same productive technique could be applied to any two patients. In business terms the hospital employs odd-lot, job order, or unit production technology.

This process, of course, is not unique to the hospital. Business terms have been used, and business firms employ similar technology with different materials and labor. Research in England, which bears directly on the aforementioned bridge between organizations, has identified a continuum of production technology extending from the cited unit production methods through various batch production techniques to continuous process production methods.[2]

These English studies indicate that two forms of organizational structure predominate, and these appear to be more applicable to specific production technologies. Batch methods of production, in their various modifications of mass production technology on the assembly line, adhere to a form of management organization which has been discussed here as being traditional. The British choose to call this form which has demonstrated significant success in these types of enterprise, "mechanistic." This term is very descriptive of the method of management itself. On the other hand, an "organic" form of structure is more likely to be associated with success in the unit and process production firms, even though they would appear to be on either end of the technology spectrum.[3]

The organic form of organizational structure differs in many significant respects from the traditional form of structure, although the requirement for management is much the same. Specifically, the organic form of structure is noted for a looseness of relationships which allows for rapid adaptation to changing circumstances, without explicit management intervention. The definitions of duties and responsibilities are less rigid than in the mechanistic organization, with the operative performer being given wider latitude in defining his own functions to fit a particular work situation. In turn, communications in the organic structure follow no established pattern but rather respond spontaneously to the situation. As a prerequisite to each of these characteristics of structure, the command hierarchy of the organic organization must be ill-defined, with consultation replacing the order-giving situation typical in the mechanistic, or traditional, structure. As reported in these English studies, the force which gives this structure a semblance of order is provided by the close working relationship which exists among the experts with common goals who compose the work force in these highly individualistic industries. It appears that a mutual dependence exists among the various participants under these working conditions, although their expertise will be highly dissimilar and their values unique.

UNDERLYING SENSE OF ORDER

The reader who is familiar with hospital administration will already have recognized that the chaos which has been described here closely replicates that which is contained in the typical hospital. But it should also be noted that this surface chaos has an underlying sense of order. This order will be indistinct, however, to the managerial mind trained in traditional concepts. What is most important for our present purpose is that the description provided has been obtained from the business situation and is associated with the employment of management techniques, however strange these techniques may be as compared with the classic textbook examples.

It should be acknowledged that the opportunities for transfer between the hospital organization and the unit production firms of industry have certain limitations. The hospital is atypical in comparison to these firms because of the relatively small size of firms employing unit production technology. While this might provide comment in regard to the optimal scale of hospital operations, it is beyond the purposes of this paper to develop this subject here. It would be suggested, however, that the affinity of organizational structure between unit and process production firms would allow the management technology of process production to be readily suited to the hospital situation. While, again, the topic cannot be discussed here, a strong case can be developed for the similarity in purpose between the process and unit production firms, with the former employing a much more advanced form of production technology. There is a real possibility, however, that the organic form of structure has its impetus only partially in the form of production technology employed, and by turning directly to the hospital for explanation the prototype characteristics of this form of structure can be deciphered.

AFFINITY THROUGH RELATIVE PROFESSIONALIZATION

The more important basis for affinity between the hospital organization and the universal structure of enterprise is the degree to which individuals of a professional persuasion find their life's work within an organizational context. While it can be said that hospitals have shared with certain industries a devotion to unit production methods and a proclivity toward process production, the professional in business is a relatively new phenomenon on any large scale. It would appear that in this area the business manager could learn a great deal from the hospital administrator. In many cases, it has become imperative for competitive survival that the business firm incorporate a method of evolving professionals into their organizational structure.

The hospital is undoubtedly a pioneer in this area. The epitome of professionalization in our society is the physician, and while it may not be correct to consider him a part of the internal structure of the institution, he has provided a model for the status aspirations of the more typical hospital worker. The pace at which professionalization has progressed within the hospital would truly mark this organization as a prototype for the universal structure. It is possible to refer to the professionalization of nursing, dietetics, medical technology, and many other more subtle fields of medicine having similar, but incipient, aspirations.

More important than the appearance of the individuals themselves in organizations, however, are the characteristics of the professional which mark the enterprises within which they are employed. In this regard the professional will be only partially involved in the activities of the institution as a life's work. The degree of organizational loyalty one could expect from an employee in the traditional industry will be unobtainable, although the degree of participation in enterprise objectives may be much the same. In addition, the professional will demand a high degree of autonomy within his functional area of competence and will insist upon independence in matters within his area of specialization. He will seek prestige and emphasize the prestige-bearing aspect of his work. In this respect, he will avoid tasks which carry a menial connotation within the minds of his professional peers outside his particular organization. Finally, but not all inclusive of the organizational ramification of professional employees, he will view the enterprise as an opportunistic area within which to pursue professional goals. But, in spite of these largely negative aspects, he will still cooperate with other enterprise members when the matters at hand are relevant to their discipline.[4]

UNIT PRODUCTION AND PROFESSIONAL CONCEPTS

It should be apparent that a great deal of similarity exists between the character of professional participation in organizations and the characteristics of the organic form of structure found in the successful unit and process production firms. Pure chance could not explain this similarity. Although the approach here has been to indicate that technology demands an organic structure in the unit and process production enterprise while the human resources employed in the professional organization dictate an "organic" form of structure, a more direct affinity unalterably links the two. Specifically, the approach of the professional dictates a unit or a process production method— the so-called "arts" of the professional forewarn a unique approach to the production situation. He will view each unit of his output as a rare entity. Considering the link between professionalization and unit and process production from the other direction, the one-of-a-kind production situation, whether the product is shaped from its raw state on a single basis or is produced by a process which allows an infinite variety of individual differences, the skills of the craftsman—and in our service and highly technical industries, the skills of the professional—are a prime necessity. There is no need to ask the chicken or egg question, for in fact, the two concepts of individualized production and professionalization are closely linked, to which the hospitals of our society are sufficient testimony.

THE FUTURE PREDOMINANCE OF ORGANIC STRUCTURES

It should be apparent that the organizational structure, which is the workbench of management, can vary to a considerable degree. The best structure may not be the stable platform described in traditional theory, particularly when the technology of production and the human resources of the organization are considered. More important, the characteristics which have been considered are common to both the hospital and selected industries. The opportunity for the exchange of management techniques is available among organizations which share these common forms of structure.

There is more to interest the management students in these observations than the simple notation that a bridge exists between two forms of enterprise which now assume a minor position in our social structure. A trend can be discerned which could lead to the prediction that more forms of enterprise are assuming these same characteristics. Considering this trend from the point of view of professionalization, one can simply predict that larger proportions of the work force will assume these characteristics as general educational levels are raised. A more complicated explanation of increasing professionalization is provided by noting the increasing complexity of our society and the manifest need of the individual to obtain order and meaning from a value system less remote than the total society or a disintegrated family or community structure. Professionalization provides this value system and in turn protects the individual from the vagaries of a social organization which is too large and complex to be dealt with individually. As a further point in favor of the prediction of increasing professionalization, one can note that, as society continues its progress in solving the economic problem, new heights of human motivation become apparent in the need hierarchy, and an advancing maturity of man in regard to psychological healthiness can be discerned. The higher levels of need which became operative in these circumstances are conducive to the mode of the professional, particularly as it concerns the self-esteem needs of independence, freedom, knowledge, and ultimately, self-realization.

This same rising of man's needs has implications for the predominant form of production technology. As man passes beyond the level of his lower needs he finds a new expression of individuality in his taste for products. Man becomes unique as he rises above the social emphasis of group and esteem needs, and as Marshall McLuhan has noted, production will become an individual service which can provide those unduplicated products required by an individualistic society. The age of mass consumption, serviced by the traditional forms of enterprise, dedicated to batch methods of technology, will pass in favor of the organic structures of enterprise which emphasize unit and process methods of production directed toward individual consumption.

NEW PIONEERS IN MANAGERIAL PROBLEMS

As more and more industries come under the sway of these factors and their managements recognize that new forms of structure are required to accommodate their changing technology and modified work force, they will undoubtedly turn for guidance to managers experienced in using these new forms. Where the hospital administrator had previously been most humble in regard to his uncertain workbench of organizational structure, he will come into his own as a specialist among managers. He will be considered a pioneer in the treatment of managerial problems which appear to defy solution. While no hospital administrator can claim solution to the complexities involved in these situations, he does bear witness to the attempt and, therefore, provides a fruitful field of study for the management theorist. To the administrator's benefit he will once again be within the mainstream of management thought and an active participant in the theory which should result. I need not add that a new concentration on the management problems associated with health care can only benefit our entire society.

FOOTNOTES

[1] Included among these discussions and representative of the literature are: Amitai Etzioni, "Authority Structure and Organizational Effectiveness," *Administrative Sciences Quarterly,* II (June 1959), pp. 43-67; Basil S. Georgopoulos and Floyd C. Mann, "The Hospital as an Organization," *Hospital Administration,* IX (Summer, 1964), pp. 23-35; and Harvey L. Smith, "Two Lines of Authority Are One Too Many," *Modern Hospital,* LXXXIV (March, 1955), pp. 59-64.

[2] Joan Woodward. *Industrial Organization: Theory and Practice.* London: Oxford University Press, 1965.

[3] The terms "mechanistic" and "organic" employed by Woodward and attributed to Tom Burns and G. M. Stalker, *The Management of Innovation.* London: Tavistock Publications Ltd., 1961.

[4] The collection edited by Howard M. Vollmer and Donald L. Mills. *Professionalization.* Englewood Cliffs, New Jersey: Prentice-Hall Inc., 1966, provides an excellent presentation of the various ramifications of professionalization in the widest context.

5.
Hospital Administration and Systems Concepts

FREMONT E. KAST AND JAMES E. ROSENZWEIG

Fremont E. Kast, Ph.D., and James E. Rosenzweig, Ph.D., are both Professors of Management and Organization at the University of Washington.

An omnipresent phenomenon of modern society has been the growth and development of large-scale, complex organizations. In most human activities there has been an evolution from small-scale, informally organized groups toward large, highly-structured, formal organizations. Hospitals, business enterprises, governmental units, educational institutions, labor unions, charitable activities, and even social and recreational endeavors have tended to become larger and more complex. These large-scale organizations have been primarily devices for rationalization of human effort and for the more effective accomplishment of many objectives. They provide a means for coping with the increased complexities and challenges of modern societies.

In spite of their prevalence, development of a general model or theory of large-scale, complex organizations has been extremely slow. Although a great deal has been written about large organizations in recent years, most of the models presented have been restricted or partial, rather than general models.[1] It is our view that at this stage, systems concepts provide the most useful general model for the study of complex organizations such as hospitals. In this article we will review general systems theory, show some broad applications of systems concepts outside the field of hospital administration, and then discuss more specifically the application of systems concepts in hospital administration.

DEFINITION OF A SYSTEM

A system is "an organized or complex whole: an assemblage or combination of things or parts forming a complex or unitary whole." The term system covers an extremely broad spectrum of concepts. The biologist Ludwig von Bertalanffy set forth a model which he called open systems.[2] The basis of his concept is that a living

---

[1] Among the most significant of these are: James G. March and Herbert A. Simon, *Organizations* (New York: John Wiley & Sons, Inc., 1958); Amitai Etzioni, *A Comparative Analysis of Complex Organization* (New York: Free Press of Glencoe, Inc., 1961); and Peter M. Blau and W. Richard Scott, *Formal Organizations* (San Francisco: Chandler Publishing Co., 1962).

[2] Ludwig von Bertalanffy, "General Systems Theory: A New Approach to Unity of Science," *Human Biology,* December, 1951, pp. 303-61.

Reprinted by permission from *Hospital Administration: Quarterly Journal of the American College of Hospital Administrators,* Chicago, Vol. 11 (Fall, 1966), 17-33. Copyright 1966 by the American College of Hospital Administrators. All rights reserved.

organism is not a conglomeration of separate elements but a definite system, possessing organization and wholeness. An organization is an open system which maintains a constant state while matter and energy which enter it keep changing (so-called dynamic equilibrium). The organism is influenced by, and influences, its environment and reaches a state of dynamic equilibrium in this environment. Such a description fits complex organizations such as hospitals. The hospital is a man-made social system which has a dynamic interplay with its environment—the community, patients, medical practitioners, governments and many other elements. Furthermore, the hospital is a system of interrelated parts working in conjunction with each other in order to accomplish a number of goals, those of the organization *and* individual participants.

The systems concept is a useful way of thinking about the function of management and administration of large-scale, complex organizations. It provides a framework for visualizing internal and external environment factors as an integrated whole. It allows recognition of the proper place and function of subsystems. But, above all, it emphasizes the importance of the integration of these subsystems into an operational whole.[3]

GENERAL SYSTEMS THEORY

General systems theory is concerned with developing a systematic, theoretical framework for describing general relationships of the empirical world. One of the most important reasons pointing to the need for a general systems theory is the problem of communication between the various disciplines. Although there is some similarity between general methods of approach—the scientific method—the results of research are not often communicated across discipline boundaries. Increasingly, there has been a development of interdisciplinary studies. Areas such as social psychology, biochemistry, astrophysics, social anthropology, economic psychology, and economic sociology have developed to integrate various disciplines. Recently, areas of study and research have developed which utilize knowledge from various fields. For example, sybernetics calls on electrical engineering, neurophysiology, physics, biology, and other fields. Operations research is often pointed to as a multidisciplinary approach to problem solving. Organization theory embraces economics, sociology, engineering, psychology, physiology, and anthropology. Problem solving and decision making are becoming focal points for study and research, drawing on numerous disciplines.

With these examples of interdisciplinary approaches, it is easy to recognize a surge of interest in larger-scale, systematic bodies of knowledge. However, this trend calls for the development of an overall framework within which the various subparts can be integrated. General systems theory may help to provide this framework.

THE HIERARCHY OF LEVELS

Kenneth Boulding has provided a useful classification of systems which sets forth a hierarchy of levels as follows:[4]

---

[3] For a more comprehensive discussion of these concepts see R. A. Johnson, F. E. Kast, and J. E. Rosenzweig, *The Theory and Management of Systems* (New York: McGraw-Hill Book Co., Inc., 1963).

[4] Kenneth Boulding, "General Systems Theory: The Skeleton of Science," *Management Science,* April, 1956, pp. 197-208.

1. The first level is that of static structure. It might be called the level of *framework;* for example, the anatomy of the universe.
2. The next level is that of the simple dynamic system with predetermined, necessary motions. This might be called the level of *clockworks.*
3. The control mechanism or cybernetic system, which might be nicknamed the level of the *thermostat.* The system is self-regulating in maintaining equilibrium.
4. The fourth level is that of the "open system," or self-maintaining structure. This is the level at which life begins to differentiate from not-life; it might be called the level of the *cell.*
5. The next level might be called the genetic-societal level; it is typified by the *plant,* and it dominates the empirical world of the botanist.
6. The *animal* system level is characterized by increased mobility, teleological behavior, and self-awareness.
7. The next level is the *human* level, that is, of the individual human being considered as a system with self-awareness and the ability to utilize language and symbolism.
8. The *social system* or systems of human organization constitute the next level, with the consideration of the content and meaning of messages, the nature and dimensions of value systems, the transcription of images into historical record, the subtle symbolizations of art, music and poetry, and the complex gamut of human emotion.
9. *Transcendental systems* complete the classification of levels. These are the ultimates and absolutes and the inescapables and unknowables, and they also exhibit systematic structure and relationship.

Obviously, the first level is most pervasive. Descriptions of static structures are widespread. This descriptive cataloguing is helpful in providing a framework for additional analysis and synthesis. Dynamic "clockwork" systems, where prediction is a strong element, are evident in the classical natural sciences such as physics and astronomy; yet even here there are important gaps. Adequate theoretical models are not apparent at higher levels. However, in recent years closed-loop cybernetics, or "thermostat," systems have received increasing attention. At the same time, work is progressing on open-loop systems with self-maintaining structures and reproduction facilities. Beyond the fourth level we hardly have a beginning of theory. It is obvious that the social sciences are operating in the last four levels of this systems hierarchy.

RELATIONSHIP TO FUNCTIONALISM

There is a close relationship between general systems theory and the development of functionalism in the social sciences. This relationship is apparent in the following statement of Don Martindale:

In the period since World War II, as Western society readjusted to the radical change in milieu that followed, with the attempt to return to something that looked like "normalcy," but in a permanently transformed world, the essential unity of the social sciences has been revealed through the flooding of the functionalistic voint of view across the boundaries of the special disciplines. This point of view has had both theoretical and methodological dimensions. Theoretically, it consists in the analysis of social and cultural life from the standpoint of wholes or systems. Epistemologically, it involves analysis of social events by methods thought peculiarly adapted to the integration of social events into systems.

The functionalistic point of view has been manifest in all the social sciences from psychology through sociology, political science, economics, and anthropology to geography, jurisprudence and linguistics. Most primary theoretical and methodological debates in postwar social science have centered on functionalism and alternatives to it.[5]

Although there are several meanings of the word "functionalism," its most important aspect is the emphasis upon systems of relationship and the integration of

[5] Don Martindale, *Functionalism in the Social Sciences* (American Academy of Political and Social Science Monograph 5, February, 1965), pp. viii-ix.

parts and subsystems into a whole.[6] General systems theory and the functionalistic point of view (including dynamic equilibrium concepts from economics) offer a theoretical framework for the study of complex organizations.

SYSTEMS CONCEPTS FOR MANAGEMENT OF COMPLEX ORGANIZATIONS

Traditional organization theory, based upon Max Weber's bureaucratic model and the administrative management model, placed emphasis upon organizational structure, hierarchical relationships, specialization, span of control, and line and staff relationships. The traditional theory did not give sufficient emphasis to the problems of interrelationships or integration of activities. Nor did the neoclassical, or human relations, approach move in this direction. Its approach was aimed at interjecting back into the mechanistic, traditional models human motivations, aspirations, and limitations. Neither of these approaches provided a basis for an integrated, systematic organizational model.

Increasing attention is being given to the notion that the most useful way to study organizations is to consider them as systems. This view tends to treat them as systems of mutually dependent parts and variables, and the complex organization is thought of as a social system within the broader, more inclusive system of society. Sociologist Talcott Parsons expresses this view:

> It seems appropriate to define an organization as a social system which is organized for the attainment of a particular type of goal; the attainment of that goal is at the same time a performance of a type of function on behalf of a more inclusive system, the society.[7]

Modern organization theory and general systems theory are closely related, with organization theory a special element of general systems theory. Systems theory and organization theory are both concerned with the investigation and performance of the organization as an integrated whole. However, general systems theory is concerned with all nine levels of systems whereas organization theory focuses primarily upon level eight, human social organizations.

Under the systems concept, the complex organization is viewed as a *conglomerate of subsystems* which include the individual, the informal work groups, the formal organization, and, finally, the environmental systems which have a direct impact upon it. Furthermore, under the systems concept, consideration must be given to the means for *interrelating and coordinating* these various subsystems. These parts are integrated through various processes such as the information and communications network, the decision system, and built-in equilibrium mechanisms which exist in every organization.

APPLICATIONS OF SYSTEMS CONCEPTS

Actually, practical applications of many of the concepts stemming from the systems approach have preceded the development of adequate models or theories of complex organizations. Several of these applications are:

---

[6] Robert K. Merton discusses various connotations of the word "function" in *Social Theory and Social Structure* (Glencoe, Ill.: Free Press, 1957), pp. 20-22.

[7] Talcott Parsons, "Suggestions for a Sociological Approach to the Theory of Organizations," *Administrative Science Quarterly*. September, 1956, p. 238.

1. The weapon-system management approach has been used extensively in the development of the nation's advanced weapon and space systems. This approach calls for the systematic organization of a vast complex of strategies, technologies, industries, human and material resources, and other subsystems into an integrated whole toward the accomplishment of objectives.
2. Program management has been utilized in many of the advanced technology industries. It is essentially a managerial approach for adapting to the systems concept. Program management calls for integration of the activities related to particular projects into explicit organizational systems.
3. Automation represents an important application of the systems concept in industry. It requires the integration of many of the operations of the business firm into a formal man-machine system.
4. Systems concepts have been applied extensively in data processing; indeed the term data processing system has widespread usage. The most sophisticated data-processing systems are represented by real-time, or on-line, systems. In these cases, the computer is an integral part of the information-decision system and it is used to provide information during the actual decision process.
5. Many of the newer approaches in management science–operations research, industrial dynamics and simulation–are based upon the systems concept. These approaches structure the operation under analysis as an integrated system tied together by a series of equations. The use of computers in symbolic system simulation allows treatment of large-scale, complex systems. Thus an analyst can develop a model of a group of subsystems, their interrelationships, and the total system.
6. PERT, SCANS, RAMPS, and other techniques of network analysis are examples of more detailed applications of systems concepts. They can be used to recognize and identify all the interconnecting links in a single system or in a series or network of systems.
7. In considering human behavior in formal organizations there is a tendency to think in terms of systems concepts. For example, Rensis Likert suggests the interaction-influence system as the means for integrating and coordinating the efforts of participants in organizations.[8]

SYSTEMS CONCEPTS IN HOSPITAL ADMINISTRATION

Anyone familiar with hospitals as organizations realizes that many of the models and generalizations taken from other organizations are not directly applicable nor appropriate. Indeed, there are many reasons for questioning the usefulness of the traditional models for any large-scale, complex organization. Essentially, the traditional approach is based upon Max Weber's ideal bureaucratic model with modifications from scientific management and the administrative management approaches of Luther Gulick, Lyndall Urwick, James Mooney and Alan Reiley, and others. The basic dimensions of the bureaucratic model are:[9]

1. A division of labor based upon functional specialization.
2. A well-defined hierarchy of authority.
3. A system of rules covering the rights and duties of positional incumbents.
4. A system of procedures for dealing with work situations.
5. Impersonality of interpersonal relations.
6. Promotion and selection for employment based upon technical competence.

Although these characteristics of the bureaucratic form may be applicable to large hospitals in certain instances, there are many factors which limit their value. Shortcomings are also apparent in the application of scientific management principles and generalizations from the administrative management approaches. Some of the key

---

[8] Rensis Likert, *New Patterns of Management* (New York: McGraw-Hill Book Co., 1961).

[9] Richard H. Hall, "The Concept of Bureaucracy: An Empirical Assessment," *American Journal of Sociology*, July, 1963, p. 33.

deficiencies in applying the traditional organization model of hospitals are discussed below.

WHY HOSPITALS DO NOT FIT THE TRADITIONAL MODEL

The traditional model calls for a definite hierarchy of authority with clear-cut superior-subordinate relationships. This may be appropriate where the administrator has superiority of knowledge and information, but it is not feasible where there is specialization of skills and knowledge on the part of participants at different levels in the organization. Particularly, there is often conflict between hierarchical authority and professional values of organizational members. This is true in organizations other than hospitals. William Kornhauser found that there was substantial conflict between the professional values of scientists in industry and the organizational requirements imposed by the administrative hierarchy.[10] Amitai Etzioni sees this as a major problem in many complex organizations.

> Probably the most important structural dilemma is the inevitable strain imposed on the organization by the use of knowledge. All social units use knowledge, but organizations use more knowledge more systematically than do other social units. . . .Students of the professions have pointed out that the autonomy granted to professionals who are basically responsible to their consciences (though they may be censured by their peers and in extreme cases by the courts) is necessary for effective professional work. It is this highly individualized principle which is diametrically opposed to the very essence of the organizational principle of control and coordination by superiors—i.e., the principle of administrative authority.[11]

THE CONTINUAL POWER CONFLICT

While this conflict between the knowledge and values of the professional and hierarchical administrative authority is apparent in many organizations, it appears most critical in hospitals. A large hospital requires effective performance by many professional and semi-professional participants who have highly specialized knowledge and skills. Yet, their functions are not performed in a vacuum; they must be integrated into an over-all operation. It is understandable that there is a continual power conflict between the various professionals and the hospital administration.[12] But, traditional management models provide no answers to these problems—they do not even recognize their existence. The systems model provides a more effective means for understanding and dealing with these relationships.

Another characteristic of the traditional model which is not completely appropriate for the hospital is the emphasis upon routinization and standardization of activities. To be sure, there are a number of hospital activities which fall within this category, but there are many others which cannot be standardized and made uniform. This is

---

[10] William Kornhauser, *Scientists in Industry: Conflict and Accommodation* (Berkeley: University of California Press, 1963).

[11] Amitai Etzioni, *Modern Organizations* (Englewood Cliffs, N.J.: Prentice-Hall, Inc., 1964), pp. 75-76.

[12] Many articles in *Hospital Administration* have dealt with these problems. Two of the more directly related are George Bugbee, "Administration and the Professional in the Hospital." Winter, 1961, pp. 26-33, and Harold L. Wilensky, "The Dynamics of Professionalism: The Case of Hospital Administration," Spring, 1962, pp. 6-24.

particularly true for activities which require interactions between the various participants in the hospital.

Eugene Litwak suggests an interesting distinction between different models for large-scale organizations:

> Weber's model is most efficient when the organization deals primarily with uniform events and with occupations stressing traditional areas of knowledge rather than social skills. The human-relations model will be most efficient for dealing with events which are not uniform (research, medical treatment, graduate training, designing) and with occupations emphasizing social skills as well as technical aspects of the job....
>
> There are several models of organization with differential efficiencies depending on the nature of the work and the types of tasks to be performed. In this regard, at least three types have been suggested: Weber's, that found in "human relations" and what may be called the "professional bureaucracy." This third model is characterized by the degree to which the organization must deal with events both uniform and not uniform, or by the need to have jobs requiring great social skills as well as jobs requiring traditional areas of knowledge. Perhaps the outstanding illustrations of the third type would be a large hospital, a graduate school, or a research organization.
>
> The chief distinguishing characteristic of the professional model is its inclusion of contradictory forms of social relations. This model is particularly relevant to contemporary society where most large-scale organizations have to deal with uniform and non-uniform tasks or with occupations that demand traditional knowledge as well as social skills.[13]

MULTIPLE OBJECTIVES OF COMPLEX ORGANIZATIONS

Other studies suggest that the traditional bureaucratic model is not appropriate when applied to non-routine, "creative" decisions and activities. They show that departments or units whose tasks are nonroutine or difficult to standardize are significantly less bureaucratic.[14] Many aspects of hospital operations are also non-programmable and require freedom from the restriction of bureaucratic mechanisms. Interestingly, the same problem is evident in many complex organizations. Universities generally have been ill-adapted to the traditional bureaucratic model because of the need for freedom, creativity, and self-expression. Increasingly, in business organizations and even in such formally structured activities as military units and governmental agencies, we find that the bureaucratic model must be modified to cope with non-programmed decision problems.

Traditional administrative models assumed well-defined, clear-cut objectives, toward which all organizational participants would strive. In the business organization the prime objective was assumed to be maximization of profits; in government agencies, it was the most effective use of funds in providing a service to the public. Increasingly, the complex organization is being viewed as a viable coalition of many interest groups who may have different and even conflicting objectives. Rather than maximization of any one overriding accepted objective, many objectives must be achieved satisfactorily in order to retain the cooperation of participants.

The large hospital is a prime example of a complex organization faced with attaining many diverse objectives. To be sure, the major objective is to satisfy the needs of the patient for treatment and care. But each group of participants—patients, the medical

---

[13] Eugene Litwak, "Models of Bureaucracy Which Permit Conflict," *American Journal of Sociology,* September, 1961, pp. 177-81.

[14] Andre L. Delbecq has conducted an interesting study concerning the relationship between the bureaucratic model, types of decision-making problems, and various leadership styles in "Bureaucracy, Leadership Style, and Decision-making," *Proceedings of the 1963 Annual Meeting of the Academy of Management, Boston, Massachusetts, December 1963,* pp. 14-38.

staff, department heads, the administrator, the trustees, and others—interpret the means for meeting this objective in terms of their own value system and requirements. And there are additional objectives, such as medical and nursing education and research, which have to be integrated into the operation. The entire organization must operate within the constraints of economic factors, the need for continued survival and growth, and the maintenance of balance and equilibrium both internally and externally. Traditional management theory assumes distinct, clear-cut objective and provides little help in dealing with the multiple objectives of complex organizations. The systems concept provides a useful approach for doing so.

THE HOSPITAL AS A HUMAN-SOCIAL SYSTEM

Large-scale, complex organizations such as hospitals should not be analyzed in terms of the traditional bureaucratic model, nor from the frame of reference of administrative management models adapted from other organizations. Rather, it should be viewed as a unique human-social system. This concept is certainly not new.

Basil Georgopoulos and Floyd Mann expressed a similar point of view as follows:

> An organization like the hospital is not merely a technological arrangement wherein people work according to the demands of the work plan, or in accordance with existing rules, regulations, and procedures, or in accordance with formal communication and authority lines and commands from above. It is a human-social system as well. It is a system whose members, unlike pieces of machinery and equipment, have (and use) the power to reason, to feel, to engage in informational relationships, and to make decisions—decisions which may be rational or nonrational, correct or incorrect, organizationally desirable or undesirable. . . .
>
> Under the impact of recent experience and research, many hospital administrators, trustees, and others are becoming convinced that a hospital is basically, fundamentally, and above all, a man-system. It is complex, human-social system: its raw material is human; its product is human; its work is mainly done by human hands; and its objective is human—direct service to people, service that is individualized and personalized.[15]

THE FUNCTION OF THE HOSPITAL ADMINISTRATOR

The function of the hospital administrator in today's hospital is to coordinate the activities of the numerous operational units and to facilitate achievement of the goals of the organization and its various participants. The administrator must understand the hospital, not as a number of isolated parts, but as a system; he must have knowledge of the relationships between the parts and be aware of their interaction. He must bring these individual, often diverse, functions together into an integrated, organized *system* with all the parts working toward common organizational goals. With growing size, specialization, and complexities of hospitals, this problem of integration has become increasingly difficult. In adapting the systems concept to hospitals the following aspects should be considered.

SUBSYSTEMS AND INTEGRATION

To illustrate the use of systems concepts, we will outline several approaches to organizational analysis based on subsystems. The age-old process of analysis and synthesis (subdivision and integration) has long been useful in theory building. It is also a useful approach for practitioners who want to understand any situation or environment in which they must operate. Any one or a combination of these approaches should be a useful frame of reference for administrators.

[15] Basil S. Georgopoulos and Floyd Mann, "Hospital Organization and Administration: Prospects and Perspective," *Hospital Administration,* Summer, 1964, pp. 25-26.

Strategic parts—It seems logical to focus attention on those parts of an over-all system which are strategic or crucial for its effective operation. Pfiffner and Sherwood describe substantive and adjective functions of organizations.[16] Substantive functions are those that must be done and done well in order for an organization to achieve its goals. Adjective functions, on the other hand, are those which facilitate the carrying out of substantive functions. Scott emphasizes systems concepts and strategic parts as follows:

The distinctive qualities of modern organization theory are its conceptual-analytical base, its reliance upon empirical research data, and, above all, its synthesizing, integrating nature. These qualities are framed in a philosophy which accepts the premise that the only meaningful way to study organization is as a system.

System analysis has its own peculiar point of view. Modern organization theory accepts system analysis as a starting point. It asks a range of interrelated questions which are not seriously considered by the classical and neo-classical theories of organization. Key among these questions are:
1. What are the strategic parts of the system?
2. What is the nature of their mutual interdependency?
3. What are the main processes in the system which link the parts and facilitate their adjustment to each other?
4. What are the goals sought by the system?[17]

Each administrator can identify the strategic parts of whatever system he is involved in. The strategic parts for a hospital administrator may be quite different from those of a plant manager in the metal fabricating industry. An administrator should understand the nature of subsystems and how they relate to one another. He should be able to identify the goals of individuals, informal groups, departments, and the organization as a whole. And he should understand the processes which integrate these various subsystems into a meaningful whole.

Flow concepts—One general approach in systems design involves identification of material, energy, and information flow. These three elements are strategic parts of every system and subsystem. Consideration of them facilitates thinking about systems and subsystems. The material aspects of any system include the facilities involved and the raw material, if any, which flows through the process. A system must be designed to ensure the acquisition of raw material and/or components necessary for processing into finished products. Whenever the operation in question involves the flow and processing of material, appropriate systems can be identified. In a sense, patients represent material flow for hospitals. For operations such as insurance companies or other commercial institutions, there may be no material flow *per se*. Rather, the material in these systems is represented by the facilities, equipment, and supplies involved. Regardless of whether there is any material flow, all business operations, whether producing a product or service, contain elements of energy and information flow.

OBVIOUS SOURCE OF ENERGY: PEOPLE

Some source of energy is present in any operating system. It may be electricity obtained from available sources or generated by the firm's own power plant. The process may require natural gas, petroleum, coal or other fuel for production purposes. A business usually requires electrical energy for operating facilitating systems, if not

[16] John N. Pfiffner and Frank P. Sherwood, *Administrative Organization* (Englewood Cliffs, N.J.: Prentice-Hall, Inc., 1960), p. 171.

[17] William G. Scott, *Human Relations in Management* (Homewood, Ill.: Richard D. Irwin, Inc., 1962), p. 138.

for the main processing operation itself. Another obvious source of energy is people. Both physical and mental energy are required to operate organizations such as hospitals. People represent a renewable source of energy, at least for the short run. And, as an energy source, people are quite variable as individuals. However, in total, the group represents a reasonably stable source of energy for the system. An organization maintains a flow of worker energy throughout its life—on a day-to-day basis and from the standpoint of a long-range cycle which includes recruiting, hiring, orientation stages, and employment until retirement.Thus, all energy can be considered as a flow process both in and of itself and as part of other systems.

Another basic element in any system is information. It facilitates inter-relationships among subsystems and provides the linkage necessary to develop systems of systems. Information flow may be developed to flow along with the routing of material to be processed, for example, production control (or patient workups). For many systems where manufacturing and material flow are not present—service, commercial, and many governmental organizations—the flow of information is the critical element. Information must flow through key decision points where action is taken with regard to a service to be performed by the organization in question. In such cases, the system can be defined primarily on the basis of the flow of information to appropriate decision points. Subsystems can be identified on this basis, and they in turn can be interrelated to define the total system.

SIX MAJOR SUBSYSTEMS

Key subsystems—There are certain key subsystems and/or functions essential in every business organization which make up the total information-decision system, and which operate in a dynamic environmental system subject to rapid change. The subsystems include:

1. A sensor subsystem designed to measure changes within the system and within the environment.
2. An information processing subsystem such as an accounting, or data processing system.
3. A decision-making subsystem which receives information inputs and outputs planning messages.
4. A processing subsystem which utilizes information, energy, and materials to accomplish certain tasks.
5. A control component which ensures that processing is in accordance with planning. Typically this provides feedback control.
6. A memory or information storage subsystem which may take forms such as records, manuals, procedures, computer programs, or human experience.

The goal-setting function will establish the long-range objectives of the organization, and the performance will be measured in terms of factors such as sales, profits, and employment, or cost reduction—relative to the total environmental system. As described, these key subsystems seem vague and impersonal. Each statement outlines a function, one which will be performed in some fashion regardless of the size and/or type of organization. Often, technical and mechanical elements are involved—automated equipment, computers, paper work forms—which are coupled with human effort to close the loop. The specific approach for a subsystem can be tailor-made even though standard "hardware" items are utilized. Customizing can be accomplished via the "software" (sometimes referred to as "brainware") elements of the system. It is particularly important that attention be devoted to the people aspects of key subsystems.

PFIFFNER'S AND SHERWOOD'S "OVERLAYS"

Individuals interact with other individuals in both large and small groups to comprise the social system that is an organization. Both formal and informal organizations are involved. The organization chart depicts a system of interdependent roles in a job-task hierarchy. This basic job-task hierarchy is modified by a number of other systems which have been called "overlays" by Pfiffner and Sherwood.[18]

These modifying subsystems include:

1. The sociometric network
2. The decision network
3. The communication-feedback grid
4. The network of functional relationships
5. The power center network
6. The network of individual personalities
7. The network of personal and institutional values

Some of these overlays parallel key subsystems as set forth above. Others identify additional, confounding elements in a typical large-scale, complex organization. Pervasive value systems should be recognized as important factors in decision making. Personalities and sociometric networks, with their attendant systems of power and influence, alter the formal system of authority based on the job-task hierarchy. These "people aspects" should be considered in any analysis of key subsystems in an organization.

Each of the subsystems has interactions within its own framework. In addition, they interact with some or all of the other systems. The complexity involved is evident. Thus managers would be well advised not to succumb to the temptation to adopt over-simplified views of organizations or "ten steps to managerial success" which are guaranteed in any situation. The administrator is better advised to attempt to understand the complexity and why straightforward, simple-minded approaches do not seem to work out in the real world.

CONCLUSIONS

Models based on systems concepts have not been designed to simplify the task of administration. On the contrary, this approach is a way of recognizing the complexity of the real world. And it facilitates anticipation of problems. By identifying the parts of a complex whole and the means of integrating such subsystems into a meaningful endeavor, approaches to solutions may become evident. As an old adage suggests: "A problem well stated is half solved."

To assume the real world conforms to the simplified, traditional models set forth decades ago is folly. Another adage states, "Ignorance is bliss!" However, such bliss is usually short lived as managers wonder why their perfectly straightforward, well--thought-out plans and programs evoke unanticipated responses. It is our contention that there is no set recipe for managerial success—cookbook approaches will not suffice in the long run. If there are ten steps to success, there are usually eleven or more critical problems in today's large-scale, complex organizations. Thus, rather than developing a list of "do's" and "don'ts," it seems more appropriate to develop a frame of mind which will help cope with current problems. Rather than trying to simplify the real world, it will be more fruitful to develop an understanding of its complexity and the concomitant need for flexibility in coping with problems as they arise. Systems concepts facilitate such understanding.

[18] Pfiffner and Sherwood, *op. cit.*, p. 207.

6.

Corporate Models in Health Care Delivery

LYNDA DIANE BAYDIN AND ALAN SHELDON

Lynda Diane Baydin, M.A., was formerly a Program Associate for the office for International Health Programs - School of Public Health - Harvard University.

Alan Sheldon, M.D., is Associate Professor - School of Public Health - Harvard University and lecturer, Harvard Business School.

In response to environmental and economic demands, the past 20 years have seen the development and growth of new types of health institutions based on corporate models; a number of these are described in this article.

The basic network for the health care delivery system has traditionally been a combination of private physicians, group practices, clinics, private and public nonprofit voluntary hospitals, proprietary hospitals, teaching and research institutions, extended care and rehabilitation facilities, and nursing homes. While the network has been maintained, these institutions are finding it increasingly difficult to operate as autonomous cost and service units. One consequence has been a trend toward various innovative types of association that range along a continuum from total merger to the sharing of a few services, such as laundry or purchasing.

Among these new ways of organizing and financing limited resources are the merger, the joint venture, the holding company concept, the investor owned national hospital companies, and management contracts. In the case of these five models, any generalizations are confounded by the great variation among the particular examples. It is important that the reader recognize that the models described in the footnote are in constant flux, e.g., certain types of associations such as the Joint Venture may be appropriate at the exploratory stages of a union, depending on the degree of commitment between two or more institutions and the viability of the arrangement, but not practical five years after talks have begun.

A hospital merger is said to take place under the following conditions: when either the assets of two institutions are pooled or a takeover or acquisition of one institution

---

Reprinted by permission from *Hospital Administration* (currently *Hospital and Health Services Administration*): *Quarterly Journal of the American College of Hospital Administrators*, Chicago, Vol. 20 (Winter, 1975), pp. 40-52. © 1975 by the American College of Hospital Administrators. All rights reserved.

by another occurs.[1] In the event of pooling assets, a new corporate structure is formed. In terms of physical structure several combinations are possible depending on the needs of the facilities involved. Sometimes a new plant is built to house the merged hospitals; sometimes, one of the old facilities is abandoned, and the other utilized. Figure 1 shows the extent of merger activity in the United States from 1947-1969.

The purposes of a merger may be many. One can be to achieve improved patient care at reasonable cost by eliminating the inefficiencies inherent in duplication of facilities and services, perpetuation of obsolete plants, outmoded methods of medical care distribution and competition for scarce personnel.[2] Whether mergers always accomplish these objectives, especially increased economies, is open to question; however, they often guarantee the survival of a hospital, and speed the process of regional planning for the delivery of health care in a community.

A merger may take place because the acquiring hospital or hospital company can achieve economies of size, such as centralized purchasing, accounting, electronic data services, etc. It may also take place because the financial condition of the acquired hospital is deteriorating, and the acquiring entity can provide needed capital for operating purposes of expansion.

In terms of legal criteria, the following have been established by the Joint Commission on Accreditation of Hospitals: the hospitals must be under a single ownership and have one governing body and one set of corporate laws; the merged hospitals must have one medical staff with one set of by-laws, rules and regulations, and the usual medical staff committees.[3]

LEGAL OBJECTIVES

The legal objectives of a merger in the nonprofit sector are:

- a recognized corporate entity with a governing body and management possessing full authority to contract and take other necessary action;
- continuation of approval by all accrediting bodies, both governmental and private, for all segments of the combined corporate entity;
- continued validity for all contractual commitments of the merging corporate entities;
- an effective appointed medical staff organization that is legally recognized by the combined entity;
- legally recognized freedom to dispose of the combined assets of the combining organizations with no restrictions on such disposition than existed before and a clear title to such assets;
- a clearly recognized status as a tax exempt organization under both state and federal law;
- a clear termination of the obligations and liabilities of the trustees of the prior entities, to the extent permitted by law; a clear avoidance of transfer taxes on real or personal property transferred by operation of law in the course of the consolidation.[4]

66   Hospital Organization and Management

Figure 1

Hospital Merger Activity in the United States
1947-1969

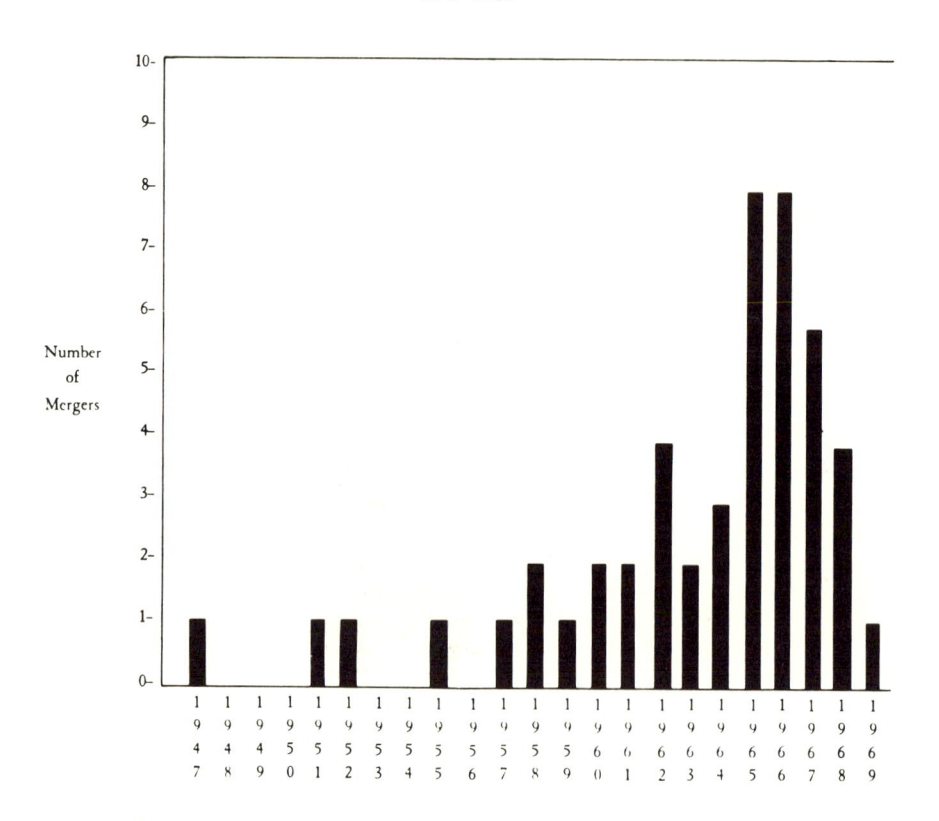

Source: Harris, Allyn Rueben, *Causes and Effects of Hospital Mergers,* August, 1969, p. 43.

WHY SOME MERGERS FAIL

Some of the major obstacles to fulfilling these requirements include: 1. ideas of autonomy, proprietorship, and loyalty to a particular institution, which die hard, especially with Boards of Trustees and communities which have supported a facility financially; 2. the fear on the part of medical staff and employees that many will be lost in the consolidation process, especially if a larger more powerful institution merges with a smaller one; 3. the possibility that certain advantageous policies and privileges will be curtailed.[5]

The advantages which frequently result include potential benefit to the community through either new facilities and equipment, or a more satisfactory deployment of those that already exist, the increased ability to attract needed medical specialists and skilled personnel, and the saving of time for physicians who have multiple staff appointments.

When mergers fail, it is usually because certain considerations and preliminary activities are not undertaken. Internal scrutiny often reveals such potential problem as:

1. Loyalty of Trustees, auxiliaries, and other volunteers.
2. The personal autonomy and security of existing medical staffs relationships.
3. The job security sought by employees.
4. Disruption of the existing management system and its ability to be integrated.
5. The initial costs of merger with regard to losses of medical staff, loss of patients and loss of key personnel.
6. Overextension of management resources.
7. Overestimation of ability of existing hospitals to provide expanded services.
8. Underestimating the difficulties of integrating basically incompatible institutions.[6]

In addition, certain decisions must be made and important issues settled by the respective boards early in the negotiation process. They include the choice of administrative leadership and of a name for the new organization, the development of a governing board structure, a detailed study of the objectives of the consolidation, and the preparation of articles of incorporation, by-laws and other necessary legal documents. Other premerger considerations include the accounting aspects, i.e., will the association be a "pooling of assets" that results in a consolidated balance sheet or will assets have to be reevaluated? What is the attitude of patients, physicians, board members, trustees? In short, the extent to which the joint agreement provides for the full integration of progam services and administrative structure will, in large part, predetermine the overall effectiveness of the new management in the merged program.[7]

JOINT VENTURE

So far the concept of "Joint Venture" has only been attempted in a limited number of hospital situations in the United States. As none of this species of consolidation is alike, the discussion will focus on two examples of joint venture.[8] One is an association of three hospitals in Boston: the Peter Bent Brigham Hospital, the Robert Breck Brigham Hospital and the Boston Hospital for Women.

How did this particular arrangement originate and why was it selected? The environmental demands on the three institutions included: (1) antiquated facilities,

(2) fragmentation of services, (3) affiliation with Harvard Medical School, (4) geographic location within proximity of each other; hence, service to the same general community, (5) multiple staff appointments within the three institutions, and (6) the desire of each hospital to maintain its identity and a certain degree of autonomy.

With the formation of a fourth entity, the Affiliated Hospital Center, Inc., a new physical structure to house the three separate hospitals and ancillary services was to be constructed. This particular corporate structure provided the opportunity for fundraising for the new entity as a whole, as well as for individual campaigns, whereby each institution could call upon its particular resources. It allowed for financing of the entire project in proportion to the number of beds each institution would occupy in the completed structure.

Increased utilization of services was expected to occur because of (1) occupation of a single site, (2) consolidation of highly specialized services and an increase in their size, and (3) a strengthened relationship between the three medical staffs due to proximity. Increased efficiency of utilization was expected to occur due to redistribution of beds according to levels of care, and greater economies through the centralization of certain supportive services such as labs, dietary, maintenance, housekeeping, radiology.[9]

MAINTAINING INSTITUTIONAL IDENTITY

In order to maintain the individual identity of the institutions, the following corporate structure had been decided upon: an Executive Vice President would be the chief operating officer of the Affiliated Hospital Center; the Governing Board was to be composed of an equal number of members from each of the constituent hospitals appointed by each of those hospitals; the Board of Governors was to name a Medical Executive Committee from the Chiefs of Services of each hospital.[10]

Each hospital would be responsible for its own financing; budget; medical staff appointments; patient care; teaching program; research; community service, except for an ambulatory care facility to be run by all three together; separate identifiable geographic location in the complex and the costs associated with that area; and all services unique to each hospital's own program. The central core area was to house shared services and facilities, the cost of which would be borne by all the partners.[11]

Clearly, a joint venture of this type is an unwieldy association not suited to many circumstances; however, it is an alternative currently being subjected to closer scrutiny for those situations where two or more institutions with very powerful identities must combine to deliver better care at lower costs.[12] In fact, the Boston example has now progressed on toward a proposed merger.

The second example of a joint venture is Metropolitan Medical Center in Minneapolis, which is a formal merger of Swedish and St. Barnabas Hospitals. Both hospitals pursuant to merger moved into a new facility in a new location under the title Metropolitan Medical Center.

In addition, the new structure houses Hennepin County General Hospital. Although there was no clinical merger with the Metropolitan Medical Center, Hennepin County General maintains a separate entrance to the hospital building.

HOSPITAL HOLDING COMPANIES

A widespread corporate structure, the holding company, long employed in banking, is another corporate model with possibilities for associating a group of health care facilities. One of the first such associations occurred when three non-profit Lutheran hospitals in the Minneapolis area consolidated on January 1, 1973 and formed a holding company, Fairview Community Hospitals. Because non-profit institutions have no ownership of stock, all property, assets, and income, as well as debts, liabilities and obligations of the constituent corporations become those of the holding company. In the case of the Fairview Community Hospitals, it was decided to maintain separate operating statements for the individual hospitals with one consolidated balance sheet.

The member hospitals selected their own representatives to sit on the board of directors of the holding company. The members were appointed in proportion to the respective assets of the constituent corporations. Each constituent hospital has its own by-laws, rules and regulations. Each institution will maintain its own staff officers and executive committees. While reciprocal admitting privileges exist among the member institutions, should a physician admit more than ten patients annually to another facility, he must apply for privileges at that hospital.

According to Carl Platou, President of Fairview Community Hospitals, the hospital holding company concept has several distinct advantages. Foremost is its usefulness for providing a vehicle for maintaining the viability of the small non-profit community hospital. This can be accomplished primarily because of the greater resources of the parent holding company, which provides management skills and services, as well as a wider economic base.

ECONOMIES OF SCALE

Within the corporate framework of the hospital holding company, large scale economies through shared services are possible without the problems of coordination which exist when several independent institutions get together to engage in joint purchasing.[13] Furthermore, Mr. Platou believes the holding company form of organization stresses the ease with which modern management techniques, such as systematic decision making, management by objectives, long-range planning by divisions, are facilitated. The central office would function to encourage group meetings and activities of subsidiary hospital management for the interchange of new management concepts and techniques; and aid in the mutual assessment of member's performance toward goals.[14] In addition, the holding company format "encourages technological advances in data processing, materials management, and budget forecasting."[15]

The advantages of centralized and corporate resources in the multihospital holding company, which offers specialized skills and services, are balanced by the emphasis on decentralized operational autonomy of the member units, which function in liaison with their particular community and as independent cost centers. The broader capital base of the holding company provides a resource of assets which the member units could draw upon for capital expenditures, such as expansion or remodeling. As a result, certain benefits would accrue to the communities which these institutions serve, such as greater stability of local units because of the strong capital base and operational standards of the holding company, its centralized research and program development; better rates because of economies from centralized purchasing and superior management; and broadened services and facilities adapted to the unique need of the community.[16] Platou feels that, unlike the merger, the hospital holding company would allow for community responsiveness because member hospitals would not only be more secure as to their future, but would be able to maintain their identity and traditions. The general trend, which is reflected by these four very different models from business, is away from the individual hospital operating in isolation while trying to cope with rising costs, a shortage of personnel, increasingly specialized and sophisticated equipment, and the need for modern management techniques.

INVESTOR OWNED HOSPITAL COMPANIES

Investor owned hospital companies are unlike the other corporate models described in that they are proprietary and public. Not all proprietary hospitals are part of these companies. However, the majority are singly owned institutions delivering short-term care, "owned and operated for profits by individuals, partnerships or corporations."[17]

In 1972, existing investor owned national hospital companies in the U.S. numbered 29 with the oldest company only started in 1960. Each owned two or more hospitals for a total of more than 300 hospitals. This represents a very small percentage of the 7,123 hospitals in the United States. The total number of beds for all hospitals reported in 1972 was 1,616,000;[18] for proprietary hospitals, approximately 40,000.[19] The two largest were American Medicorp., Inc., owning 31 hospitals, and Hospital Corporation of America with 48 hospitals.[20] The growth of these companies had been primarily through the acquisition of existing proprietary hospitals, rather than the construction of new hospitals. Recently, however, the emphasis has been primarily on new construction. Generally, stock in the company is offered in exchange for ownership, and the market history of chains up through 1968 and 1969 has very rapid gains with a sudden drop in prices in 1970. In general, these national companies have transformed the individual proprietary hospital into a corporate owned hospital. The most recent development is the construction of new hospitals in middle-class communities by these corporations.[21]

CHARACTERISTICS OF THE PROPRIETARY HOSPITAL

Certain characteristics of proprietary hospital companies make them distinguishable from other multi-hospital groups, such as Veterans' Administration hospitals, non-profit hospitals operated by religious orders, or from proprietary hospitals in general.

1. They are not necessarily or totally owned by physicians.
2. They employ corporate staffs trained in management skills.
3. They can raise necessary capital through the issuance of equity shares, convertible bonds and regular bonds.

Some of these hospital companies also operate nursing homes, hospital supply subsidiaries, and extended care facilities. Below is a brief summary of the assets of three companies which own and operate acute hospital chains.

American Medicorp (AM), formed in 1968, in 1972 operated 60 hospitals, 3 skilled care nursing centers, and a school of nursing. As the largest proprietary operator in terms of revenue, AM's sales in 1969 were $77.6 million, and in 1972 $191.4 million.

American Medical International operates 45 hospitals in the United States, England and Switzerland, as well as medical laboratories and other services. In 1972, sales for these activities were $131.4 million, after tax earnings were $8.4 million (before extraordinary expense).

Hospital Corporation of America (HCA) operates 48 acute care hospitals nationwide with 7,300 beds. Sales in 1972 were $172.6 million, up from $55.1 million in 1969. During the same period, after-tax earnings increased from $3.3 million to $10.4 million, or from $.58 to $1.14 per share. Total assets at the end of 1972 were $273 million.[22]

In addition to centralized purchasing, the corporate management of these national hospital companies frequently emphasizes the benefits that accrue from "efficient, centralized financial controls." Because these companies are publicly accountable for profits and losses, annual reports generally devote considerable space to explaining the financial information and the internal audit procedures of the company. While the organizational structure of companies owning hospital chains varies, the following description from the 1970 stock prospectus of the Hospital Corporation of America, which owned 26 hospitals at the time with a total of 2,845 beds, shows how one company has organized for greater economies.

Each hospital has a Management Committee, at least two-thirds of whose members are persons connected with the hospital, usually physicians on the staff of the hospital, and the remainder of whom are appointed by the company to supervise the medical, ethical, and professional affairs and the daily operations of the hospital. The company supplies management services to each of its hospitals, including the furnishing of accounting forms and controls and of technical personnel to assist in hospital administration and management. Each hospital records its financial and statistical information on a standard chart of accounts which enables the company to aid in the control of expenditures and to compare operations of the various hospitals.

The company has instituted a program of centralized purchasing which, it believes, has resulted in economies. It has short-term contracts with a number of major suppliers for the purchase of various types of hospital supplies and equipment, including intravenous solutions, surgical dressings, X-ray machines and supplies, non-perishable foodstuffs, kitchen and other food service equipment, and medical and anesthetic gasses. In addition, the company has centralized the purchasing of substantially all equipment and furnishings for its new hospitals.[23]

LOWER OPERATING COSTS

Like other investor-owned hospital companies, HCA believes that the average operating costs for each of its hospitals are less than those experienced by most neighboring non-profit institutions because (1) it provides fewer infrequently used services of a highly skilled and technical nature, which require expensive equipment and facilities,[24] (2) it is company policy not to engage in extensive research or educational programs, and (3) it does not initiate services which would unnecessarily duplicate those offered by neighboring hospitals.[25]

With respect to medical staff and employees, none of the 5,200 physicians on the staffs of its hospitals in 1972 were employees of the company except certain officers. Many physicians have staff privileges at other hospitals as well. As of the fall of 1970, HCA had no contracts with labor unions. It is a company policy when constructing new hospitals to standardize design and equipment when possible; this policy makes possible bulk purchasing and more economical operations.

A final mixed corporate model would be that of a hospital deciding to achieve better management/purchasing economies/centralized services, etc., through making a contract with another hospital organization, which could be either non-profit or investor owned.

For example, over the past two years the investor-owned hospital companies have signed management contracts with about 25 voluntary hospitals, and many more are being negotiated. Financial pressures usually are the cause of voluntary hospitals deciding to do this, and, in many cases, part of the management contract agreement is that working capital is provided as part of the arrangement.

The voluntary hospital, in doing this, has as its basic premise the opinion that economies will result from this arrangement, such as mass purchasing, tighter controls and clearer accountability.

It has been suggested that this might result largely from the fact that doctors, who make many, if not most, of the decisions affecting cost, understand that they are always accountable to management in the investor-owned hospital, whereas in many non-profit hospitals accountability gets diluted, if not dissolved, in the murky currents of the trustee-staff-administrator relationship. One executive, John A. Hill, past president of Hospital Corporation of America and a long-time trustee of several voluntary hospitals, agreed that this could be the case and added that management methods were the same in both types of hospital but that investor-owned hospitals appeared to be free of the deep cleavage that has so often developed between the medical staffs and managements of voluntary hospitals.

CONCLUSIONS

These five approaches share a concern with using scarce resources, especially management skills, more effectively. They reflect a growing willingness in the health care field to experiment with new forms, an attitude both necessary and valuable at a time when traditional approaches have been found lacking. They reflect also a growing willingness to *share* resources, rather than go it *alone.* This is an even more radical departure from traditionally autonomous values, and one to be applauded.

FOOTNOTES

[1] Salley E. Knapp, Ed.D., and Robert R. Lovejoy, *Hospital Mergers in New England: Organizational Perspectives* (Durham, N.H.: Systems Educators, Inc., 1973).

[2] Ibid.

[3] Ibid., p. 10.

[4] Ibid., pp. 8, 9.

[5] Ibid., p. 10.

[6] Ibid., p. 5.

[7] Ibid., pp. 147-53.

[8] Other examples of associations of hospitals which might qualify as joint venture include the Iroquois Hospital Association in Rochester, New York; the Fairview Hospitals in Minneapolis; Downstate Medical Center in Brooklyn; Harper Hospital in Detroit; and the affiliated hospitals of Marquette University in Milwaukee.

[9] Knapp and Lovejoy, *Hospital Mergers in New England,* pp. 136-38.

[10] Ibid., p. 134.

[11] Ibid., p. 33.

[12] Early in 1973, it was decided to abandon the idea of a joint venture for the Affiliated Hospital Center in favor of a complete merger mainly because of the difficulties outlined above.

[13] Carl N. Platou and James A. Rice, "Multi-hospital Holding Companies," *Harvard Business Review,* May-June 1972.

[14] Ibid., p. 4.

[15] Ibid.

[16] Ibid., p. 13.

[17] For a review of the quantity, quality and economics of proprietary hospitals in the U.S., see A. Bruce Steinwald and Duncan Neuhauser, "The Role of the Proprietary Hospital" in *Health Care,* ed. Clark Havighurst (New York: Oceana Press, 1972).

[18] American Hospital Association, *Hospitals, J.A.H.A. Guide Issue* 45, no. 115 (1 August 1971): 463-67.

[19] Ibid., pp. 445-93.

[20] Steinwald and Neuhauser, "Role of the Proprietary Hospital."

[21] American Hospital Association, *J.A.H.A. Guide Issue,* p. 32.

[22] Eoin Trevelyan, "Supplemental Reference Data on the Health Industry in the U.S.," mimeographed (Cambridge, Mass.: Harvard University, 1973).

[23] Hospital Corporation of America, 1970 Stock Prospectus, p. 10.

[24] Ibid.

[25] Ibid., p. 13.

Governing Authority

The composition and responsibilities of the hospital governing authority is presented next. *Selection 7,* "THE BOARD OF TRUSTEES" by Temple Burling, Edith M. Lentz, and Robert N. Wilson, provides background on who trustees are and what they do. The information presented, especially in terms of relations between governing authority and physicians and administrators, is a framework within which the other articles in the section are presented. Although trustees are usually found only in voluntary, not-for-profit hospitals, the term is synonymous with governing authority for purposes of the section. In *Selection 8,* "CURRENT PERSPECTIVES ON HOSPITAL GOVERNANCE," Lawrence D. Prybil and David B. Starkweather describe hospital governance and management as a joint venture. After discussing new developments in hospital governance the authors conclude that the hospital industry's future is dependent upon the leadership and performance of the hospital's governing authority.

In *Selection 9,* "SHOULD DOCTORS BE ON YOUR BOARD?" C. Jerome Jorgenson discusses the desirable and undesirable aspects of physicians serving on the governing authority. He concludes that while greater physician involvement does not necessarily mean improved hospital performance, it is an important first step. This section ends with *Selection 10,* "GOVERNING BOARDS," by Anthony R. Kovner. The writer identifies and discusses the major issues in hospital governance today, including composition, performance, structure and function, and reform. He warns that undue emphasis on improving accountability of governing boards, rather than hospital performance directly, may have negative results.

7.
The Board of Trustees

TEMPLE BURLING, M.D., EDITH M. LENTZ, PH.D. AND ROBERT N. WILSON

The responsibility of the hospital trustee for the general policy of the institution cannot be understood without some conception of the voluntary nature of the role. The spirit of voluntarism in America has traditionally supported the idea that men can willingly band together for a common purpose without governmental controls. Thus outstanding citizens freely devote time and energy to a nonprofit enterprise from which they can derive no personal gain except community prestige and inner satisfaction. Trustees serve, for the most part, because they are genuinely interested in the quality of hospital care and feel some obligation, as favored members of the society, to give their voluntary service. When a loose association of men governs a complex organization, innumerable problems of authority, specialization, and definition are created. The advantage of such control is that it is responsive to local community interests and preserves the flexibility essential to meet a swiftly changing situation.

WHO ARE THE TRUSTEES?

Trustees are usually chosen from among the more prominent members of the community, and in the hospitals we observed they tended to have attained high status in business or the professions. Representatives of old families with inherited wealth are often found on hospital boards. More recently, however, trustees seem to be chosen more for community influence or unique ability than for social position alone. A businessman who can lend his prestige to fund appeals or policy decisions is valuable. So is an advertising executive who can contribute expert talents in the field of public relations. The strategic position of a prospective board member in the community at large is generally given first consideration. Does he hold a place from which power can be wielded in the hospital's favor? Is he likely to be able to influence the press, the city government, or the private donors to hospital funds? In one hospital the local newspaper editor and the president of the women's auxiliary of the hospital were elected to the board although neither was wealthy nor conspicuously successful. The editor was chosen because he could arrange favorable treatment to news stories and provide much free publicity through editorials. The president of the auxiliary was chosen because the board thought that her presence would insure liaison between the trustees and the volunteer hospital workers, and add a feminine voice to an otherwise male board.

Reprinted by permission of G.P. Putnam's Sons from *The Give and Take in Hospitals* by Temple Burling, *et. al.*, pp. 39-50. Copyright 1956 by G.P. Putnam's Sons.

The vice president of a board in a small hospital explained the membership composition of the board in this way:

> I feel the board should include representatives from the top business and professional people and those that can really do something for the hospital. Some people think we should get some boys from the other side of the tracks, but if we did, they would just talk and not *do* anything, because they haven't any influence.

Another board president, after describing his work in fund raising for the hospital and explaining how important a personal chat could be in obtaining a large gift, said:

> Our auxiliary does well too. Their main trouble is that they don't ask for *enough* money when they try to raise funds.

Although certain board members recognize the need for bringing the young community leaders in, it is probable that boards tend to be heavily weighted with older citizens because of the qualifications demanded for membership. It takes time to develop into a successful, prominent community leader and in a man's early career he is perhaps too busy getting ahead to occupy himself with public service. Since age and high income tend to be associated with conservatism, it is to be expected that a board of trustees is usually conservative. Many harassed administrators and eager research-minded medical men would agree that one of the functions of the board seems to be to "drag its feet," especially when finances are an issue.

It is not always easy to get good members for the board. The hospital in a small town, especially, may be handicapped by scarcity of citizens qualified for and interested in board service. Many otherwise outstanding people do not have the largeness of view, particularly in fiscal matters, which a board needs if it is to set far-reaching policy.

The composition of a hospital board almost inevitably reflects the characteristics of the surrounding community, since the members are leading products of that setting. A board can be a mirror of community social relationships. It cannot assume a character or set goals which are radically different from those of the city in which it is enmeshed. This is not to say that trustees cannot exercise creative leadership, but the hospital is closely bound up with other institutions and with prevailing patterns of behavior.

RESPONSIBILITIES

The board holds the hospital in trust. A private voluntary hospital is a gift of private donors to serve a community need. It is the responsibility of the board to provide and maintain an institution which will serve these needs according to the wishes of the donors. It has a responsibility both to the terms of the trust and to the community which the hospital serves. In order that it may fulfill this trust, it must be the ultimate source of authority. Individual trustees differ widely in the amount of responsibility that they exercise. Some attend the board meetings once a year merely to confirm policies which have been determined by others, while some take an active, detailed interest in hospital problems. Boards as a whole also differ from one hospital to another in the degree to which they participate in the formation, as compared to the ratification, of policy.

We pointed out in the introduction to this section that much of the initiative for major policy comes from outside the board itself, because so many choices are grounded on specialized knowledge which the trustees do not have. This seems to be an increasing trend. But because they are in a sense outsiders to the hospital system, they are able and are often called upon to mediate between the goals of competing groups within it. The board's relation to hospital policy can be of three sorts:

(a) initiation of policy
(b) transmission of policy
(c) mediation of policy

(a) There are times when the board must *decide* upon some important change and work to carry it through. Excellent examples occur in the reorganization of smaller hospitals which have fallen on grim days. The major difficulty may be financial, but just as frequently it is an internal disorganization of one sort or another, especially the sort found when the administrator and medical staff are at loggerheads. At one such institution the president described his first steps after being chosen to head the board:

> First I fired the superintendent and brought in somebody I thought could do a good job. This place was saddled with debts. There were many months of bills outstanding and some creditors were getting worried about the hospital's ability to pay. The first thing I did was to go down to the bank and borrow $25,000 to pay off the worst debts. The doctors had been fighting among themselves. There were two factions on the medical staff, and their battles had split the whole town. Our hospital had a bad reputation and the public was beginning to lose confidence so I called the leaders of the factions together – they're both younger than I am – and told them that they would have to get together and end this open warfare. Then I started a fund raising campaign and forced the doctors to contribute first. I told them they were benefiting from the hospital as much as anyone else.

(b) The board may be called upon to transmit policy when an outside agency puts pressure on the hospital to improve its standards or run the risk of losing accreditation.[1] The various accrediting agencies do not actually determine policy but the penalties for losing their stamp of approval are serious for the hospital. The trust imposed upon the board members cannot be fully met if minimum standards are not maintained. The trustees pay attention to these agencies and will fight hard for suggested changes that did not originate with the board.

(c) When a suggested policy change is developed from within the hospital, as it often is, the trustees must monitor the proposal and attempt to resolve divergent aims. One interesting type of conflict involves the relative emphasis to be placed on research on the one hand and regular medical care on the other. Here, although the root of the difference is probably a philosophic disagreement as to the hospital's proper function, it may be brought to the trustees as a technical argument; e.g., whether a particular type of research investigation is feasible. The board must then attempt to choose on information supplied by others. A group of generally informed laymen is thus called upon to decide between technically informed experts.

---

[1] Accrediting agencies are voluntary in character. Member hospitals submit to regular inspection as a means of self-discipline. In this way, adequate standards are maintained and regular improvements are encouraged.

RELATIONS WITH THE ADMINISTRATOR

In a large industry, the board of directors exerts its authority mainly through a hired president or executive. The situation of the hospital administrator differs from that of the company president in two ways. First, hospital administrators are usually given much less discretionary power than a corporation president. They have been on the whole much more closely tied to the board and its wishes, and consult with it more frequently in decision-making. In the second place, the board of directors of a factory is in a position to delegate to the president authority over all workers, but, as we have pointed out in Chapter IV, the hospital board is not able to delegate effective authority over the doctors.

The board itself occupies a unique position in hospital affairs which sharply distinguishes it from the business situation. While it lacks the proprietary interest of directors who have a financial stake in an organization, there is often a feeling of responsibility exceeding anything found in other enterprises. A hospital board has a keen sense of pressure stemming from responsibility for human life. This makes for difficulty in the delegation of authority, as trustees responsive to patient needs strive eagerly to be certain those needs are met. Reluctant to assign authority in matters which may touch life-or-death, they sometimes become directly involved in hospital operations.

The amount of discretionary power which the board does delegate to the superintendent varies widely. Many administrators feel strongly that the board should limit its activities to the formulation of general policy, but should stop short of detailed supervision in the day-to-day life of the hospital. Yet they express a desire that the board be interested and involved. Perhaps one cannot have deep persistent commitment without inviting occasional "meddling."

The board president whose sympathetic understanding of the difficult position of his hospital superintendent was noted earlier,[2] when he remarked on how hard it is for a full-time executive to be supervised by part-time trustees, nevertheless said at a later time:

> Did you notice the color Jenkins [the administrator] put on the front hall? He went right ahead without asking anybody. I should have kicked his pants for it, but I didn't because it's unimportant.

One administrator writes as follows about the general problems:

> On the negative side there is something more to expect. I want my trustees to know what not to do. Many of my colleagues dread the interference of trustees in the routine administration of the hospital. This interference is generally conceded to be the greatest single threat to the authority of the administrator.[3]

A very important feature of the obligation of the board both to the donors and to the public is to insure the permanence of the hospital and its services. This imposes on the board a very clear responsibility for financial management and most people probably think of this first, as the trustees' job. A prominent feature of nearly every report from the hospital administrator or his staff to the board is a balance sheet showing what part each specific department or activity plays in the hospital's economic structure.

---

[2] Introduction to Part Two, p. 36.

[3] E. M. Bluestone, M.D., "What I Expect of My Board," *Hospital and Modern Society,* Bachmeyer and Hartman, eds. Cambridge: Harvard University Press.

The board considers the effect of every proposed policy decision on the financial stability of the institution. If it failed to do so, it would be unfaithful to its trust. This is obvious, but the necessary concern of the board with means is one of the commonest sources of misunderstanding between it and those who are primarily concerned with ends. It should also be pointed out that attention to financial problems of the hospital has its constructive side. Very often it induces the administrator or the medical staff to re-examine certain of their goals and to clarify their own thinking. The board is the great asker of questions in the hospital. Why build a new wing? Why purchase new equipment? Why raise the salary of maids? The close questioning often irritates enthusiastic proponents of an idea, but it can be a safeguard against hasty or ill-examined actions. Furthermore, close attention to the budget is more than a banker's concern for neatly balanced ledgers. The board may use financial management as a means of directing the hospital to certain goals, rather than make it simply an end in itself. Money problems often symbolize underlying cross-purposes in conflicts which seem at first to have little relation to dollars and cents.

Though all boards in discharging their responsibility must concern themselves actively with financial matters, they differ widely in their attitudes toward hospital finances, as the following quotations indicate:

> We have developed a research philosophy in this hospital. Our trustees once were very anxious about the balance sheets but they have educated themselves to accept the deficit as the price for intensive research work. They recently expressed remarkable attitude and insight for a group of businessmen. We were considering a candidate for the administrator's position, since I will soon retire. This young fellow came up here and brought with him the books from his current hospital. He was very efficient and very proud of his balanced books. Our board rejected him as a candidate because he showed *too much black ink* in his books. They felt that he couldn't be recording these beautiful surpluses if his hospital were doing all that it *ought* to in the way of medical care and research.
>
> —An administrator

> All that board cares about is how much will it cost. They pondered and pondered over the problem of buying a new deep therapy machine. I explained to them that if they bought the equipment and didn't like it they could turn around and sell it at a profit the next day....Finally they put up the funds. They just can't look ahead of the immediate costs and what a hole it makes in their books. They don't see the long-range value of spending money in certain ways.
>
> —A staff surgeon

Human relations inside the hospital are influenced by the attitude of the top policy-makers toward monetary decisions. In a hospital where the board allowed the administrator fairly wide discretion in the purchase of equipment, nurses spoke in warm terms about how promptly their most urgent needs were met. Little doubt seemed to exist that money policies were well tailored to medical requirements.

RELATIONS WITH DOCTORS

The board and the organized medical staff seldom deal with each other directly as formally constituted groups, although liaison committees may be created to act in an advisory capacity, and as we pointed out, informal relations between individual doctors and individual board members often have far-reaching effects on the hospital.

Although it was once common for one or two older physicians to be appointed to the board, both trustees and doctors have come to feel that this practice is generally undesirable. It is held that such an arrangement fosters a possible conflict of interests, since the doctor is himself subject to the judgment of the board, and his membership on it might give him an undue economic or policy-making advantage. As a noted surgeon put it:

> We doctors have no part in management, and I am sure that that is only right. We do plenty of griping about management but it is better that we should not have responsibility in management.

Since the board has little direct authority over the doctors except its power to appoint or refuse to appoint them to the staff and since even this authority is limited in practice, it must to a considerable extent depend on the self regulation of the medical group. However, when this fails the trustees often try to push the doctors toward accepting a new code of standards and practices. Sometimes they try to do so through the administrator, instituting regulations which he is expected to enforce. At times they persuade the medical staff to tighten its own self regulation. Dealings between the trustees and the doctors were greatly facilitated in the hospitals we studied if the medical staff itself was well organized. A board has no effective, established way of exerting pressure unless it can do so through a chief of staff who has definite authority. A board president took note of this in the following comments:

> Discussion of cases with our liaison committee usually ends up in a pleasant evening's conversation. The doctors say, "Oh, we'll take care of that," but that's as far as it goes. There is no clear line of responsibility shown. I was asking the staff about a new anesthetic that had been used on a patient who had died on the table. They couldn't give me a good explanation. I feel that if there were a head of surgery appointed by the board of managers, we could go to him and say, "Look, you're responsible for this case, we want to know what happened."

Just as in its relations with the administrator, the line between guidance and meddling by trustees in medical problems cannot be clearly drawn. No one can say just how deeply the trustees should penetrate into medical affairs. The medical staff can often use its special competence as a lever to extend its influence into nonscientific areas and to block trustee investigation. A board president recounted that in discussions with the doctors about economic practices, as in the case of salaried medical specialists, a certain physician always lectured the trustees about interfering with "the sacred doctor-patient relationship."

Yet medical topics are legitimately reserved for those qualified to discuss them. The dividing line cannot be drawn in advance but must be worked out in give and take between the two groups and this calls for mutual understanding of the other's point of view. But that this understanding is not always complete is shown by the following quotations:

> I don't like the way the board always goes so slow. We should have a full-time pathologist, but you have to get them used to the idea gradually. It's the same with equipment. How do you get them to see the medical necessity?

> —A doctor

> The board must watch expenses. Doctors will buy anything, all sorts of new gadgets, and never care how much it costs. Once they were all excited about those glass boots for stimulating circulation. We bought them, and I'll bet you can still find a few around the hospital, but they were never once used to my knowledge.

> —A board president

Many trustees believe they must take a broader view of hospital affairs than doctors can be expected to. These board members tend to see the medical staff as a group of experts whose interests are largely confined to medical matters. The comments of two different board presidents are illustrative:

> Doctors you might say are technicians. What we need are not technicians but coordinators. People who bring all the different techniques together. As I see it, that's what the board of managers is supposed to do at the hospital. The first duty of the trustee is to help preserve the patient's identity. Doctors get case-hardened, can't see the patient as an individual.
>
> Our publicity committee has to censor the things doctors say for publication. Doctors will do foolish things in public if you don't watch them.

RELATIONSHIPS WITHIN THE BOARD

Trustees vary greatly among themselves. Any single board, despite the common characteristics described earlier, will have members who differ in the interest and the amount of time they devote to the hospital. An "active board" is not necessarily one in which every member digs eagerly into hospital affairs. One board president stressed that certain trustees who don't participate fully should nevertheless be retained:

> Some members who don't appear at meetings can still be very important. I know their telephone numbers. I called on a business executive the other day and before we were through he had given me $10,000 for the hospital out of a clear sky.

A major problem is age and retirement. Unless individuals are elected for a specific tenure, the board may become weighted with inactive members.

> Some of them don't do anything. I'm sure some haven't been inside the hospital for over a year. We have one old lady who has been an invalid for five years, but still hangs on. They stay until they die. I am trying to get some of the dead wood off of the board. We have a committee set up now to ask one member per year to retire.
>
> —A board president

Factionalism may of course interfere with the board's effectiveness. The members, perhaps because of their success in the outside world, tend to be individualists and to hold their opinions with some firmness. The stress which they place on values may diverge at many points. The familiar conflict between financial means and humanitarian objectives which is a source of stress among other hospital people sometimes divides board members as well.

Since trustees have the major task of threshing out a working philosophy for the institution, it is not rare for them to disagree, particularly on the policies to be adopted toward the other two powers, the administrator and medical staff. One board president described his effort to induce the other board members to have chiefs appointed to the medical departments. His board refused to back him in this proposal, arguing that, "We cannot do medicine. You can't get away with that." Similarly we have known boards which debated long and hard the problem of replacing an authoritarian director of nurses with a more democratic one.

RELATIONS WITH THE PUBLIC

Trustees are an important link, perhaps the most important, between the hospital and the community. They are normally active in the community and can exercise much influence by explaining the hospital's position on controversial issues such as costs. They (and the patients) *are* the public within the hospital.

While the trustees represent the public interest, they serve without compensation. This adds weight to their impartial position. However, their very eminence as community leaders, which makes them alert to certain key values and attitudes, may separate them from the average citizen. The board is in some sense insulated from the currents of mass opinion, and may have to make special attempts to discern that opinion.

Trustees recognize that part of what the board holds in trust is the hospital's reputation and they are usually zealous to preserve its good name. They work toward this end in two ways. First, there is a formal explicit effort to hold public favor. There is often a publicity committee of the board which concentrates on this problem. One such committee was set up under the leadership of an advertising executive and charged with the supervision and censorship of all news releases. It is interesting that in this case the committee began to act only after a premature release of research findings had brought censure to the hospital.

Perhaps more vital than planned effort to promote understanding is the informal influence of the board. Through their day-to-day activities in the community, trustees can learn what the public opinion is and do much to sway influential persons. A casual word dropped by a powerful trustee can often accomplish much more than months of routine work.

The hospital's position and policy have become the object of so much public attention in recent years, and its problems are so enormous, that some board members have nearly a full-time job smoothing public relations. Constant interpretation of the hospital's situation to the surrounding community is essential for both financial support and intelligent public use of hospital resources. Then, too, the growing public awareness of medical standards has made the board more sharply aware of responsibility for explaining those standards, and defending hospital practices in the forum of community opinion. In particular, complaints about the high costs of medical care and anxieties about its quality as compared to the ideal or to standards in other cities have forced trustees to become self-conscious about the relation of hospital to community. Finally, the board has come to protect the hospital against unwarranted pressures of outside groups eager for a policy-making voice.

The success of the board in its public relations has a direct bearing on human relations within the hospital. The employees soon learn the local reputation of the hospital. Their pride and spirit are strongly influenced by what others think of their job. These in turn have a significant effect on their attitudes and relationships to one another.

SUMMARY

The board of trustees is the bridge between the hospital and the local community. Its members are the responsible public guardians of the hospital organization. Beyond their corporate trust in the financial realm, the board members act as general policy-makers. Their degree of supervision over the administration varies, but it is generally agreed that they should not concern themselves with the details of routine management. The division of the responsibility between the two varies widely from one hospital to another. The board deals chiefly with the administrator and the medical staff. In both cases, the relationship poses the fundamental problem of lay versus expert authority. The board members' prestige and formal power in the community are usually at least as great as that of the physician and therefore they are better able than anyone else to maintain a balance between technical scientific claims and other interests. Relations between board, medical staff, and administrator are complex and rest finally on mutual understanding and accommodation rather than formal lines of organization. This triad of human relations affects more than the three top agents. It profoundly influences the internal relations of the hospital as a whole, as well as its ties with the outside world.

8.

Current Perspectives on Hospital Governance

LAWRENCE D. PRYBIL AND DAVID B. STARKWEATHER

Lawrence D. Prybil, Ph.D., is Professor and Chairman - Department of Hospital and Health Administration - Medical College of Virginia - Virginia Commonwealth University.

David B. Starkweather, Dr. P.H., is currently Associate Professor of Public Health and head of a group of graduate curricula in Administrative Sciences - The University of California, Berkeley.

During the past decade, the hospital industry has become one of the nation's most closely-regulated industries. The hospital's performance is subject to continual review by a host of private, quasi-governmental, and governmental agencies at the local, state, and federal level. Yet, at the same time, society expects hospitals to adapt rapidly to technological, socio-economic, and demographic changes and to demonstrate creativity in their organizational responses to changing health care needs and demands. This paradox, in combination with the intrinsic difficulties involved in operating one of the most complex forms of large-scale organization, has created many problems and challenges for those who have responsibility for hospital governance and management.

It is certainly true that, in the 1970s, hospital governance and management is a "joint venture" and that the future of the nation's hospitals depends upon the effectiveness of their mutual efforts.[1] However, it is the hospital governing board which is ultimately responsible, legally and morally, for the institution and all services it provides.

BOARD FUNCTIONS AND PERFORMANCE

In the not-for-profit hospital, as in every corporation, overall responsibility for the institution's operations and services is vested in a board of directors. The board's responsibility is a fiduciary obligation and cannot be divested through delegation.[2]

This paper will relate primarily to the governance of public and private not-for-profit hospitals, although many of these issues also pertain to the governance of investor-owned institutions.

Reprinted by permission from *Hospital and Health Services Administration: Quarterly Journal of the American College of Hospital Administrators,* Chicago, Vol. 21 (Fall, 1976), pp. 67-75. Copyright 1976 by the American College of Hospital Administrators. All rights reserved.

To fulfill this responsibility, it is widely accepted that the board should perform certain corporate functions including:

- Establishing corporate goals and major institutional policies.
- Ensuring that plans and programs are developed and implemented to meet corporate goals.
- Establishing and maintaining sound procedures for conducting the business of the governing board.
- Providing for the hospital's long-range financial stability.
- Selecting and maintaining a qualified medical staff and ensuring that the staff is properly organized to fulfill the responsibilities that the board delegates to it.
- Evaluating all phases of hospital performance, including the quality of medical care, and ensuring that established standards are met.
- Selecting the chief executive officer, defining duties and responsibilities, and evaluating performance.
- Reviewing and approving the hospital's overall organizational structure.
- Ensuring that the community the hospital serves is well informed about the hospital's goals and performance.[3]

These are complex and vital functions, and one important issue in the hospital industry today is how effectively boards are really performing them. The literature contains both praise and substantial criticism for hospital governing boards. It has been suggested by several authorities that many governing boards, as presently structured and composed, are unable to perform their functions in a timely and effective manner.[4,5] Unfortunately, few studies have been conducted regarding what hospital governing boards actually do and how well they do it.[6] There is a real need for careful research to evaluate the actual performance of governing boards and determine the factors that influence their effectiveness (e.g., size, composition, policies and procedures). The results of such studies would not only improve knowledge and understanding of the boards' performance, but also provide an objective basis for instituting changes in board structure and operations that would improve their performance and, thereby, the performance of the hospitals for which they are responsible. Meanwhile, each governing board should periodically re-examine its fundamental responsibilities and assess its own performance. Self studies of this sort are difficult but can yield worthwhile results and lead to improvements in board awareness, motivation, and performance.

STANDARDS OF CONDUCT AND ACCOUNTABILITY

Extensive litigation over the years has defined the standards of conduct that must be exercised by directors of business corporations to avoid liability; however, there is not a comparable history of case law to provide specific, well-established guidelines for directors of not-for-profit corporations.[7] The principal sources of law regarding the legal authority and responsibilities of governing boards are state incorporation statutes and articles of incorporation; however, these do not specifically define standards of conduct for directors of not-for-profit corporations.[8] An important issue of concern in hospital governance, therefore, has been the absence of clearly-established standards of conduct that members of hospital boards should demonstrate to properly perform their duties and avoid liability.

This matter was clarified to some extent in the Sibley Hospital case which was concluded in the District of Columbia in 1974.[9] Since litigation involving the governing boards of not-for-profit hospitals has been infrequent to date, this case is likely to have considerable impact. The decision in this case provides some clarification regarding the standards of conduct that directors of not-for-profit hospitals should exercise, particularly in regard to management of the institution's financial and investment affairs.[10] Knowledgeable legal authorities and hospital officials should endeavor to further develop and disseminate sound performance guidelines for the trustees of not-for-profit hospitals; these would be extremely useful for hospital administrators and governing boards and, very possibly, reduce the likelihood of future litigation due to improper or inadequate performance by board members.[11]

Consideration of standards of conduct leads to a closely related matter: accountability. The hospital's chief executive officer, selected and appointed by the board of directors, is accountable to the board for performance in carrying out the functions that are delegated. Moreover, as a result of several important legal decisions during the past decade, it is increasingly accepted that the hospital's medical staff is also accountable to the governing board for its performance in accomplishing delegated functions.[12] However, it is the board of directors that is ultimately responsible for the institution and all services it provides.

Who is responsible for evaluating the performance of the governing board? To whom and for what are governing boards accountable? In recent years, much has been written about corporate accountability in the hospital industry and this has been useful in defining and explaining the concept.[13] However, it is the responsibility of each governing board to translate this concept into concrete action. Every board of directors should carefully assess the nature and limits of its institutional accountability and take the actions that are necessary to properly and fully discharge these obligations.

IMPACT OF PL 93-641 ON BOARD'S ROLE AND FUNCTION

Rapid changes in society-at-large and in the health industry pose many important issues for hospitals and their governing boards. One such issue is the probable impact of Public Law 93-641 on hospitals and, specifically, on the responsibility and authority of their governing boards. Under this Act, health systems agencies (HSA) are being established across the country. The Act states that these bodies will have responsibility within their designated areas for "the provision of effective health planning and the promotion and development of facilities, manpower, and services to meet identified needs and reduce documented inefficiencies." Among the many functions these agencies will be expected to perform are the development of an area-wide health systems plan including health care goals and priorities, development of plans and projects to achieve these goals, and periodic assessment of the appropriateness of all existing institutional services in their area.[14]

It is certain that the new planning law and structure will have substantial impact on the hospital industry as a whole—and on every institution and its governing board. Some authorities believe that HSA will serve to limit the responsibilities and further constrain the authority of hospital boards. Others believe that this new planning structure will require hospitals to sharply improve their planning and decision-making processes, and thereby challenge the governing boards to perform more effectively.[15]

Careful studies, conducted over a period of time, will be needed before the actual impact of Public Law 93-641 on the hospital industry is known. National and state-level hospital associations as well as hospital administrators and board members should encourage and support such efforts. Meanwhile, members of governing boards and administrators should become thoroughly familiar with the new planning legislation and requirements. They should also assess the probable impact of the new planning process and requirements on their institution and determine the actions, if any, that should be taken within the institution to adapt to them.

GOVERNANCE IN MULTIPLE-UNIT HOSPITAL SYSTEMS

In recent years there has been a definite trend toward the development of multiple-unit systems. According to recent data compiled by the American Hospital Association, more than 1900 non-federal hospitals are included within multiple-unit systems that include at least two operating institutions managed by a single corporate entity.[16] These multiple-unit systems, both investor-owned and not-for-profit, are being created through mergers, consolidations, and the use of mechanisms such as management contracts and holding companies.

The development of multiple-unit systems throughout the United States raises many important issues for the governing boards and administrators of single-unit institutions. The most basic of these issues is whether or not they should become part of a multiple-unit system through some form of affiliation or expansion. To resolve this issue, hospital officials need to assess the alternative approaches that are feasible in their particular situation and determine, to the best of their capability, the costs and benefits of these alternatives in relation to maintaining the status quo. A movement from single-unit to multiple-unit operations, regardless of the organizational approach, will affect many aspects of the institution—including the role and functions of the governing body—and the responsible officials should prepare carefully for these changes.[17]

The governing boards that are responsible for existing multiple-unit systems have other important issues to address. In some instances, hospital organizations have expanded into multiple-unit systems without significant adjustments in the structure of the governing boards or in the manner that the boards operate. This may be very appropriate; in other situations, failure to modify the traditional pattern of hospital governance may prove dysfunctional to the organization and the community it serves.[18] In any event, the governing board of any corporation that has moved toward multiple-unit operations should periodically evaluate its structure and composition as well as its performance in fulfilling its expanding role and responsibilities. It is likely that the governance of multiple-unit systems will require relatively greater attention to long-range corporate planning and strategic decision-making as compared to close involvement in institutional operations. This, in turn, will necessitate careful review of the functions and authority that the board delegates to management and to medical staff.

BOARD COMPOSITION AND STRUCTURE

Traditionally, the governing boards of not-for-profit hospitals have been primarily composed of individuals who are neither employed by the institution nor affiliated with its medical staff. The governing boards have been composed predominantly of "outside directors" who serve without remuneration as a service to the institution and the community. In recent years, there has been a trend toward including physicians and hospital administrators on governing boards. Several recent studies have found that more than half of all boards now include physicians and a substantial proportion include administrators (and, in some instances, other members of the administrative staff).[19] In other words, there has been a shift toward including more "inside directors" on hospital boards. At the same time, some individuals and groups have advocated the inclusion of "consumer representatives" on hospital boards.[20]

An important issue that each governing board and/or its sponsoring body should address is the appropriate size and composition of its membership including the mix of outside and inside directors. Interestingly, this is also an important issue in other industries where many firms and business leaders are re-examining the traditional patterns of board composition, selection, and evaluation.[21] There is concern that the boards of directors in many business corporations are not performing their functions effectively and, according to some authorities, public policy is turning against the concept of heavy reliance upon inside directors who have close links with the corporations for which they are serving as directors.[22]

Unfortunately, there is little evidence that relates board size, composition, or policies to board effectiveness or hospital performance. There is a need for more studies directed toward determining the factors that influence the performance of governing boards.[23] Nonetheless, in the context of their particular circumstances and constraints, boards of directors and administrators should periodically assess their present size and composition as well as their current policies and procedures regarding selection, evaluation, and replacement of board members. They should also give consideration to alternative approaches to provide the board membership, especially outside directors, with all the information necessary for them to perform their functions properly. Management audit programs,[24] a standing audit committee of the board,[25] and information systems tailored to meet the needs of the governing board[26] are among the mechanisms that are available to improve the board's knowledge and understanding of the institution for which they are responsible.

The U.S. hospital industry is facing serious problems and great challenges and, in a very real sense, the industry's future is dependent upon the leadership and performance of the hospitals' governing boards. The boards, with the support and participation of hospital administrators and professional associations, should consider complex issues. Whether or not these issues are addressed, and the manner in which they are addressed, will have a direct bearing on the future performance of governing boards and of the hospitals for which they are responsible.

The Cooperative Information Center for Hospital Management Studies, M2240 School of Public Health, The University of Michigan in Ann Arbor, helped in compiling the bibliography and references for this article.

FOOTNOTES

[1] H. Robert Cathcart, "Governance and Administration: A Joint Venture," *Trustee* 28 (October, 1975):19.

[2] Catholic Hospital Association, *Guidelines on the Responsibilities, Functions, and Selection Criteria for Hospital Boards of Trustees* (St. Louis: CHA, 1974):7.

[3] See, for example, W. J. Hickey, "The Functions of the Hospital Board of Directors," *Hospital Administration* 17 (Summer, 1972):43-53, R. D. Willits, "What Boards of Trustees Do," in *The Hospital Trustee Reader* (Chicago: AHA, 1975): 3-9; and Lawrence Prybil, "Accountability Vested in Trustees," *Hospitals, JAHA* 50 (April 1, 1976):48.

[4] See, for example, Ray E. Brown, "Strictures and Structures," *Hospitals, JAHA* 44 (August 16, 1970):79; and Richard L. Johnson, "Governance Seen As Weak Link," *Hospitals, JAHA* 48 (June 1, 1974):47.

[5] Interestingly, the general management literature shows that leaders in other industries are also concerned and critical about the actual performance of corporate boards in carrying out their legal responsibilities and functions. See, for example, Myles Mace, "The President and the Board of Directors," *Harvard Business Review* (March-April, 1972):37; and Marvin Chandler, "It's Time to Clean Up the Boardroom," *Harvard Business Review* (September-October, 1975):73.

[6] Anthony R. Kovner, "Governing Boards," *Hospital Administration* 20 (Winter, 1975):65.

[7] Myles Mace, "Standards of Care for Trustees," *Harvard Business Review* (January-February, 1976):14.

[8] Arthur Southwick, "The Trusteeship Function," *Hospital Progress*, 52 (September, 1971):76; and Arthur Bernstein, "Legal Liability of Hospital Trustees," *Hospitals, JAHA* 48 (April 1, 1974): 192.

[9] Stern v. Lucy Webb Hayes National Training School for Deaconesses and Missionaries, 367 F. Supp. 536 (D.C., D.C., Nov. 30, 1973) and 381 F. Supp. 1003 (D.C., D.C., 1974).

[10] Arthur Bernstein, "Judging Hospital Trustees," *Hospitals JAHA* 49 (January 1, 1975):83. Also see Myles Mace, "Standards of Care for Trustees," *Harvard Business Review* (January-February, 1976):14.

[11] For an interesting discussion of the difficulties and the benefits of establishing such guidelines, see Myles Mace, "Legal Guidelines for Directors," *Harvard Business Review* (September-October, 1975):18.

[12] Eric Springer, "The Darling Case: Ten years later," *Trustee,* 28 (July, 1975):17; and Stephen Blaes, "The Legal Perspective," *Trustee,* 29 (May, 1976):9.

[13] See K. J. Williams, "Beyond Responsibility: Toward Accountability," *Hospital Progress,* 53 (January, 1972):44; and Robert Cunningham, *Governing Hospitals: Trustees and the New Accountabilities* (Chicago: AHA, 1976).

[14] Public Law 93-641, The National Health Planning and Resources Development Act of 1974. For a summary of the major provisions of this Act, see Robin MacStravic, "Provisions of the National Health Planning and Resources Development Act," *Hospital Progress* 56 (April, 1975):48.

[15] Symond R. Gottlieb, "What Trustees Should Know About the Planning Law," *Trustee* 28 (July, 1975):12.

[16] Montague Brown, "Multiple Unit Systems Under Single Management," *Hospital and Health Services Administration* 21 (Spring, 1976):88.

[17] For example, see Montague Brown and Howard Lewis, "Small Hospitals Contract for Management Help," *Harvard Business Review* (May-June, 1976):8.

[18] For further discussion, see Carl Platou and James Rice, "Multi-Hospital Holding Companies," *Harvard Business Review* (May-June, 1972):14; Samuel Tibbitts, "Multiple Hospital Systems," *Hospital Administration* 18 (Spring, 1973):10; and Carl Platou et al., "The Consector Theory of Hospital Development," *Hospital Administration* 18 (Spring, 1973):61.

[19] See, for example, Kay Gilmore and John Wheeler, "A National Profile of Governing Boards," *Hospitals, JAHA* 46 (November 1, 1972):105; Edgar Mansfield, "Physicians in Management: Report on a Survey," *The Hospital Medical Staff* (April, 1972):17; and Armand Checker and Richard Knapp, "A Profile of Teaching Hospital Board Members," *Trustee* 28 (August, 1975):20.

[20] See, for example, Lowell E. Bellin, "Changing Composition of Voluntary Hospital Boards: An Inevitable Prospect for the 1970's," *HSMHA Health Reports* 86 (August, 1971):674.

[21] See, for example, Peter Vanderwicken, "Change Invades the Boardroom," *Fortune* (May, 1972):156; Christopher Stone, "Public Directors Merit a Try," *Harvard Business Review* (March-April, 1976):20; and Joseph Ban, "The Role of the Professional Director," *Harvard Business Review* (May-June, 1976):18.

[22] Marvin Chandler, "It's Time to Clean Up the Boardroom," *Harvard Business Review* (September-October, 1975):73.

[23] One such study is Jeffrey Pfeffer, "Size, Composition, and Function of Hospital Boards of Directors: A Study of Organization-Environment Linkage," *Administrative Science Quarterly* 18 (September, 1973):349.

[24] Marshall Gavin and Paul Kessler, "The Development of a Management Audit Program for Hospitals," *Hospital Administration* 20 (Fall, 1975):20.

[25] William Freitag, "The Hospital Audit Committee," *Trustee* 28 (July, 1975):26.

[26] Myles Mace (ed), "Management Information Systems for Directors," *Harvard Business Review* (November-December, 1975):14.

9.

Should Doctors Be on Your Board?

C. JEROME JORGENSEN

C. Jerome Jorgensen is Executive Director of Stormont - Vail Hospital in Topeka, Kansas.

Recommendations for involving physicians more directly in hospital management are being heard with increasing frequency and greater force from national and state medical societies and hospital associations, from the Joint Commission on Accreditation, from such authoritative groups as the Barr Committee which reported its findings on hospital effectiveness directly to the President.

Some agencies suggest involvement of doctors in the highest decision level—the hospital governing board. Others merely say, "We encourage more meaningful involvement of doctors in policy-making councils of the hospital." But the reasons for the recommendations seem more important than the suggestions themselves, for they reflect changing attitudes and the use of new concepts of management.

The clamor for more physician involvement has not necessarily arisen because the physician is *not* "involved" in most hospitals but because there are contemporary demands for rethinking this concept. It appears that there is a need for *renewal* of present relationships and the role that physicians must play within the hospital setting and in revising the form of delivery of health care services.

REASONS FOR PARTICIPATION

Let's explore some of the reasons given for greater doctor participation and what objectives may be achieved. Presumably, doctors should become more involved in the *hope* of helping to improve the health-care system and because without them some problems cannot be solved.

One primary problem is spiraling hospital costs. Because quality and cost of care decisions are inseparable, governing boards and management will find it difficult to bring about fundamental changes or effective controls without including the patient's purchasing agent—the doctor—someplace in the deliberations. More frequently, hospitals and physicians on many issues are not judged separately but as a single entity.

Reprinted by permission from *Hospital Administration* (currently *Hospital and Health Services Administration*): Quarterly Journal of the American College of Hospital Administrators, Chicago, Vol. 15 (Fall, 1970), pp. 6-13. Copyright 1970 by the American College of Hospital Administrators. All rights reserved.

The increased cost problem cannot be taken lightly. It threatens to profoundly change the entire voluntary health-care system which hospital leaders want to see continue. This dual system of responsibility for patient care can no longer be continued. We must all get on the same team. As a further aggravation, technological improvements in medical care usually do not reduce costs—they increase them. This is contrary to the technological change in most industries. Numerous examples can be cited of expensive duplications of highly complicated and expensive equipment and personnel. There also are duplications in unsophisticated services. Cooperation, not competition, must be emphasized in planning and physicians will be needed to bring about sound decisions.

THE CHARLESTON CASE

The second reason for greater physician participation in hospital management is the legal principle established in the Charleston Case—that the hospital board is responsible for the quality of professional care provided by the institution. The hospital is now seen as *one* organization designed to deliver the highest quality of care which clearly points out that the division of medical staff and administration objectives has been conceptually and legally eliminated.

The development of professional care standards is a shared responsibility. Hospitals and boards of trustees are legally required to maintain the medical staff structure for advising and recommending professional standards of care and to insure that these standards are enforced. This does not dilute control for medicine because this is a shared responsibility between administration and medical staff. To insure that the institution effectively controls care, it will be necessary to integrate the physician even more completely within the authority and responsibility structure of the hospital.

The third major reason is that federal and third-party interest in health care is creating greater public scrutiny. Medicare, comprehensive areawide planning, Regional Medical Programs, and various commissions and committees established to evaluate the delivery of care can be cited as compelling areas of activity requiring greater doctor involvement.

The fourth reason is the need for fundamental changes in the delivery of health care, such as progressive patient care, neighborhood health centers, areawide planning councils, and expanded preventive health programs. If these fundamental changes are to be made in the near future, participation by all providers is essential. Physicians should be included to help shape the process.

A fifth point is the medical centering of the hospital. It has been said that the hospital will no longer be merely a facility but will become a facilitating agency providing the leadership and direction for the development of comprehensive and continuous services. Most likely it will play a central role in the organization of health services, not necessarily providing them, but providing centrality to a nebulous system of health care delivery. It must provide functional and organizational relationships to the farious facets currently providing health care.

INCREASED USE OF EMERGENCY ROOMS

One example of the centrality of this role is increased utilization of hospital emergency rooms all across the United States. The solution to this problem is complex and will require all of the skills and thinking of the entire health care establishment to provide proper solutions. The physician must lead the way in assisting with solutions.

Another factor is most basic to all—the patient-physician relationship. After all, the relationship between the patient and the physician will remain regardless of the organization of health service. It is only natural that those serving the patient most directly should be involved in structuring the setting for delivery.

The complexity of hospital operations is another factor. Hospitals can no longer afford monolithic decision processes. The successful hospital will use participative management and integrative organization theory to administer the health care program. Elimination of separatism, establishing mutual trust, and developing a clear understanding and appreciation of the role of all individuals within the hospital operation must be a common goal.

These reasons are all substantial. There may be more. There are also reasons cited why physicians shouldn't be involved. Fear of diminishing the role of the hospital administrator, having one more group or person to counsel, lack of trust, alleged lack of improvement in the decision-making process are a few that might be cited. I would suggest renewed thinking about present and more effective participation by physicians be considered before judgments are made regarding its success.

ACHIEVING MEANINGFUL INVOLVEMENT

How can this be done? How can more meaningful involvement be achieved? In many hospitals good physician representation within the organizational structure already exists. The question is, "Is this meaningful participation?" Increased involvement is a two-way street. There must be an interest in having physicians participate and physicians must be interested in participating in a positive fashion. I would suggest that there are three steps to achieve meaningful involvement of physicians within hospitals: (1) education and information, (2) present performance, and (3) future participation.

Let's examine each step.

EDUCATION AND INFORMATION

First, education and information. In order for anyone to become effective in his performance or participation, he must be educated regarding the nature of the problem and what can be done to help. I suggest there is not enough education of medical staff or of individuals within the staff toward the problems faced by the hospital. How many administrators have conducted cost seminars? How many have really tried to explain why hospital costs are what they are, and found some way to justify their increased spiraling? What innovative and creative ways have been tried to bring this message across? Physicians must be brought into the picture to the extent that they become aware of their influence on unit cost and total patient cost. The physician must be equipped with proper information, not only to assist in making judgments but to assist in interpreting hospital and medical problems to his patients and to the community. I was recently informed that one hospital adminstrator sends copies of the patient's bill to his attending physician upon dismissal. The effects were astounding. Immediately, staff physicians became acquainted with the costs of the services they were ordering and became concerned about the high prices the hospital had to charge. I am not suggesting this be done to open the door to criticism but it is a technique that can develop enough interest to open ears so the message regarding costs will be heard.

Education about the management function is also important. Costs cannot be viewed separately and apart from planning, management, and financing of hospital care. Informal day-to-day communication by the administrator with individual doctors and in-depth discussions with staff leaders also can be extremely helpful in bringing to bear the opinions and judgments of physicians on any single problem. There must be a formal education program aimed at board and staff—seminars, medical staff meetings, reading material, retreats, and national conferences for physicians and trustees.

PRESENT PERFORMANCE

The second step I labeled "present performance." Currently there exist within the hospital framework many legitimate areas for effective and meaningful physician involvement. It seems to me that performance of these activities ought to be improved before we begin talking about new patterns or new relationships to be superimposed upon an already complex situation. The management structure for physicians is the medical staff organization. It is not separate from the hospital organization. You say you have that? But, is it effective? Does it function using good principles of organization and management? It is, after all, the agency of the *board* for managing medical practice.

Professional practice within the hospital in the future will need to hold up under public scrutiny. Frequently there are weaknesses of hospital staff organization, bylaws, meetings, discipline, patterns of practice, etc.

Within the medical staff organization several committees are concerned with hospital costs and can provide the physician with an opportunity to become involved in the management process.

Utilization review is an excellent area for committee function evaluating and controlling the quality and use of hospital services. Under the purview of this committee any department of the hospital or any patient activity can be scrutinized on some regular basis. Many tools are available to permit this committee to function effectively and it can become a real strength for management if used properly—tools such as HAS, PAS, and MAP. Blue Cross-Blue Shield and state hospital associations can also provide useful hospital data.

The Nursing Liaison Committee is another example of where new services can be evaluated, with reference to both improved patient care and costs. The Adjunctive or Professional Services Committee involving physician evaluation and direction to pharmacy, physical therapy, inhalation therapy, and other paraprofessional departments is an excellent opportunity for physicians to assist in the process of drug inventory and control, understanding the problems of quantity purchasing, and becoming involved in cost and quality-related decisions in patient care departments.

And not to be forgotten is the Joint Conference Committee which in many hospitals is made up of either the officers of the staff or other selected physicians to meet on a regular basis with members of the board of trustees. If these committees are viewed properly and the functions defined, all of them can be reoriented and *renewed* with broadened objectives and new emphasis and functions to provide for a more direct relationship between physician-patient decisions and effective management decisions based upon cost information.

FUTURE PARTICIPATION

The third area I labeled "future participation." Numerous references indicate it is no longer enough to merely have physicians sitting in various meetings of the hospital. They argue that in order to be truly effective in decision- and policy-making there must be a full and complete involvement which would include voting privileges.

What about having physicians on the board? At our hospital we have had a physician on the board for many years. Personally speaking, it is very helpful and in the future will be even more essential. He is selected just as any other member of the board. In addition, the president of the medical staff attends all meetings of the board and reports on activities of the staff. When considering the various ways in which physicians can become involved directly in policy- and decision-making, this is the most direct and least difficult since the board of trustees is a legally constituted body which is formed for policy- and decision-making. Decisions made by other groups within the hospital can cause problems.

It is suggested in the Barr Report that physicians be *involved in the development* of the budget and operating plan and in the achievement of financial and service objectives as budgeted and planned. Presumably, at some point, the recommendations of the Barr Committee may become the law of the land. Also, already within the State of Kansas the Department of Health, in its new regulations soon to be published, has specified that "the governing authority shall demonstrate evidence of liaison and close working relationship with the medical staff."

Another area of physician participation can be the long-range planning committee of the board. This group can be constituted with members of the medical staff or physician members of the board or both. Certainly the Joint Conference Committee is an effective mechanism in existence in most hospitals to achieve close liaison with the medical staff.

NOT THE WHOLE ANSWER

Greater physician involvement is not the whole answer to improving the hospital cost picture, but it's a beginning. The case for involvement will not necessarily result in improved effectiveness. The dichotomy of the present approach must be diminished and physicians must have more responsibility.

Education and information are the forerunners to more effective physician involvement and this should lead the way to improved staff performance in the present organizational patterns. Meaningful involvement cannot be achieved without an understanding of the complexity of hospital management and a delineation of the role the medical staff as well as individual physicians must play. Once this is achieved, the way is paved for involvement in other levels of hospital policy-making situations. With this approach and informed perspective, the physician can make his greatest contribution to the balance of quality care and costs. Physicians' involvement is a change in attitude and process rather than a change in pattern or structure.

THIS IS THE BOX SCORE FOR KANSAS

A 1968 survey by the Kansas Hospital Association, based on replies from 122 of 154 hospitals in the state, reveals the extent of physician involvement in Kansas hospitals:

	Yes	No	No Answer or Answer Unclear
1. Do you have one or more physicians on your Hospital Board?	16	106	0
(The 16 indicating "Yes" reported a total of 23 doctors as Board Members.)			
2. Do you have one or more physicians on your Hospital Advisory Board?	26	88	8
3. Do you have a Joint Conference Committee?	69	48	...
4. Do physicians who are not Board Members attend your Board Meetings?	52	63	...
5. Does your hospital have the medical staff or a physician group review any of the following:			
a. The Budget?	16	100	6
b. Cost and/or Financial Statement?	27	87	8
c. Staffing Needs?	63	51	8
d. Need for New Services?	100	21	1

REFERENCES

1. Crosby, Edwin L., M.D. "The Physician's Place in Health Care Administration," *Hospitals, J.A.H.A.,* Vol. 42, Part I (August 1, 1968), pp. 47-49, 121.
2. Eisele, C. Wesley, M.D. "How Changing Times are Changing Staffs," *The Modern Hospital,* Vol. 108, No. 5 (May, 1967), pp. 127-128.
3. Kansas State Board of Health, Hospital Facilities Division. *Hospital Regulations,* 4th ed., 1958.
4. U.S. Department of Health, Education, and Welfare. *Report of the Secretary's Advisory Committe on Hospital Effectiveness* (Washington, D.C., U.S. Government Printing Office, 1968).

FURTHER READING SUGGESTED BY THE AUTHOR

"The Physician's Place in Health Care Administration," Edwin L. Crosby, M.D. (*Hospitals, J.A.H.A.,* Vol. 42, Part 1, August 1, 1968, pp. 47-49, 121).
"How Changing Times are Changing Staffs," C. Wesley Eisele, M.D. (*Modern Hospital,* Vol. 108, No. 5, May, 1967, pp. 127-128).
Report of the Secretary's Advisory Committee or Hospital Effectiveness. (U.S. Department of Health, Education, and Welfare, Washington, D.C., U.S. Government Printing Office, 1968).
"The Practicing Physician's Role in Hospital Management—a consultant's view," Albert W. Snoke, M.D. (*Hospital Progress,* Vol. 50, No. 11, November, 1969, pp. 57-59, 84).

10.

Governing Boards

ANTHONY R. KOVNER

Anthony R. Kovner, Ph.D., is currently the senior health care consultant, International Union of Automobile, Aerospace, Agricultural Workers (UAW) and was previously Director of the Graduate Program in Health Care Administration - The Wharton School - University of Pennsylvania.

Governance in hospitals is increasingly challenged and questioned. Whether the pressure is from consumers and taxpayers and their governmental representatives or from managers and physicians, dissatisfaction is increasingly voiced with the policy-making process in hospitals. The critics argue that the tripartite authority structure of governing board, administration and medical staff is no longer relevant to the organizational needs of hospitals. The present governance structure of the typical voluntary, not-for-profit hospital is usually as follows: governing boards make overall policy; medical boards and chiefs recommend and implement policy concerning medical services; and administrators recommend and implement policy concerning support and financial services, the relation of medical to support services, and the relation of the hospital to other organizations and interest groups.

Research on hospital governance is relatively undeveloped for several reasons: restricted access because of policy implications, inadequate methodology to isolate cause-effect relationships; and a lack of agreed-upon operational definitions for hospital performance or output. This survey attempts to focus on major research concerning governing boards of hospitals and other organizations which has been published during 1969-1974. Important issues addressed include: (1) role in the decision-making process; (2) composition and methods of selection; (3) structure and function; and (4) accountability.

Kovner has defined four roles for hospital governing boards: the making of policy or important decisions; gaining access to needed resources, such as capital and professional manpower; representation of the interests of stakeholders in the organization such as consumers, physicians, and government; and advising top management in areas

---

Reprinted by permission from *Hospital Administration* (currently *Hospital and Health Services Administration*): *Quarterly Journal of the American College of Hospital Administrators,* Chicago, Vol. 20 (Winter, 1975), pp. 65-72. Copyright 1975 by the American College of Hospital Administrators. All rights reserved.

of special expertise, such as construction, law, labor and consumer relations.[1]

In a study of boards of directors of manufacturing, mining and retailing companies, Mace found that the governing boards did: (1) advise and counsel the chief executive; (2) act as a source of discipline to top management; (3) act in times of crisis. Mace found that governing boards *did not:* (1) establish objectives, strategies and policies; (2) ask discerning questions of top management; and (3) select the corporate president except in times of crises.[2]

In part following up on Mace, Kovner found, in a study of 47 hospitals of 200 beds or larger in the greater Philadelphia area, that hospital governing board members said they *did* advise and counsel the chief executive, make major decisions in the event of a crisis, establish objectives, strategies and broad policies, ask discerning questions of top management and suggest and select board members.[3] Weaknesses of the Kovner and Mace studies are reliance on questionnaire responses and oral interviews with those involved and a lack of empirical verification of what trustees and executive officers said happened.

USING STATISTICAL TECHNIQUES

Applying statistical techniques in establishing the relationship between board composition and organizational access to key resources, Pfeffer found that when business boards do not function as instruments to deal with the environment, the firms pay a price in terms of reduced profits.[4] Similar results were obtained when Pfeffer applied this methodology to 57 midwestern hospitals. Hospitals were more likely to be effective in obtaining resources (the number of medical programs, beds, and growth in facilities and physicians) to the extent that the board was seen as a linkage with the environment, rather than as management of the hospital. Linkage was reflected in the selection of board members for their influence in the community and political connections, rather than their knowledge of hospital administration.[5]

Governing boards perform multiple roles. Which role should be stressed at any given time depends upon historical and present circumstances, such as commitment to providing services to the poor or the need to attract additional capital or physicians. Top management and governing board members should formally examine role, assess alternative role emphases, and adapt board role in response to a changing set of environmental pressures.

COMPOSITION

Studies by Goldberg and Hemmelgarn, Berger and Earsy, Kovner and by Gilmore and Wheeler have revealed a remarkable similarity in the composition of community hospital governing boards.[6] Roughly 60 percent of board members are businessmen, bankers and lawyers.

Vance and the Catholic Hospital Association have specified desirable traits or criteria to use in selecting board members.[7] With reference to industrial firms, Vance argues for technical expertise, management expertise, specific economic service, broad economic sophistication, image, asset impact by virtue of serving on other boards, interlock (meaningful associations) and owner's equity. The CHA suggests personal qualifications such as commitment to community health and welfare and the ability to conceptualize; professional qualifications, such as technical competency and managerial experience; sponsoring group interests; political realism; and community visibility.

Vance suggests that the portfolio concept be applied to board selection in order to gain for the organization "a maximum return with a high degree of security." In other words, a hospital should evaluate the expertise and qualifications of its present board against criteria which reflect the hospital's current problems and opportunities, and then attempt to add or replace board members in the areas where gaps are most significant.

Kovner found that the typical hospital board member was male, from 50-69 years old, served on three or more other boards, had been on his hospital board for more than five years, and spent five or more hours per month on board activities. Kovner related board member occupation to perceived qualifications for decision-making in eleven policy areas, e.g., cost and quality of care.[8] Relative to other occupations, in areas perceived by all board members as highest priority (cost and quality and relations with third party payors), administrator and physician board members rated themselves most highly. About 12 percent of hospital board members in this study were either physicians or administrators.

BOARD COMPOSITION VIS à VIS HOSPITAL PERFORMANCE

There is little valid evidence which relates board composition to hospital performance. First, there is lack of agreement on comprehensive measures of hospital performance, and, second, causal relationships between board composition and performance outcomes have not yet been isolated. There is, therefore, no research justification for the recent governmental practice of adding "consumer" representatives to the governing boards of medical care organizations; that is, unless the role of governing boards is solely to "represent" community groups or the interests of artificial age, income, race and other groups. Such representativeness implies some as yet lacking structure of accountability tying representatives to group constituencies. Of course, a governing board itself may wish to add consumer representatives. This is appropriate for hospitals seeking to attract certain consumer groups as purchasers of services or to enhance identification with the hospital by certain groups. It also implies sharing of power with such representatives. However, most hospital governing boards have important roles in addition to representing or attracting certain consumer groups. Appropriate board composition is, thus, related to the desired and changing emphasis on the four roles previously mentioned.

STRUCTURE AND FUNCTION

In addition, little research has been done concerning board structure and function. A 1969 survey of 22 large industrial corporations revealed that the typical board had 15 members and met once a month for half a day.[9] Pfeffer found that the larger the hospital board, the greater the fund raising and support capability, and the smaller the board, the more hospital management was emphasized as a board function.[10] Kovner found that the typical hospital board had 16 or more members, met 6-15 times a year for one to two and one half hours per meeting, meetings were attended by 70 percent or more members with attendance records being kept by the hospital, and there were no age restrictions on board members.[11]

Research should be undertaken to ascertain what governing board members actually do, to include their participation in the various stages of policy-making and implementation, both in and outside of board meetings. It may be important also to examine whether there are any important differences among boards relating to the size of the board, the number and length of meetings, the remuneration of board members and so forth. It would be interesting to examine as well the expectations of board members and of hospital management and physicians regarding board member performance.

As has been stated earlier, the late 1960s and early 1970s had seen an increasing focus on the accountability of governing boards, especially in the health services sector. Part of the argument has focused on the desirability of placing consumer representatives on governing boards. Findings do not conclusively argue for or against such representation. Schwartz found no significant differences in operations of consumer sponsored prepaid health plans and provider sponsored plans.[12] Bellin and others have found important behavior changes, such as hiring a director of ambulatory care, associated with tying hospital funding by the New York City Health Department to the functioning of consumer advisory committees; Falkson, in a study of three neighborhood health centers, found that clients did not place a high priority on board participation by fellow consumers; Wise has argued that in the ghettos community participation in health center governance is not relevant because of the mobility of the population (50 percent turnover of residents every five years) and the lack of client participation in organized groups of any kind.[13]

BOARD REFORM

Vance has emphasized reforming the structure and function of boards toward improving accountability. This includes meaningful disclosed minutes of board meetings which indicate how each director responded on important issues. Vance also suggests recording attendance, and frequent, and fairly lengthy meetings. Other approaches include limitations of tenure and a structured self-evaluation of board activities by a committee established for this purpose. The committee may include non-board members and use outside consultants. Mace's suggestions also emphasize structure and function rather than performance outcomes. Mace argues for a governing board which is composed of outsiders rather than corporate officials, with the chief executive officer the only corporate official serving on the board. He suggests specifying the functions of board members in writing and similarly the criteria used to evaluate the chief executive officer. Mace also urges adequate compensation of board members to motivate active and responsible participation.[14]

ACCOUNTABILITY

Accountability is becoming more important for hospital survival and growth, as well as for perceived responsiveness by consumers. Consumers, as Falkson indicates, want improved performance rather than control *per se*. And so, it is dissatisfaction with the quality and cost of hospital services which is fueling consumer and taxpayer proposals to change hospital governance. It should be recognized, moreover, that undue emphasis on improving the accountability of governing boards, rather than hospital performance directly, may unduly limit board autonomy and flexibility, and thereby actually impact negatively on hospital performance.

FURTHER READINGS SUGGESTED BY THE AUTHOR

Bellin, Lowell, et al. "Phase One of Consumer Participation in Policies of 22 Voluntary Hospitals in New York City." *American Journal of Public Health* 62 (1972): 1370-78.

Cathcart, H. Robert. "Including the Community in Hospital Governance." *Hospital Progress*, October 1970, pp. 72-76.

Catholic Hospital Association. *Guidelines on the Responsibilities, Functions and Selection Criteria for Hospital Boards of Trustees.* St. Louis, Mo., 1970.

Goldberg, Theodore, and Hemmelgarn, Ronald. "Who Governs Hospitals?" *Hospitals*, 1 August 1971, pp. 72-79.

Koontz, Harold. *The Board of Directors and Effective Management.* New York: McGraw-Hill Book Co., 1967.

Kovner, Anthony R. "Hospital Board Members As Policy Makers: Role, Priority and Qualifications." *Medical Care*, Vol. 12, No. 12 (December, 1974), pp. 971-982.

Mace, Myles. *Directors: Myth and Reality.* Boston, Mass.: Harvard University Press, 1971.

Pelligrino, E. D. "The Changing Matrix of Clinical Decision-Making in the Hospital." In *Organization Research in Health Institutions,* edited by Basil S. Georgopoulos, pp. 301-54. Ann Arbor, Mich.: Institute for Social Research, University of Michigan, 1972.

Perloff, Earl. "For the Trustee, Deepening Responsibilities." *Hospitals*, January 1970.

Pfeffer, Jeffrey. "Size, Composition and Function of Hospital Boards of Directors: A Study of Organization-Environment Linkage." *Administrative Science Quarterly*, 1972, pp. 349-64.

Vance, Stanley C. *The Corporate Director: A Critical Evaluation.* Homewood, Ill.: Dow Jones-Irwin, Inc., 1968.

Zald, Mayer. "The Power and Functions of Boards of Directors: A Theoretical Synthesis." *American Journal of Sociology* 75 (1969-70): 97-110.

FOOTNOTES

[1] Anthony Kovner, "Hospital Board Members as Policy-Makers: Role, Priority, and Qualifications," *Medical Care*, Vol. 12, December, 1974, pp. 971-982.

[2] Myles Mace, *Directors: Myth and Reality* (Boston: Harvard University Press, 1971).

[3] Kovner, "Hospital Board Members."

[4] Jeffrey Pfeffer, "Size and Composition of Corporate Boards of Directors: The Organization and the Environment," *Administrative Science Quarterly*, 1972, pp. 218-28.

[5] Jeffrey Pfeffer, "Size, Composition and Function of Hospital Boards of Directors: A Study of Organization-Environment Linkage," *Administrative Science Quarterly*, 1974, pp. 349-364.

[6] See Theodore Goldberg and Ronald Hemmelgarn, "Who Governs Hospitals?" *Hospitals* 1 August, 1971, pp. 72-79; Ian Berger and Robert Easry, "Occupations of Boston Hospital Board Members," *Inquiry*, March 1973, pp. 42-6; Kovner, "Hospital Board Members," and Kay Gilmore and John R. Wheeler, "A National Profile of Governing Boards," *Hospitals*, 1 November 1972, pp. 105-08.

[7] See Stanley C. Vance, *The Corporate Director: A Critical Evaluation* (Homewood, Ill.: Dow Jones-Irwin, Inc., 1968); and The Catholic Hospital Association, *Guidelines on the Responsibilities, Functions and Selection Criteria for Hospital Boards of Trustees*, St. Louis, Mo., 1970.

[8] Kovner, "Hospital Board Members."

[9] *Survey of Boards of Directors–Practices and Procedures* (New York: General Electric Company, 1969).

[10] Jeffrey Pfeffer, "Function of Hospital Boards."

[11] Kovner, "Hospital Board Members."

[12] Jerome L. Schwartz, *Medical Plans and Health Care* (Springfield, Ill.: Charles C. Thomas, Publisher, 1968).

[13] See Lowell Bellin et al., "Phase One of Consumer Participation in Policies of 22 Voluntary Hospitals in New York City," *American Journal of Public Health* 62, no. 10 (1972): 1370-78; Joseph L. Falkson, *An Evaluation of Alternative Models of Citizen Participation in Urban Bureaucracy* (Ann Arbor, Mich.: Program in Health Planning, University of Michigan, 1971); and Harold Wise, *A Closer Look at Community Control*, 4th Annual Report (Bronx, N.Y.: Martin Luther King Health Center, 1971), pp. 32-44.

[14] Myles Mace, "The President and the Board of Directors," *Harvard Business Review*, March-April 1972, pp. 37-49.

The Administrator

Charles J. Austin in *Selection 11*, "WHAT IS HEALTH ADMINISTRATION?" and Everett A. Johnson in *Selection 12*, "THE LESSONS OF A PROFESSION," cover a broad spectrum of information and issues about the hospital's chief executive officer. The articles are especially good in showing the development of hospital administration and the environment and problems currently confronting the hospital manager. They concentrate on the chief executive officer as an individual who must deal and work effectively with other individuals if the job is to be done properly.

11.

What is Health Administration?

CHARLES J. AUSTIN

Charles J. Austin, Ph.D., is Dean of Graduate Studies and Professor of Health Care Administration, Trinity University. He was previously study director for the Commission on Education for Health Administration (sponsored by the W.K. Kellogg Foundation).

Administrative leadership is an essential, but often neglected, ingredient in the search for solutions to the serious problems of equity, quality, and efficiency in the delivery of health and medical services in this country. This paper examines the major roles and responsibilities of health administrators, and suggests that: health administration is unique, both as a specialty field of administration and as a function within the health and medical care industry; health administration may be viewed theoretically in a systems context but must also be looked at as an emerging profession that is taking on the attributes as well as the self-limiting features of professionalism; and health administration as an area of practice has the potential for steering the larger health and medical care industry into patterns of responsiveness, responsibility, and reconciliation.[1]

THE UNIQUENESS OF HEALTH ADMINISTRATION

Although health administration's commonalities with other kinds of administration are acknowledged (particularly in other service industries), and its interrelationships with other kinds of health and medical care activities are assumed, it also has unique characteristics which set it apart and afford special opportunities for both practice and education.

Most of the unique characteristics of health administration derive from the idiosyncrasies of the health and medical care "industry," one of the human service industries which comprise the larger service industry complex in our society.

Adapted from a staff working paper prepared for the Commission on Education for Health Administration, Washington, D.C. The Commission's report and related background papers were published by the Health Administration Press, Association of University Programs in Health Administration and the University of Michigan in 1975.

Reprinted by permission from *Hospital Administration* (currently *Hospital and Health Services Administration*): *Quarterly Journal of the American College of Hospital Administrators*, Chicago, Vol. 19 (Summer, 1974), pp. 14-29. Copyright 1974 by the American College of Hospital Administrators. All rights reserved.

DELIVERY OF INDIVIDUALIZED SERVICES

A unique feature of the health and medical care industry is the extent to which its services must be individualized—usually to a greater extent than those of other human services industries, regardless of whether delivered in large, complex, impersonal settings or in smaller, more intimate ones. Whatever the size and function of the organizational setting, management and organization in the health field must be combined with provision of services personally designed for each client of each organization. Personal health and medical care services simply cannot be mass-produced and sold, as are the products of many modern industries; even community health and medical services delivered on an agency-to-group basis must be tailored to the needs of particular groups and their members.

PROFESSIONALISM IN THE HEALTH AND MEDICAL CARE INDUSTRY

The health and medical care industry is the most highly professionalized industry in our society. Members of a number of professions, accredited in a variety of ways (academically, by licensure, and by peer association membership) work within the industry, both as providers of direct services and as directors of institutions, agencies, and programs. However, all other professionals involved in direct patient care activities one way or another, are responsive and responsible to the most prestigious of professionals, the physicians.

The U.S. health and medical care system has been dominated by the medical profession throughout its more than 200 years of development. Only within the last decade or two has there been evidence that this balance of power can, should, or probably will shift. However, this shift will be neither sudden nor rapid, as illustrated by the following report of positions taken by the American Medical Association at its 1973 Annual Convention:

> While noting that conflicting legal decisions have been made on the question of accountability, the AMA deplored the actions of some hospital boards in attempting to set medical policies and strongly reaffirmed that accountability for patient care in hospitals is the responsibility of attending physicians.
>
> Among its actions, the AMA in effect turned down the American Hospital Association's peer review plan, known as the Quality Assurance Program (QAP), by expressing "grave reservations" because of "its potential for lay control of medical practice."[2]

Since professionals tend to identify more closely with professional goals than with organization, subsystem, or industry goals, the major problems of the health and medical care industry receive minimal attention from the professional groups or their individual members—wherein lies one of the main sources of challenge and opportunity for the emerging health administration profession.

COMPLEXITIES OF THE HEALTH AND MEDICAL CARE INDUSTRY

A third major characteristic of the health and medical care system in the United States is its extreme complexity. This complexity is referred to again and again in the health and medical care literature.[3] The system's three major components—its users, its providers of direct services, and the many mechanisms for bringing users and providers together—interact in myriad and complex ways.[4]

Factors contributing to this complexity are several: (1) the pluralistic, "mosaic" nature of the mechanisms (institutions, agencies, programs) involved in bringing the system's users and providers together; (2) the interface of public service objectives with private ownership interests and obligations within the industry; (3) the heavy dependence upon indirect financing from both private and public third-party sources; and (4) the complicated intra- and inter-system relationships which must be developed, rationalized, and maintained.

THE WIDE RANGE OF DELIVERY FACILITIES

The industry's pluralistic nature is manifested in service delivery settings ranging from huge academic health centers providing comprehensive care to small single-service units. Between these extremes are a wide variety of organizations, such as teaching hospitals, state mental hospitals, extended care facilities, voluntary special disease agencies, comprehensive health planning agencies, group practices, community mental health centers, solo and partnership physician practices, commercial and nonprofit health insurance plans, regional health authorities, and others. All too frequently, the health services provided by this large group of agencies are fragmented and uncoordinated from the user's vantage point. Such pluralism requires a diversity of administrative approaches unequaled in other specialty fields.

Administrative complexity is also increased by ownership patterns in the health and medical services industry with the predominant pattern still based in the private sector (voluntary, not-for-profit organizations, such as community hospitals, and proprietary, entrepreneurial activities, such as private medical practices and most long-term care facilities). Should health administrators in the private sector be considered quasi-public servants accountable to the communities which they serve? If so, can they subordinate the interests of their private owners in meeting this broader set of goals?

FINANCIAL REIMBURSEMENT ARRANGEMENTS

Financing arrangements also increase administrative complexity in the health and medical care system. Payments for services are derived from a variety of sources: direct payment from patients; capitation payments from pre-paid insurance plans; reimbursement from commercial insurance companies, Blue Cross/Blue Shield agencies, Medicare and Medicaid, and several other sources. Such a varied mix of financial arrangements not only upsets classical supply and demand market conditions, but also creates administrative layers between provision of, and payment for, services with attendant delays, regulations and other frustrations for the administrators of health service agencies.

All of the above leads to the need for a very high degree of inter- and intra-organizational coordination between units of the health and medical care system, and to a complexity of professional and administrative relationships unrivaled by most other industries.

Some may argue that none of these factors (individualized services, professionalism, system complexities) are really unique, and will point to similar examples in other fields—particularly fields providing other human services. However, in no other field do all of these factors converge as they do in the U.S. health and medical care system. For example, the welfare system is also concerned with the provision of highly personal services (although not as individualized as most personal health care), but these services are rendered mostly by tax-funded public agencies, not by privately owned organizations with indirect payment mechanisms as in the health system.

ADMINISTRATIVE AND ORGANIZATIONAL THEORY

Administrative roles and functions in the health system are best examined in a broader framework of administrative and organizational theory. The brief discussion which follows traces the development of several theories of management and their application to problems of health administration.

The classical school of management (early 1900s) sought general principles that could be universally applied to any organization. These principles focused on internal operations within an organization and emphasized strict attention to method, measurement, and work standards. This "gospel of efficiency," preached by such advocates as Frederick W. Taylor, Henri Fayol, Luther Gulick, Lyndall Urwick, and others, resulted in many of the "principles" of management still in wide use today—work specialization, separation of line and staff activities, and hierarchical organization, to mention just a few.[5] Attempts to apply some of these principles blindly to health services organizations are frequently unsuccessful because of the highly personal nature of the services involved and the professionalized work force which renders the services.

World War II helped to produce a broader appreciation of the administrative process as a system of policy formulation, decision-making among alternative policies, programming work to carry out such policies, and evaluation of program outcomes. This model stressed purpose more than method. Simon, for example, conceived of administrative organizations as decision-making structures, with efficient organizations narrowing the scope of decisions to be made.[6]

THE BEHAVIORAL APPROACH TO MANAGEMENT

The behavioral approach to management developed at approximately the same time. The human relations "pioneers" (Elton Mayo, Mary Follett, Douglas McGregor,

Chester Barnard, and others) viewed organizations as social systems possessing complex values, motives, and attitudes, with considerable attention paid to employee motivation and cooperation using "democratic" strategies of management and organization.[7] The effects of the human relations school of management theory can be seen in participative management and management-by-objectives strategies practiced in many of our health care institutions today.

The three major approaches described above (scientific management, decision theory, human relations) all focus inwardly on organizational structure, both formal and informal. Rigid application of such approaches often results in considerable goal displacement. The more recent development of the neo-classical, or structuralist, school of management theory (Gouldner, Parsons, Etzioni, Blau, Scott, Bennis, and others) takes a different approach.[8] Administration is viewed as a system of responsibility or accountability, with emphasis shifting to external organizational relations. Attention focuses on the responsibilities of an institution to its constituencies and the arrangements by which such responsibilities are met. In cases where external forces inhibit the ability of an organization to meet these responsibilities fully, the organization may take on the role of change agent in the community, working toward needed changes in attitudes, values, and social policy. Accountability is used as a primary control mechanism within the organization, and program emphasis—emphasis on ends rather than means—is a major weapon in combatting goal-displacement.

Principles of accountability and program (i.e., client) emphasis are beginning to have their effect on the delivery of health services, but they still frequently conflict with the goals of private owners and professional providers in the system. Resolution of the conflict between administrative authority, directed toward public accountability, and professional authority, often preoccupied with professional prerogatives, may be the single most important challenge facing the health system today.

COMPONENTS OF THE HEALTH ADMINISTRATION SUB-SYSTEM

No single model could hope to describe the complex set of relationships between health administration and the many other components of the health and medical care system. However, administrative functions within the system can be described using general systems theory.

In simple terms administration in the health delivery system can be viewed as the process of converting a set of inputs (needs, demands, resources and others) into a set of outputs (services rendered to clients, plans for new services and others), with success and/or failures at the output stage influencing future input through positive and negative feedback. The system is an open one, in the sense that the input, conversion, and output components are heavily influenced by a variety of environmental factors—socio-economic, political, and technological—which sometimes facilitate and often constrain the process of delivering services.[9]

Inputs to the health administration sub-system are several and include: needs and demands for health services determined through planning, analysis, evaluation and advocacy; resources required to provide services including manpower, capital and operating funds, and necessary technology; behavioral variables (both individually and culturally determined) which affect utilization of services; community values (including those of special interest groups) which influence both service outputs and the mechanisms for providing them; formal regulations which are imposed by external authorities; and "power inputs" which are largely determined by political processes. Finally, given the complexity of the system as mentioned previously, a high degree of administrative invention is an essential input factor.

THREE TYPES OF OUTPUT

Outputs are of three types: specific health services rendered to clients and related outcomes of these services; evaluation of health services rendered and related plans for new and/or modified services; and symbolic messages transmitted to the clientele and the community at large through the attitudes, gestures, and statements of those providing care. These determine the "image" of the health services organization in the community. As mentioned above, the effectiveness of services rendered will feed back to the input stage and will influence future needs, demands, and resources.

The conversion process requires organization of resources (men, money, material, and technology) into a set of formal and informal procedures for the delivery of health and medical care. Administrative and organizational theory, as discussed previously, has particular applicability to the conversion process. However, it must be applied with full realization of the limitations of all such theories when applied to a set of problems which are largely situational in nature. Furthermore, much of this theory has been developed by experimentation in the material goods production industries, and such theory does not take into account the "uniqueness" of health administration.[10]

ENVIRONMENTAL FACTORS

Environmental factors which influence the health administration sub-system are several. Economic conditions influence the market value of goods and labor required to provide health care. Community attitudes and values help to determine the level of resources that will be made available for community health services. Political factors affect the level of regulation which is levied on health organizations in the conduct of their business. A variety of third party organizations representing consumers (e.g., the "people's health movement"), employees (labor unions), professional providers (county medical societies), as well as third party payment agencies all constitute elements of the environment for health administrators.

The model reinforces the concept that health administrators cannot be viewed as internal managers only. They participate directly in the policy-making process by virtue of their positions as leaders of administrative units, with complex relationships to consumers, providers, and the several environmental forces mentioned above.

THE TEAM APPROACH

Finally, two points seem to flow from this discussion of systems theory as applied to health administration. First, administra*tors* are not the only participants in the process of health administra*tion.* System complexity mandates team approaches and shared responsibility among administrators, physicians, nurses, other health professionals, politicians, community leaders *et al.* in the allocation and application of resources to effect successful health outcomes. Second, administrators are by no means in total control of their own activities, let alone all aspects of the larger health and medical care system, and to date their impact on changing that system has been marginal.

PLURALISM AND COMPLEXITY OF DELIVERY SETTINGS

As mentioned above, personal and community health services are planned and delivered in a variety of settings, ranging from large complex organizations, such as university medical centers, to very small organizations with complex purposes and activities, such as a five-man comprehensive health planning agency responsible for planning and coordinating all personal and environmental health services for a large metropolitan area. Hence the complexity of the administrative task is related to both organizational size and mission.

In addition to organizational complexity, health administrators are responsible for coordinating the delivery of a broad array of services, some requiring complex technology and others dependent upon careful attention to personal, social, and cultural factors.

Despite the complexities of the task, administration within the health care system has traditionally been viewed as a function of less significance, and in some way subordinate to, the direct provision of services. In fact, however, the delivery of health services to individuals and to groups of individuals is inherently an administrative process dependent upon planning, allocation of scarce resources, evaluation of performance, and other tasks basic to management. This is not to say that administrators can carry out the task alone. Obviously, team efforts are required involving physicians, nurses, and other health professionals as well as administrators, and it is important to note that responsibility for effective administration is shared by all members of this team. The fact, however, that health administrators do not "lay on hands" does not diminish the importance of their broader functions in the system; an analogy would be to consider the functions of administrators and planners in the space industry less important than those of astronauts, since the former group has never landed on the moon. In fact, of course, health administrators must take final responsibility for all activities which take place in the organizations which they manage, and this includes quality of care as well as efficiency in the allocation of resources.

ADMINISTRATIVE ACCOUNTABILITY IN THE HEALTH SYSTEM

As mentioned previously in this paper, health administrators frequently find themselves on the horns of a dilemma with regard to public accountability because of the competing demands placed upon them. A simple taxonomy of administrative accountability in the health field would include six elements: owner accountability, community accountability, consumer accountability, resource accountability, regulatory accountability, and third party accountability.

Administrators are formally responsible to the sponsors or owners of their organizations, e.g., the board of trustees of the community hospital, the board of health for the local health agency, the governor of the state for the state health planning agency. Administrators cannot ignore patterns of formal accountability, even when the issues involved may be in conflict with their own personal value system or what they perceive to be the values of the public being served.

Administrators are also accountable to the communities which their organizations serve. Problems arise when the community does not have a well-identified representative body to speak for it (which often is the case). Consumer accountability accrues to the patients served by the administrator's organization or program. Conflicts sometimes develop between consumer accountability and community accountability, particularly when the client group is a small, stratified segment of the larger community (e.g., an inner-city hospital serving a suburban, upper middle-class clientele, rather than the residents of the surrounding neighborhood).

In a sense administrators are also accountable to (or at least very dependent upon) the scarce resources essential to accomplishment of organizational goals. Resource accountability accrues to the professional providers of care who operate as private entrepreneurs in most health delivery settings, as well as to other scarce employment categories and to providers of funds for capital and operating purposes.

Administrators are also responsible to the public and private agencies which exercise legal or voluntarily-yielded control over their organizations, such as the State Health Department and the Joint Commission on Accreditation of Hospitals. Finally, administrators must respond to organizations which serve as intermediaries, or third parties, in the provision of financial and other resources necessary to the accomplishment of organizational missions. Examples include Blue Cross and other private insurance carriers, employee unions, and county medical societies.

ADMINISTRATIVE ROLES

How, then, do health administrators respond to this complex set of demands which are often in competition with one another? A variety of role-responses are possible including one or some combination of the following: (1) Super Clerk—retreating to the position of one who oversees a complex process of paperwork, designed primarily to facilitate the activities of the private entrepreneurs providing medical care within the organization; (2) Efficiency Expert—adopting the role of one whose only purpose is to "optimize the allocation of resources," thus leaving the more difficult problems of policy to others; (3) Magician—the "Houdini of the health system," bridging the gap between unlimited demands for health services and scarce resources; (4) Ombudsman—spokesman for the clients or consumers of health services; (5) Negotiator—super arbitrator of the conflicts between special interests; (6) Empire-Builder—"grabbing as big a piece of the action as possible"; (7) Philosopher-King—the benevolent despot, with ultimate policy authority.

The list of possible roles is almost endless: educator, fireman, change agent, scapegoat, czar, and so forth. Although most administrators would probably acknowledge playing some of these roles on some occasions, none of them would appear to be an accurate or sufficient description of administrative processes. Administrators must aspire to a broader role which emphasizes proper balance between accountability to all the special interests mentioned, tempered with an overriding sense of moral accountability. They must constantly strive to develop and maintain proper perspective between means and ends, between organizational imperatives and a broader community perspective. To do this, they have to become power brokers; not neutral brokers, but "tilters," facilitators of the public interest within their organizations and community. Assumption of such a role requires a high degree of administrative invention, flexibility, and change-orientation.

EMERGING PROFESSIONALISM IN HEALTH ADMINISTRATION

Health administration can be viewed as an emerging profession. Historically, the early development of this field placed the emphasis on business management functions with program and quality control in the hands of physicians. During the last 15 to 20 years, the era of the "lay" administrator has arrived with current emphasis being placed on the management of large and complex medical care organizations using management and systems techniques. If this fledgling profession is to continue to mature, then future emphasis will need to be placed on extra-organizational responsibilities for assessment of community health needs and demands, and active participation in the policy-making process to insure that adequate community health services are provided. Hence, two important ingredients in the further professionalization of health administrators will be policy orientation and health, rather than medical care, orientation:

> The modern health care manager will be expected to function in several newly-emerging roles that were not demanded as often of his predecessors in the forties and fifties. These are:
>
> 1. To serve as an organizational change agent and innovator in terms of process and productivity.
> 2. To serve as a systems integrator and regulator.
> 3. To serve as a mediator in external relationships with the community, with other providers, with third party payers, and government.
> 4. To exhibit strong leadership.[11]

The history of professional development in other fields is not all favorable. In too many cases, professional goals and codes of ethics which originally were intended to be client-serving degenerate over time and tend to become self-serving to members of the profession. If this is to be avoided in the emerging profession of health administration, members of the profession must continually be guided by Strauss' "3R's"—responsiveness to the needs and demands of users of the health system; responsibility for the functions of planning, organizing, controlling, and coordinating services; and reconciliation of the vast array of knowledge, attitudes, and skills that interact in the functioning of the system.[12]

There are many ingredients for the successful development of a new profession with the positive characteristics which have been suggested. These include formal education, directed experience, commitment, and ability—all parts of professional competence. Active and effective relationships between clients, practitioners, and educators is a further important element of professionalism.

All of the preceding suggests a complex set of problems and related opportunities available to the field of health administration, provided that the field can rise to the challenges which are presented. The normative definition which follows assumes that health administration can and must play an important role in the solution of problems of inequitable distribution and access, uneven quality, and inefficiency in the provision of health services. Through improved administration, the health of the total community can be promoted in a more equitable, comprehensive, high quality, and efficient manner. Accordingly, the following definition is offered:

> Health Administration is planning, organizing, directing, controlling, and coordinating the resources and procedures by which needs and demands for health and medical care and a healthful environment are fulfilled by the provision of specific services to individual clients, organizations, and communities.[13]

The definition implies leadership in community policy decisions, as well as organization and management of resources gathered together in increasingly complex organizations. The administrative process must be carried out in socially responsible ways under conditions of continuous change and increasing uncertainty in the social, economic, political, technological, and professional environment.

IMPLICATIONS FOR PRACTICE

The definition suggests that health administrators can become a major force in solving many of the problems of our health care system. As mentioned previously, the problems to be solved are really only amenable to an administrative solution through improved planning, organization, financing, and performance evaluation of health and medical care. Some believe that the solution to all of these problems lies solely in provision of more professional manpower or better financing mechanisms. However, the complexities and pluralism of the delivery system as discussed in this paper suggest that provision of increased manpower or new financing mechanisms without attention to broader administrative matters may only aggravate the problems in our system.

In essence, some group within the system must pull it together. Administrators may be the logical group, provided that they can be both sensitive and pragmatic, responsive, and responsible. Anne Somers calls for positive leadership in the system with the following attributes: clear vision, intelligent strategy, adequate resources, determination, and courage.[14]

Of primary importance, the definition suggests that extremely competent individuals will have to be attracted into the field if administrators are to "bite the bullet" and provide the leadership needed to bring about changes in the health and medical care system. Since formal educational programs serve a gate-keeping function for entry into the field, universities will need to attract students with a wide array of backgrounds, including minority groups and women, and with the native intelligence and personal attributes essential to future leadership roles.

The paper also suggests that educational programs must continue to pay attention to principles and techniques of modern management and systems theory, but must also prepare individuals who can operate effectively in the arena of public policy. Future administrators will need a solid understanding of health as health, rather than health as medical care (or sick care) planning and delivery.

Finally, close cooperation between educators and practicing administrators appears to be an essential ingredient. Researchers and educators must constantly question the way things are currently done and search for solutions to problems of the health services delivery system. Practitioners must participate by constantly reminding educators of the "art of the possible" and by providing the laboratory of real life experiences for students and faculty to utilize. Such a shared agenda will greatly facilitate the overriding goal of providing leadership in response to complexity.

FURTHER READINGS SUGGESTED BY THE AUTHOR

American Public Health Association, Committee on Professional Education. "Educational Qualifications of Management Personnel in Health Agencies." *American Journal of Public Health,* February 1970, pp. 345-350.

Brown, Douglas R. "A New Administrative Model for Hospitals." *Hospital Administration,* 1967, no. 1, pp. 6-24.

Etzioni, Amitai. *Modern Organizations.* Englewood Cliffs, N.J.: Prentice-Hall, Inc., 1964.

Georgopoulos, Basil S., ed. *Organization Research on Health Institutions.* Ann Arbor: University of Michigan Institute for Social Research, 1972.

Gross, Bertram M. *The Managing of Organizations.* (Two Volumes) New York: Free Press, 1964.

Levey, Samuel and Loomba, N. Paul. *Health Care Administration: A Managerial Perspective.* Philadelphia: J. B. Lippincott Co., 1973.

Mintzberg, Henry. *The Nature of Managerial Work.* New York: Harper and Row, 1973.

Ross, Austin, "Trends in Clinic Administration." *Medical Group Management,* January 1972, pp. 9-11.

Wilensky, Harold L. "The Dynamics of Professionalism: The Case of Hospital Administration." *Hospital Administration,* 1962, no. 2, pp. 6-24.

FOOTNOTES

[1] Janet A. Strauss, *Future Trends in Health Care Delivery, A Forecast* (Washington, D.C.: Commission on Education for Health Administration, 1973), p. 46.

[2] "Hospital Board Actions Worry Delegates," *American Medical News* 16 (July 1973):3.

[3] See Anne R. Somers, *Health Care in Transition: Directions for the Future* (Chicago: Hospital Research and Educational Trust, 1971); Julius B. Richmond, *Currents in American Medicine* (Cambridge, Mass.: Harvard University Press, 1969); and W. L. Kissick, "Health Policy Directions for the 1970's," *New England Journal of Medicine* 282, no. 24 (11 June 1970): 1343-54.

[4] See Avedis Donabedian, "Models for Organizing the Delivery of Personal Health Services and Criteria for Evaluating Them," *Milbank Memorial Fund Quarterly* 50, no. 4 (October 1972): 103-54; and Barbara Starfield, "Health Services Research: A Working Model," *New England Journal of Medicine* 289, no. 3 (19 July 1973): 132-36.

[5] For a further description of this school, see the classical work by Frederick W. Taylor, *Principles and Methods of Scientific Management* (New York: Harper & Row, 1911); or the reviews by Amitai Etzioni, *Modern Organizations* (Englewood Cliffs, N.J.: Prentice-Hall, 1964), chapter 3; and Bertram M. Gross, *The Managing of Organizations* (New York: Free Press, 1964), vol. 1, chapter 6.

[6] Herbert A. Simon, *The New Science of Management Decision* (New York: Harper & Row, 1960).

[7] For reviews of the human relations school of management, see Etzioni, *Modern Organizations*, chapter 4; and Gross, *The Managing of Organizations*, chapter 7.

[8] See Peter M. Blau and W. Richard Scott, *Formal Organizations* (San Francisco: Chandler Publishing Co., 1962); Warren G. Bennis, *Changing Organizations* (New York: McGraw-Hill, 1966); Etzioni, *Modern Organizations*, chapters 4 and 5; and D. Katz and R. L. Kahn, *The Social Psychology of Organizations* (New York: John Wiley & Sons, 1966).

[9] For a good description of systems theory applied to administrative processes, see Ira Sharkansky, *Public Administration* (Chicago: Markham Publishing Co., 1970).

[10] Some good work is beginning to emerge in health administration research. See, for example, Basil S. Georgopoulos, ed., *Organization Research on Health Institutions* (Ann Arbor: University of Michigan Institute for Social Research, 1972).

[11] Samuel Levey and N. Paul Loomba, *Health Care Administration: A Managerial Perspective* (Philadelphia: J. B. Lippincott Co., 1973), p. 588.

[12] Strauss, *Future Health Care Trends*, pp. 46-7.

[13] This is the official definition of health administration adopted by the Commission on Education for Health Administration to guide its work.

[14] Anne R. Somers, "The Hospital in the Evolving Health Care System" (First Mark Berke Memorial Lecture delivered at the Mount Zion Hospital and Medical Center, San Francisco, November 21, 1972).

12.

The Lessons of a Profession

EVERETT A. JOHNSON

Everett A. Johnson, Ph.D., is President, the Dunes Group-Dune Acres, Indiana.

For more than two decades hospital administrator-watching has been an order of business in my daily work. I have observed both the student and the practitioner, as worker and boss, follower and leader. These observations have spanned hospital changes from the institutional freedoms of the fifties to the disciplines and restraints of the seventies.

When prospective students for graduate programs in hospital administration ask questions about the life and work involved in the administrative profession, they want to know exactly what work is done, and what quality of life they can expect as an administrator. Too often, unasked questions in the student's mind concern happiness, contentment, fulfillment, and service. Answers to these questions, if asked, would be difficult, because they are personal. However, my twenty years of administrator-watching may be useful to potential colleagues in describing how the career hospital administrator feels.

AN ADMINISTRATOR'S WORLD

The student first needs to understand that an administrator's world is his own. Its agonies and ecstasies are totally private. His personality is unique, singular, and beyond the complete understanding of another. He is at once both a man of silence and public utterance, of motivation and apathy, of straight-forwardness and confounding of prediction in judgment and action.

A hospital administrator is a decision-maker, a risk taker and an intellectual about the good of society. He is a person of love, concern and tenderness—a pragmatist who molds, moves, and decides other peoples' futures.

Beyond the human quality of the man, an administrator is a mixture of competence

---

Reprinted by permission from *Hospital Administration* (currently *Hospital and Health Services Administration*): *Quarterly Journal of the American College of Hospital Administrators,* Chicago, Vol. 17 (Summer, 1972), pp. 9-17. Copyright 1972 by the American College of Hospital Administrators. All rights reserved.

and incompetence, of great ability and skill and maddening blind spots and insensitivities. As a hospital administrator he knows much and yet very little. He is a generalist among a mass of specialists.

He is seen by some as an earth-shaker, by others as a definer of goals or as a busybody without accomplishments. He can be both devil and saint, simultaneously or over a period of time, as well as by issue or through the relationship of perceiver to hospital.

A VARIETY OF EXPECTATIONS

A society is a potpourri of expectations. Organizations function as vehicles of expression for personal worth, for identification purposes, for masking of hidden failures with accolades of public success, and as a raison d'être for making life worth living.

A hospital serves many expectations for many people: It serves the young nurse who has not found her own niche in life and is privately working out her scheme of usefulness, the mature nurse who is complete in her family life and reaching for greater goals by serving man, the newly-certified medical specialist, sure of his skills and sense of the world, and the experienced senior physician, aware of the limits of the science of medicine and the limits of those who care about the future of medicine and its total usefulness.

WORKING WITH TRUSTEES

Since an administrator directly serves the expectations of hospital trustees, their desires must also be measured. In working with this group, he finds pressures abounding, pushing and demanding new programs and conveniences from the hospital. He finds that administrative life is a constant series of changes, one after another—the only predictable point in his career.

On the other hand, the administrator will find that most trustees do not really desire change. Their position typically will be that if the administrator can find the money, persuade all key parties that it is a worthwhile improvement and keep all dissonant voices to a murmur then he may proceed. If the stakes begin to rise—and particularly if the change appears to be generating active opposition from the medical staff—then the administrator must adjust, delay, modify or postpone to a more appropriate time. The student will later learn that most necessary fundamental improvements in patient care have floundered on this particular shoal.

In previous times, as well as today, it has always been an article of faith with hospital administration that boards of trustees are necessary and highly useful. When the student sees local government hospitals with patronage and other political problems, he will know that they are a less workable system than one with a board of trustees. Looking at the rigidities of operation that exist in state and federal hospitals, the student similarly will be disenchanted.

SEEING TRUSTEES' MOTIVATIONS

When he sees many private hospitals with trustees continually involved in daily operations, he will be aghast. He will wonder, and wonder again, about the notion of trusteeship. As student life fades into first active administrative work the individual will need to reinforce his faith that hospital trustees typically are motivated by good intentions and seriousness of purposes. He will learn to suffer privately the understanding that dedication and intelligence are no substitute for experience, specific knowledge, and appropriate behavior.

When the new administrator experiences the hospital boardroom becoming a center ring for local power struggles, he will see how rarely patient care is a primary consideration. When the local physicians close ranks and lay it on the line, he will generally watch the local élite quickly ride off into the hills. Too often he will see the chief administrator, left at the pass to cover the retreat, get wiped out.

The fledgling administrator must learn the rationality and irrationality of an organized medical staff and its constituent parts, the physicians of the community. He will learn that whenever change occurs in a hospital, physicians will typically be slow to accept it, require personal attention to insure understanding and generally offer comments about how to spend hospital funds more profitably. Medical staffs almost never believe that new boilers are a necessity; they believe that administrative offices are mostly personal aggrandizement, that too much space goes into storage areas and that home-type ranges ought to be satisfactory in the main kitchen.

The frustrations of unreasonable opinions need to be counterbalanced with an understanding that the physician's life and interest spins around clinical concerns. His great sense of assurance and independence, his lack of awareness that medical care is now a process involving many people rather than only himself and his unwillingness to accept the expertise of administrators will block or make difficult an easy accommodation to change.

When administrative innovations aimed at improving medical affairs in hospitals are tried, the rigidities of attitude and behavior of trustees and physicians are joined. Yet, the administrator's future will be filled with one pressure after another for using the hospital to force adjustments in traditional medical practices.

ADMINISTRATION OF A MEDICAL STAFF

Past administrator-watching has taught me that only foolish or independently wealthy chief executive officers have ever seriously believed that they could direct and administer a medical staff. Even though most administrators have been concerned seriously with medical administrative practices that abuse patients, they have been unable to do more than skirmish on the fringes of concern.

Conformity and endless continuation of these existing practices have been part of past administrative life. The unvarnished lesson, that the organizational triad of trustee, medical staff and administration is the best way to run a hospital, is a myth. It is a fair weather device that quickly buckles under a light breeze.

When trustees hire and set conditions of employment for administrators and when physicians direct the hospital's financial future by controlling patient admissions and dismissals, it is only the starry-eyed neophyte that believes all three parts are equal. In a major hospital crisis, when stakes are high and both physicians and trustees make a hospital momentarily their primary concern, administrative leverage is lost.

In situations where physicians squeeze a board of trustees, the chief executive officer learns that the usual outcome is for trustees to accede to physician pressure. Trustees do not have the daily administrative experiences which lead to understanding the nuances of hospital issues of deciding how much of a gamble can be run with some safety and the importance of alternative outcomes. When one administrator must try to hold a board of trustees in line against an assault of fifty or two-hundred and fifty physicians it is understandable for the trustees to opt for the prestige and goodwill of medicine and to ignore the reasoned judgement of their employee, the administrator.

A young hospital administrator will probably learn another lesson: only in rare circumstances does a board of trustees really exercise control for the quality of medicine practiced in the hospital. Early in his career he will discover that this is a joint operation between medical staff and hospital administration and that this state of affairs bothers physicians. Not that trustees don't understand or aren't part of the picture, but rather administrative types have a nasty habit of recognizing medical problems being swept under the rug or remembering which closets hold which skeletons.

AN ADMINISTRATIVE DILEMMA

The hospital-based, full time medical staff specialist generally requires special advice for the inexperienced administrator. To wit, when one of these medical types is quite competent and has a personality like a friendly local car salesman, it is almost a guaranteed tamper-proof administrative dilemma. Older administrative heads know for sure, that if it comes down to a take it or leave it situation, the medical staff will choose to support one of their own—and the patient be damned. While trustees may get indigestion over these problems, they typically fold their tents and accede to the wishes of the medical staff rather than take the bull by the horns; and that's what an administrator is left with—a bum steer.

In the tumult of daily administrative-medical interaction, a fundamental perspective can easily be lost. The administrator should remember to respect physicians as individuals who are delighted, well-meaning, hard-working people, who carry some of the toughest loads in our society.

Too often today, progress toward improving patient welfare depends upon an unusually competent chief executive officer. When he leaves an administrative post, the drive for improvement in his institution and the skills and the acceptance he has developed necessary for accomplishing that improvement are lost. Because of the subtleties in medical staff and trustee relationships, the succeeding administrator will spend several years in developing a position strong enough to win the successes of his predecessor. The need for hospital administration to achieve a more secure status was once covered in a remark by Walter Lippmann, "The genius of a good leader is to leave behind him a situation which common sense, without the grace of genius, can deal with successfully."

Frustration is the handmaiden of hospital administrators. The daily grist of hospital operation is often shackled by stodginess and the mediocrity of its institutional setting and structure. However, the administrator's status is reflective of the practices of our times and the restraints all organizations tolerate as part of a society with multiple inter-relationships.

USE OF EMOTIONAL UNDERSTANDING

The prospective student for hospital administration at some point will need to sort out and develop an understanding of the basic relation between emotion and intellectual understanding and conceptualization. In many administrative activities, demands of the situation seem to contra-indicate a successful assimilation of both styles of operation. Unfortunately most nonadministrative people experience a hospital organization emotionally. They become irked when, upon asking housekeeping to move furniture or maintenance to replace a light bulb, it is not done immediately. When a nurse errs on a medication, a physician's reaction often is anger, rather than an effort to help figure out what went wrong and how it can be avoided tomorrow.

Too often, a physician, department director or other person arrives at the administrator's office door in a state of agitation, because he is reacting to some activity in the organization. These people express a sense of justice, righteousness, and an impeccable logic on their side with a ready-made conclusion that hospital operation is stupid, inept, and poorly run.

To be rational and logical at this time is to create even stronger feelings. An administrator has the dilemma of figuring out the cause of a problem, yet he must respect another person's feelings, no matter how irrational or unwarranted. He must react to those feelings without losing control of his emotions and still find a way to explain and regain their support of the organization. To have feelings and sympathy, without losing one's own emotional control, is a never-ending administrative struggle.

THE SKILL OF RAPPORT WITH OTHERS

At some point in an administrative career one must develop the aptitude of concealing one's own administrative skills and maintaining rapport with other people in the organization. It is not an easily developed habit.

The administrator's use of self-control and intellectual abilities to handle feelings and emotions of others assures that there will be many times when, at day's end, he will finally turn off the lights, lock the door, leave the office, and go home—low in energy and convinced that he is mad to remain in hospital administration.

Probably the most difficult administrative skill is the art of delegation. Habits, psychological needs, self-discipline, ability to work with others, and individual analytical abilities are some of the personal factors that affect one's ability to use this mode of administration. As size of organization and complexity of operation increase, an administrator's time span is outgrown in his attempt to expand his efforts centrally to control all important, and sometimes unimportant, decision-making in the hospital.

Delegation involves accepting responsibility for other people's judgment and abilities. It means the administrator's acceptance of a quality of work that may be somewhat less than his own, because he was not free to totally handle a particular matter. A lack of flexibility and difference in others' thought processes also causes an instinctive rejection of another's work.

In the world at large, adequate administrative delegation of work seems to be the rarest of skills. It is discussed in graduate programs in management, but it is largely left unpracticed. Yet, its essence is to be able to delegate in situations of much stress and confusion. Probably the only way delegation can be mastered is in the hustle and bustle of daily administrative events.

What then is the answer to a potential administrator's unspoken question: "What are reasonable expectations in a hospital administration career for happiness, contentment, fulfillment, and service?" The answer lies within another question: "What kind of life do you think you will need to live to be happy at forty years of age?"

If you seek fame or fortune, hospital administration is a poor choice. If you need a strong sense of security, a well-structured work situation and some spare time to contemplate the world at large, you should look elsewhere.

LESSONS OF ADMINISTRATIVE PROFESSION

In hospital administration, happiness is having more work than time, greater demands than ability to respond completely, and a sense of continually helping other people. Happiness is to enjoy painting a wall at home for immediate satisfaction, because instant accomplishments are almost never experienced at work. Fulfillment is knowing that at the end of a career you will have lived and served as you would have wished throughout a lifetime of work.

The lessons of this profession are never found in textbooks. To experienced hospital administrators, these caveats have been lived at one or another place and time. To trustees, physicians and friendly psychiatrists, they will appear as one person's effort to rationalize and work out totally personal struggles. It is in truth, though, a message of realism for the coming generation of hospital administrators: an invitation to join the fray—to do so with their eyes open and their minds informed about the real world in which a great profession works. It is a profession facing major problems, coping with some, failing with others—but sure of a demanding, exciting time ahead.

As hospital administrators, our issue is to move from being operators of support systems for medical care into becoming managers of medical care systems. I believe it can happen. No other health profession is more central to our developing notions about the total medical care process than today's hospital administration.

TODAY'S ADMINISTRATIVE MILIEU

To move from today into tomorrow, hospital administrators must now accept the responsibilities and perils of leading a medical staff, trustees, hospital staff, and community that must be led before tomorrow arrives. Administrators now face a time to stand up while the house is counted. They have passed the day when boards of trustees could be looked to for local leadership, and administrators could gracefully pass the buck. Today, the buck is in the hands of hospital administration, and because it is there, sufficient leverage exists for major accomplishments.

If today's administrative milieu appears foreboding, frustrating, and turbulent, it should be remembered that the Hellespont could only be crossed by vigorous swimming.

A GRATIFYING COMMITMENT

Our sense of well-being and happiness as hospital administrators in the tumult of today was said in Kahlil Gibran's *The Prophet* when he wrote about work: "Then a ploughman said, speak to us of work. And he answered saying: work is love made visible. And if you cannot work with love but only with distaste, it is better that you should leave your work and sit at the gate of the temple and take alms of those who work with joy. For if you bake bread with indifference, you bake a bitter bread that feeds but half man's hunger. And if you grudge the crushing of the grapes, your grudge distils a poison in the wine. And if you sing though as angels, and love not the singing, you muffle man's ears to the voices of the day and the voices of the night."

Talent, commitment, and ability are needed in hospital administration. If a young person believes that it is important in life to be stretched to the toes, to strive to touch the untouchable, then join us—now, and for the days ahead. But do it with the point of view once expressed by Martin Luther, "If I rest, I rust."

The Medical Staff

In *Selection 13*, "MEDICAL STAFF FUNCTIONS AND LEADERSHIP," William W. Jack describes the organization and major activities of the medical staff. The writer suggests organizing the medical staff into councils for the various activities to be carried out. The following selection by James D. Harvey, "THE HOSPITAL MEDICAL DIRECTOR: AN ADMINISTRATOR'S VIEW," presents a candid description of the medical director, a role which is critical to the modern hospital. Emphasis is placed on the accountability of this individual. Finally, *Selection 15*, "HOSPITAL MEDICAL STAFF ORGANIZATION: STRUCTURE, PROCESS, AND OUTCOME," by Stephen M. Shortell, raises a number of issues and philosophical questions about the medical staff and concludes that adaptability of hospitals and providing medical staffs with meaningful roles are essential to success.

13.
Medical Staff Functions and Leadership

WILLIAM W. JACK, M.D.

William W. Jack, M.D., is a practicing physician in Grand Rapids, Michigan.

In the functioning of the medical staff of the modern hospital, leadership is the single most important factor. The leadership and administration of the medical staff are provided by the executive committee. This committee is normally composed of the officers of the medical staff and the various department chairmen, although the actual composition of the committee may vary from hospital to hospital.

The chief of staff (or the highest elected officer of the committee) and the members of the executive committee must possess essential leadership requirements if the purposes of the medical staff are to be realized. The chief of staff must be the peer of both the hospital administrator and the president of the hospital's governing board. He must be thoroughly familiar with the internal operation of the hospital, as well as with all local, regional, or national influences that affect the hospital and/or the medical profession.

In order to effectively fulfill his duties, the chief of staff needs a strong executive committee whose members are as dedicated to good staff government as he is. The physicians who make up the executive committee are department heads, and it is their responsibility to make their leadership felt at the department level. Good patient care, good continuing education programs, and good administrative practices are all essential functions of their jobs.

In addition to the members of the executive committee, the chief of staff also needs the help of the administrator if he is to carry out the duties of his position. The administrator is the real professional in the area of hospital administration. Cooperation between the chief of the medical staff and the administrator is vital because, without it, divisive fragmentation occurs. Such a dichotomy between medical staff and administration has been somewhat eased by the integration of the medical staff and the governing board. In many hospitals, at least one member of the hospital board is now a physician.

This kind of integration is highly desirable because the chief of the medical staff needs the action and informed help of the governing board. This board is normally composed of capable and sincere citizens who are legally responsible for the total

---

Reprinted by permission from *Hospital Progress: Journal of The Catholic Hospital Association*, St. Louis, Vol. 51 (November, 1970), 76-79. Copyright 1970 by The Catholic Hospital Association. All rights reserved.

operation and activity of the hospital. However, many members of governing boards come to their tasks with little background and little understanding, if any, of what is expected and desired of them. Continuing education of board members is necessary if they are to be able to contribute effectively to the operation of the hospital and to the medical staff as an important element of the hospital structure.

In order to make the administration of medical staff activities more efficient, it is advisable to combine certain traditional staff functions into three main categories or "councils." These three councils cover the broad areas of patient care, continuing medical education, and care evaluation.

PATIENT CARE

The council on patient care comprises a group of interrelated functions including pharmacy and therapeutics, infection control, emergency room, outpatient department, special care, and disaster. Each of these functions is oriented toward the care of the patient and each requires the cooperation of and support from administration and/or nursing. A doctor should be assigned responsibility for each of these functions and should work with his counterparts from administration and nursing in coordinating the particular function for which he is responsible with other hospital activities.

All the physicians assigned responsibility for the various functions that comprise the council on patient care constitute the members of that council. They should meet regularly in an attempt to familiarize each other with their views about each of the particular functions of patient care. In so doing, they should seek to coordinate these functions so as to achieve better patient care.

The chief of the medical staff should chair the council on patient care for various reasons: He is closely associated with the administrator and with the nursing director, both of whom are vital to any consideration of patient care. In addition, his position as chief of staff and head of the executive committee enables him to help resolve problems concerning patient care as quickly as possible.

PATIENT CARE COUNCIL

Pharmacy-Therapeutic

1. Advise the medical staff and hospital pharmacist on matters pertaining to the choice of drugs.
2. Recommend drugs available under emergency conditions.
3. Evaluate clinical data and report to the medical staff on new drugs suggested for use in the hospital.
4. Authorize the use of experimental drugs under well-defined rules.
5. Maintain a registry of adverse reactions.

Infection Control

1. Make recommendations regarding the control of all patient infections within the hospital.

2. Make recommendations regarding the hospital's isolation techniques.
3. Conduct epidemiological surveys of infections occurring in the hospital.

Emergency Room/Outpatient
1. Recommend policies regarding the care of patients in the emergency room and outpatient clinics and, after approval, supervise the implementation of these policies.
2. Make certain that the emergency room and the outpatient clinics are always ready to take part in mass casualty situations.
3. Supervise the proper record-keeping in the emergency room and outpatient clinics.
4. Aid in integrating the emergency room and outpatient clinics into the teaching program.

Special Care
1. Assume responsibility for the development of the medical policy for proper and efficient management of the intensive care unit, the pediatric intensive care unit, the coronary care unit, and such other special care units as recommended by the staff executive committee.
2. Develop policies for the admission, duration of stay, and discharge of patients in the special care units.
3. Serve in an advisory capacity for the nursing service in joint problems involving the special care units.

Disaster
1. Assess constantly the hospital's preparedness for any disaster which might strike the community at large or the hospital itself.
2. Re-evaluate the hospital's disaster plan periodically to eliminate defects, improve the plan, recommend improvements, and supervise practice sessions.

CONTINUING MEDICAL EDUCATION COUNCIL

Education
1. Develop a broad program for continuing education within the hospital, and, after approval, be responsible for its implementation.
2. Make recommendations for improving the program.
3. Assume responsibility for recruiting and appointing house staff.
4. Assume responsibility for recruiting outside speakers and integrating their presentations into the general continuing education programs.

Library-Publications
1. Recommend the purchase of books, periodicals, tapes, and visual aids.
2. Make recommendations regarding the operation of the medical library.
3. Make plans and recommendations regarding staff publications and, after approval, implement these policies.
4. Offer assistance to members of the staff who may wish to submit an article for publication.

Oncology

1. Offer a consultation service in the diagnosis and treatment of malignancies.
2. Provide leadership in the cancer teaching program.
3. Establish regular conferences for discussing cases of hospital patients with malignancies.
4. Supervise the operation of the tumor registry.

Research

1. Stimulate and guide critical investigation or experimentation that has for its aim the discovery and correct interpretation of new facts.
2. Aid or improve existing techniques or skills for patient care within the hospital.

Program

1. Develop programs for general staff meetings within the broad policies of continuing medical education.
2. Coordinate departmental and interdepartmental programs.
3. Integrate reports of the various committees and departments into the educational program.

CARE EVALUATION COUNCIL

Tissue Evaluation

1. Review and evaluate all surgery performed in the hospital on the basis of agreement or non-agreement with the pre- and post-operative and pathological tissue diagnoses, and on the basis of acceptability of the procedure undertaken.

Utilization Review

1. Offer assurance that the hospital stays and inpatient services are medically necessary.
2. Analyze and identify factors that may contribute to unnecessary or ineffective hospital stays or ineffective use of inpatient services and facilities.

Medical Records

1. Assure satisfactory completion of medical records within the time allotted.
2. Advise and recommend policies for maintaining medical records.
3. Supervise medical records to insure that details are recorded in the proper manner and that sufficient data are present to evaluate the care of the patient.
4. Advise and develop policies, with the aid of legal counsel, to guide the medical record librarian, the medical staff, and the administration insofar as matters of privileged communication and legal release of information are concerned.

Medical Audit

1. Evaluate the quality of patient care as reflected in the clinical record.
2. Audit complications that occur in the hospital.
3. Evaluate the efficacy, value, or harm of treatments and procedures used in the management of patients.
4. Audit all deaths occurring in the hospital.

CONTINUING MEDICAL EDUCATION

The council on continuing medical education also includes a number of interrelated functions. Education; library; publications; oncology; research; and various educational programs.

Post-graduate medical education is almost unbelievably complicated and competitive. The amount of printed material and the number of meetings every week, month, and year that vie for the physician's attention staggers the imagination. Almost everything that is offered is worth considering, and much is actually worth studying or attending. However, since time will not permit the individual physician to take advantage of everything that is offered, compromise is inevitable. Articles in special interest journals, meetings of selected organizations, and attendance at informal discussions on a regular basis must suffice.

Reading and attendance at outside meetings prevent parochialism. Assimilation and perspective are gained through small group discussions, and it is in this area that the hospital has a definite role. By providing physicians with an opportunity to discuss topics of current interest, the hospital enables them to keep informed.

The council on continuing medical education should be organized in much the same manner as the council on patient care, with a specific physician being assigned responsibility for each specific function. The director of medical education for the hospital should chair this council, and the council itself should provide direction and coordination for the hospital's entire educational program. Hopefully the director of medical education would also be a member of the medical staff executive committee, so that the educational function of the medical staff would be directly represented in this administrative body.

The hospital that has a house staff will find that the council on continuing medical education will have a larger role to play than it does in the hospital without a house staff. Interns and residents provide a source of stimuli for all physicians on the staff so that, in planning for their education, the hospital also plans for the education of all its medical staff members.

However, in another sense, the hospital without a house staff perhaps has an even greater need of a continuing education program, since the physicians in such a hospital do not benefit from the stimulus provided by the influx of interns and residents. At any rate, quality patient care cannot be achieved without an adequate continuing medical education program.

CARE EVALUATION

The council on care evaluation includes such functions as tissue evaluation, utilization review, medical records, and the medical audit.

This council is not designed primarily to seek out the incompetent and unskilled, but rather to pinpoint areas where patient care can be improved through continuing education. Education is the proper solution to the problem of lack of skill and/or judgment. If situations arise in which there is an uneducable lack of skill and/or judgment, they should be documented in the deliberations of the council. For this reason, the chairman of the medical staff's credentials committee should also chair the council on care evaluation.

The need for the council on care evaluation points logically to another need, that of discipline. Disciplinary rules and procedures should be written into the medical staff by-laws. They should be delineated in detail and checked thoroughly by legal council. The section on discipline should, of course, be publicized to the entire medical staff.

QUESTIONING CURRENT PRACTICES

Aside from the traditional medical staff functions of patient care, continuing medical education, and care evaluation, two additional functions must be added in order to meet the demands of modern health care. The first of these additional responsibilities is that of questioning the effectiveness of current programs and practices. No traditional practice should be allowed to continue without examination. The medical staff must ask itself if the practice is necessary, if it is being performed in the most effective and efficient manner, if it is worth the effort being expended, and if it contributes to quality care. Medical staff leaders must seek the answers to these and similar questions, hopefully with consultation and cooperation of the administration and the governing board.

AWARENESS OF NEW TRENDS

The second additional responsibility of today's medical staff is to be aware of national trends and developments and to plan local implementation of them.

Health Care Delivery. For over 50 years, the major focus in the delivery of health care has been the hospital. However, at the present time, there are not enough physicians and, at the current rate of production, there will not be enough in the foreseeable future. Vast numbers of people in the United States do not have ready access to quality health care. Yet, how many hospitals have seriously considered alternate ways of delivering health care? Is it enough for hospitals to boast that they will provide care for those who seek it at their doors? Or, must they become more actively involved in deciding how to decentralize health care delivery in order to be able to make their "product" more accessible to the public?

Planning. Another development currently receiving much attention is that of area planning. How many hospitals participate in inter-hospital cooperative programs? How many medical staffs have seriously considered the advisability of establishing a committee or council to coordinate the medical education programs of the various hospitals in the community, of centralizing the medical records and medical audit activities of the community hospitals; of establishing an acute care bed registry, common storage, common purchasing, and common food services? How many hospitals and medical staffs are willing to close their obstetrics service, pediatrics service, or newborn service in the interests of economy, efficiency, and quality care?

Allied Health Manpower. Good medical care is care provided by an initially well-trained and continually retrained physician. However, every patient condition does not require care at this level; some conditions can be cared for by a person at a different level of knowledge and skill. How many hospitals and medical staffs have seriously considered the possibilities which such an innovation presents? Efforts to make this innovation standard procedure are being made throughout the country.

Those involved in the delivery of health care should ask themselves whether the use of allied health manpower is possible in the outpatient department, the emergency room, the physician's office, the neighborhood health center. They should discuss this concept with legal counsel, insurance carriers, legislators. It is too exciting a possibility to be ignored and too promising to be disregarded.

Liability Insurance. One continuing development in which members of medical staffs should be particularly interested is that of liability insurance. Most claims arise as a result of hospital care. Is the answer to preventing or decreasing liability claims really so simple as peer review, a bigger and better tissue committee, audit committee, etc.? Medical staffs must begin seeking answers to the problem of rising medical care costs; they must not be satisfied with naive and oversimplified solutions, such as the creation of better utilization committees. Can the problem be solved merely by reducing a hospital stay to four days rather than five? Does the challenge to solve this problem lie only at the doorstep of medicine and nowhere else?

Political Influence. Responsible statesmanship seems to have given way to political opportunism, and health care has become the politician's golden opportunity. The issues and problems associated with health care and its delivery seem to mean a quick ticket to Washington, or a front-page story, or television coverage.

The national trends and developments listed above are some of the problems that face the health care system in general and the physician in particular in the 70's. They require serious consideration from every medical staff, every administrator, and every governing board. For those involved in the delivery of health care to say that everything about medicine is right and pure and innocent is just as ridiculous as to say that all detractors of the system are wrong, evil, and dishonest.

SYSTEM NEEDS LEADERSHIP

The present decade demands that the health care system provide more and better care for more people. To fulfill this demand, the system needs more doctors, nurses, and allied health personnel who are trained in such a way that they can provide more care, more efficiently and effectively at a lower unit cost. The system needs more hospitals in more locations providing care to more people at a lower unit cost. To achieve such goals, the system must encourage innovation and experimentation.

Physicians and hospitals must remember that they will have to work together if the demands of the public are to be met. If fragmentation ever existed, it must go. Medical staffs, administrators, and governing boards must find new ways of working more closely together. Physicians must not regard hospitals as their private workshops. Board members must not convince themselves that attending one meeting a month fulfills their obligations. Administrators must accept their roles as catalysts between the board and the medical staff. The key to all these requirements is the chief of the medical staff. His leadership is a single most important aspect of effective staff functioning.

14.
The Hospital Medical Director: An Administrator's View

JAMES D. HARVEY

James D. Harvey is Administrator of Hillcrest Medical Center in Tulsa, Oklahoma.

The whole health care system is "under the gun" because of its inability to cope with the needs and demands of the public at a fair price. The press, television, periodicals, and non-fiction magazines chronicle the extent of the public's disillusionment with the current system.

The concept of effectiveness gained high public visibility when the Barr Report, the popular name for the Secretary's Advisory Committee on Hospital Effectiveness, was published in 1968. In this context, effectiveness means an optimal combination of efficiency, appropriateness of service, accessibility to the service, acceptability of the service from the public's point of view, and the quality of the service as measured by professionals working in the health care system. This definition of effectiveness suggest that proposed solutions to the health care delivery problem must include a solution to the problem of poor organization. In attempting to solve the organizational problem, the system should examine its existing resources and facilities to see if they can be more effectively used or arranged before spending more money, recruiting more people, or looking elsewhere for an answer.

Paradoxically, although hospital attending staff physicians direct the use of a majority of hospital resources, they are not usually organized in a way that promotes optimal use of their power. This situation exists as a result of the organization of early-day hospitals in which a doctor and nurse constituted the entire patient care team and in which either the doctor or nurse organized and managed the institution.

However, as medical research and skill have increased, hospital operation has become more complex but hospitals' organizational patterns—particularly those of the medical staff—have not changed significantly. This is not to say that management techniques and modern organizational trends have not developed in hospitals. For example, the increasing complexity of hospital operation has created the need for a hospital administrator whose work requires him to apply modern management techniques.

Reprinted by permission from *Hospital Progress: Journal of the Catholic Hospital Association*, St. Louis, Vol. 51 (November, 1970), 80-84. Copyright 1970 by the Catholic Hospital Association. All rights reserved.

However, the application of such techniques has developed much more slowly within the medical staff. Hospital medical staffs are not organized to cope with the responsibilities which have been thrust upon them. The use of multiple physicians, as well as teams of supportive personnel, in the treatment of a single patient indicates a need for better organization of the medical staff. In addition, the general accountability of medical staffs for the practices of individual members has increased greatly because of legal precedents and decisions. Also, physicians are being faced with conflicting demands. They are becoming busier and busier, taking care of more and more patients, and consequently giving each one less and less time. At the same time, the demands of medical staff activities are mushrooming to the point where "something's gotta give."

Most medical staffs have what might be described as "sometime"—or "overtime"— leaders. Although physicians should be commended for giving their time to various elected or appointed staff offices, it is, indeed, an overtime job for them to undertake such responsibilities.

Ironically, the hospital administrator is often the first person to recognize the need for medical staff reorganization, probably because it is his job to think about hospital affairs on a full-time basis. Usually, after a series of fruitless attempts to coordinate activities with designated medical staff leaders, the administrator concludes that what is needed is a full-time, appointed medical staff "leader." Often, key doctors are not present at key meetings where important decisions are to be made. Those doctors who do give appreciable time and energy to their medical staff responsibilities do so at great personal sacrifice. Even though administrators appreciate such dedication they realize that such physicians "burn out."

Many doctors feel that full-time medical staff leaders represent a threat to the "clinical freedom" now enjoyed by attending medical staff members; many hospital administrators also consider the medical director as a personal threat. Such fears are unfounded.

One reason for apprehension on the part of both doctors and administrators is that the accountabilities of neither the administrator nor the medical director are understood—either by themselves or others. An examination of these accountabilities reveals the specific roles of those involved. The medical director must be recognized as a member of the institution's top management team. The medical staff does not exist in a vacuum; rather, it influences and is influenced by other activities within and outside the institution. Consequently, the medical staff's leaders must operate at the top management level so that these relationships can be dealt with effectively.

ADMINISTRATOR'S ACCOUNTABILITIES

In dealing with the positions of administrator and medical director, it is much more pertinent to ask, "What do we expect?" rather than, "What do they do?" In other words, their output should be of more interest than their input. By first asking what is expected, it is easier to identify the activities necessary to produce the desired end results.

"Accountabilities" is another word for end results. An examination of the administrator's accountabilities shows the relationship between them and the accountabilities of the medical director. His most basic and essential accountability is to make certain that his institution achieves and maintains full accreditation by the Joint Commission on Accreditation of Hospitals. This accreditation accountability is linked closely to medical staff activities.

Second, he must assure that an environment exists in which doctors can and do practice at optimum effectiveness. This accountability is one reason why the administrator should want a medical director with whom he can work. Another important accountability is to see to it that the institution maintains a viable financial condition. He must also make certain that the governing board of the institution receives enough information to enable it to make sound policy decisions. These are his primary accountabilities.

Other accountabilities which support those listed above include establishing and interpreting the goals of the institution and representing its interests and activities to the public. Changes within the institution may change the administrator's primary accountabilities to some extent; for example, the priority placed in research, education, rehabilitation, etc., may cause or be caused by some change in the institution itself.

MEDICAL DIRECTOR'S ACCOUNTABILITIES

Several of the medical director's accountabilities help an administrator fulfill his accountabilities. For one thing, the medical director must assure that the quality of medical care is appraised and maintained. Second, the medical director must attempt to improve communications between the medical staff and the institution, including the administration, the governing board, and the other operating departments of the institution. As a top management person and leader of the most important hospital department, the medical director has a significant impact on all hospital departments. Third, he must make certain that there are enough physicians on the medical staff to fulfill the philosophy and objectives of the institution.

Fourth, the medical director must strengthen the medical education program of the institution. The priority of this accountability depends, of course, upon the philosophy and objectives of the institution and the extent to which education plays a role.

An administrator would expect a medical director to institute new patient care programs if there is a demonstrated need for them and if the resources of the institution can sustain them. He would also expect the medical director to be proficient in management and administrative skills.

These accountabilities are admittedly stated in broad terms. However, they represent end results, not activities.

ACCOUNTABILITY MEASUREMENT

Such broad statements are not meaningful unless the administrator and the medical director can agree on certain measurements by which they can determine whether the end results are being accomplished. For example, in appraising the quality of medical care, the medical director and the administrator should ask questions which lead to specific answers, such as "What would indicate that good quality appraisal be carried out?" They should search for several percentage or quantum figures that indicate the degree of quality of medical care. Regardless of what statistical measure is used, it is essential that the administrator and medical director agree on what the indicators should be. In mutually establishing measures or indicators to the medical director's accountabilities, the administrator and medical director are really establishing the standards of performance which the medical director should meet.

Such standards are met by performing "minding the store" activities; that is, those things which the medical director must do daily in order to fulfill his accountabilities. He should periodically raise his standards on the assumption that improvement is always desirable. Such improvement is acomplished through the establishment and achievement of goals. The achievement of such goals constantly changes the situation. Thus, an accountability standard is one thing, while a goal may be to improve the standard by some quantifiable measure. For example, if the administrator and the medical director agree that this year "X" number of single unit transfusions is acceptable, but that next year "X minus Y" is their aim, they will have come up with a combination of a "minding the store" standard and a goal. This is a true system of results-centered management—or management by objectives.

It is essential that the medical director's accountabilities have high visibility, so that the staff clearly understands what they are. Obviously, it is necessary for the medical staff to be involved in accomplishing results if the medical director is to "measure up." Thus, his talent for planning, organizing, implementing, and evaluating becomes of paramount importance. The medical director's job description should be amplified by an inclusion of his accountabilities. If the results expected of the medical director are attached to his job description, he will have a working document and can proceed to achieve the results for which he was hired.

If a medical director is going to achieve specific end results, he must work with other doctors, administrators, and governing board members. There can be no place for authoritarianism in his methods. Admittedly, he must have authority and top management prerogatives in order to get things done. However, he will not last long if he imploys high-handed tactics in appraising the quality of medical care, or if he uses terse communiques containing cold, calculated statements concerning activities of the staff. The results desired simply will not be achieved by using despotic techniques.

One of the medical director's first undertakings should be to eliminate unnecessary work previously required of medical staff members. He and his office staff should be able to prepare meetings and limit discussions only to those topics on which doctors must act. In addition, a full-time medical director should be able to communicate clearly with the medical staff about various hospital activities. This is important since his accountabilities require him to improve medical staff understanding and cooperation. As a result of his efforts, staff participation should gradually become much more meaningful and important to the institution. When this happens, attendance at meetings will increase and doctors' involvement in the issues that the institution faces will become more valuable. Measures of the medical director's accountabilities will be measures of the medical staff's progress. Because performance criteria will be well-established, goals will become self-evident and much easier to achieve.

NO ROOM FOR ONE-YEAR LEADERS

The medical director's incumbency should last over an extended period of time rather than rotate from year to year. An institution's fortunes do not change drastically in a year's time, yet far too many staff leaders are in office only for that period. The long-range implications of institutional stewardship are so profound as to nullify the notion that effective medical staff operations can be achieved when leadership responsibilities are passed around on a a yearly basis. Physicians should demand a change in this system.

A NATURAL CHANGE

Doctors practice in a results-centered profession: Their task is to make patients well, to make them more comfortable, to increase their longevity. It should follow, then, that in the organization and management of the medical staff, physicians should demand a results-centered management. However, this can be achieved only by a full-time, top-level medical executive skilled enough and on the job long enough to use the same results-centered approach to staff affairs as his colleagues use in their private practices. This kind of management has proved its effectiveness in industry, and physicians should be not only willing to accept it, but should demand that it be introduced in their institutions.

It is regrettable that many hospital administrators do not yet employ this kind of leadership. A medical director would certainly be hampered if he tried to introduce this kind of management when the administrator did not operate in the same way. However, the medical staff is so important to the institution's success that the medical director, as a member of top management, could initiate a results-centered approach and try to bring his administrator along with him into a full management by objectives program.

CONCLUSION

It is much better for the medical staff to voluntarily undertake this change to management by objectives than to be forced into it. When such a system is imposed, it will not work well, because it is much more difficult to achieve someone else's goals.

To those who are worried about socialism in medicine, what has been described in this article is capitalism in its most precious form. In this system, the rewards go to the people who produce the results and achieve goals. If the hospital system can be operated and managed in the way described above there will be nothing to worry about. In addition, physicians will be fulfilling their role in society—they will be marshalling resources and producing service at an optimal level and doing it in the most efficient way possible. Moreover, they will have maintained their freedom to act. However, they can keep this prerogative only so long as the results they produce are higher than those which can be reasonably expected from any other system.

15.
Hospital Medical Staff Organization: Structure, Process, and Outcome

STEPHEN M. SHORTELL

Stephen M. Shortell, Ph.D., is Associate Professor and Director, Center for Health Services Research, Department of Health Services - School of Public Health and Community Medicine - University of Washington.

Is the present structure of medical staff organization capable of meeting the political, economic, and social changes confronting the hospital component of the health care industry? In addition to such a global issue, administrators are increasingly asking themselves (and others) the following types of questions: How can I get my medical staff to conform to government and other third party utilization and quality review requirements, without being accused of practicing medicine or interfering in professional prerogatives? How can I get them to consider issues of efficiency and cost control when they are not subject to economic accountability for their actions in the hospital?

Although these questions are framed in somewhat general terms, each administrator can readily add his own particular set of concerns. As Hall noted years ago: "It seems that doctors because they act like doctors are hard to fit into hospital organization."[1]

Due mainly to problems of gaining entry into hospitals to study medical staff organization, there have been few systematic, analytical efforts which address the above questions. This paper will review the major work which has been done. Key elements involved include the *structure* of staff organization in terms of size, departmentalization, formal methods of coordination, etc.; the *process* of its activities or the work which it performs, including decision-making and the resolution of conflict; and the *outcome* of this process, in terms of efficiency and quality of care.

There are essentially three major empirical assessments of medical staff organization related to the questions and issues posed in the previous section. These are Georgopoulos and Mann's study of 41 community general hospitals published in 1962,[2] Roemer and Friedman's study of the relationship between medical staff organization

---

Reprinted by permission from *Hospital Administration* (currently *Hospital and Health Services Administration): Quarterly Journal of the American College of Hospital Administrators,* Chicago, Vol. 19 (Spring, 1974), pp. 96-107. Copyright 1974 by the American College of Hospital Administrators. All rights reserved.

and hospital performance published in 1971,[3] and a monograph by Duncan Neuhauser dealing with the relationship between administrative activities and hospital performance also published in 1971.[4]

GEORGOPOULOS AND MANN

The principal interest of Georgopoulos and Mann was to examine the degree of coordination between various hospital components and, in turn, the relationship between coordination and organizational goal attainment or effectiveness. The 41 hospitals studied were all community general hospitals stratified by size, type of ownership, and geographic region. During the course of the study, interviews were completed with 960 physicians, 1,081 nurses, and 378 administrative personnel.

With regard to physicians and medical staff organization, the principal findings were that: (1) "key" medical staff members (specifically officers of the staff, chiefs of service and committee chairmen) generally gave more highly favorable responses than did the general medical staff in regard to degree of work coordination;[5] (2) a low percentage of key staff members (17 percent) and general staff members (32 percent) felt the community's knowledge of the hospital was very or completely adequate;[6] (3) hospitals experiencing less tension among departments, and with greater understanding and appreciation by physicians and nurses of each others roles, provided higher quality patient care (as judged by different hospital groups); (4) 50 percent of the key staff members expressed confidence in their administrator's ability to effectively represent their interests while 75 percent expressed such confidence in their chief of staff; (5) administrators markedly underestimated the medical staff's perception of its influence while the trustees and hospital department heads estimated it quite accurately; (6) medical staff members wished to see their influence increased; (7) doctors believed that trustees and nurses had a better understanding of their work problems and needs than they had of the work problems and needs of the trustees and nurses; and (8) despite the tension and misperceptions that existed between the medical staff and various other groups, tension was found to be highest among the doctors themselves, as reported not only by the doctors, but by administrators and nurses as well.

THE NEED FOR A CLOSER RELATIONSHIP

In regard to item four it is not at all surprising that the chief of staff should be perceived as better able to represent the medical staff's views than the administrator. After all, this is one of the chief of staff's primary responsibilities. But the finding does, perhaps, suggest the need for a closer relationship between administration and medical staff leaders in terms of understanding one another's views. For example, a recent study of role conflict involving hospital administrators showed that physicians were the most divergent group in their perception of the administrator's role compared with hospital employees and members of the board of trustees.[7]

One of the most significant findings is the high degree of tension that existed among medical staff members themselves. Apparently, current medical staff organization structure is unable to handle the tension that arises as a result of conflict between specialties, between older and younger doctors, between salaried and attending doctors and related sources of staff friction. In fact, Mann suggests that the existing highly departmentalized structures may themselves be a source of much of the conflict.[8] He suggests that better coordination and handling of conflict can be achieved through establishing interlocking coordinating roles between departments and committees whose interests overlap. Some evidence in support of this contention is provided by a recent study of utilization review activities in Connecticut hospitals.[9] The investigators found a strong relationship between the presence of communication and overlapping membership among staff committees and the attitudes of utilization review committee physicians concerning the effectiveness of the utilization review process. For example, of those utilization review committee physicians who felt that the review process could positively affect quality and efficiency of care, 61 percent had formal or informal relationships with other staff committees, while among those who felt that utilization review could affect neither efficiency nor quality, 86 percent possessed no relationship with other committees. The concept of overlapping committee memberships could be applied in relationships with nursing service and administration as well. Mann also suggests that key leaders establish group patterns of communication and interaction rather than dealing with problems on a man-to-man basis.

In sum, the work of Georgopoulos and Mann focuses mainly on the relationship between structure and process. But, while the changes in structure, in particular those suggested by Mann, may lead to better coordination and reduction of staff tension, will they have any effect on outcome in terms of the nature and quality of services rendered? This is the issue addressed by Roemer and Friedman.

Doctors in Hospitals actually contains two studies. The first examines the relationship between the percentage of contractual physicians a hospital has and various indicators of scope of services for a national survey of 2,434 hospitals conducted in 1959. Findings revealed that the higher a hospital's contractual physician score (percentage of physicians under contract weighted by type of remuneration), the greater its number of approvals, facilities, services and functions, even taking into account hospital size, type of ownership, and geographic region.

The second part of the book involves a case study of ten hospitals in California and examines the relationship between degree of structuring of the medical staff organization and various indicators of hospital performance. Their basic thesis was that the more highly structured the medical staff organization, the more effective the hospital's performance as measured by scope of services provided and case severity-adjusted death rate (hospital's actual death rate adjusted for case mix severity by using average length of stay and also taking into account occupancy).[10] Degree of structure was measured by the following seven items; importance weights assigned by the authors are given in parentheses: (1) composition of the medical staff (10 points), (2) nature of the appointment process (10 points), (3) contractual physician score

(25 points), (4) extent of departmentalization (20 points), (5) extent and diligence of control committees (15 points), (6) use of rules, regulations, and formal reports (10 points), and (7) communication patterns (10 points). Findings revealed that more highly structured medical staff organizations were better able to meet the needs of severely ill patients and had more supportive ancillary medical services, while nursing services were found to be more abundant in hospitals with less structured medical staff organizations. More structured staffs also had generally lower case severity-adjusted death rates, even after controlling for hospital size. Finally, overall staffing and total expenditures per patient day were lower in these hospitals. The authors were careful to note that the above relationships are only of an associational nature and say nothing about the possible causal mechanisms involved. While there are some important methodological problems associated with the study,[11] it, nevertheless, remains the first systematic attempt to measure the structure of medical staff organization and relate the differences found to particular aspects of hospital operation.

While a more highly structured medical staff, especially in regard to the percentage of physicians under contract, appears to be related to scope of service, economy and quality, findings from Georgopoulos and Mann suggested that they have problems coping with conflict and tension. However, Roemer and Friedman found that staff tension was highest in hospitals with "mediumly" structured medical staff organizations and lowest in those with very little structure or a high degree of structure. It should be noted that Georgopoulos and Mann were primarily focusing on tension among medical staff members themselves and, in this area, a high degree of departmentalized structure may, indeed, be unable to cope with the problems involved.

In contrast, Roemer and Friedman were primarily concerned with tension between the medical staff and hospital administration and, in this area, a staff with a high degree of structure, especially more fulltime contractual physicians, may be better able to relate to the overall goals of the hospital than a "mediumly" structured staff still in transition. Roemer and Friedman explain the lack of tension found in loosely structured staffs as being due to the fact that each physician pretty much went his own way with few intrusions or attempts at control by either administration or fellow staff members.

NEUHAUSER

Using data collected from 30 medium-sized community general hospitals in Chicago, Neuhauser proposed that in such a highly complex area of hospital operation as the medical staff, a high degree of specification of procedures (rules, regulations, etc.) would be negatively related to quality of medical care, while a high degree of visibility of consequences (extent to which owners and managers are aware of the consequences of their decisions) would be positively related to quality of care. It was felt that specification of procedures would be negatively related because complex tasks cannot be easily programmed through rules and regulations but, rather, require the judgment of professionals (in this case, doctors) who must be free to exercise a considerable degree of discretion in their behavior.

Specification of procedures was measured by whether the hospital made use of a formulary; the extent of required admission tests; the extent to which consultations were required for caesarean sections, D and C's, therapeutic abortions and sterilizations; the extent to which the hospital placed constraints on the range of activities each physician could perform; whether admitting privileges were suspended for having too many incomplete medical records; and, the chief of staff was asked to rate the degree of influence that he felt doctors had in hospital affairs. There were three principal measures of quality of care: evaluation by five outside physician experts; evaluation by the Joint Commission on Accreditation of Hospitals (JCAH); and Roemer's case severity-adjusted death rate. It was expected that all specification of procedure measures except perceived physician influence would reduce effectiveness.

PERCEIVED PHYSICIAN INFLUENCE

Perceived physician influence was expected to improve effectiveness as measured by positive JCAH and expert evaluations and lower severity-adjusted death rate. The results, however, only partially supported the predictions. In particular, "requiring admission tests" and "setting limits on physician activities" improved performance. In addition, "perceived physician influence" was associated with higher rather than lower severity-adjusted death rates. A possible explanation for the contrary findings in regard to admission tests and setting limits on physician activities is that medical staff members themselves largely establish these rules and regulations. Thus, it is not merely a matter of how specific various rules and procedures are, but also of who does the specifying. Longest found similar results in his study of ten Georgia hospitals where both a perceived index of regulatory coordination and actual extent of coordination through reports and control mechanisms were positively related (although not statistically significant, given the small sample size) to the same measures of quality used by Neuhauser.[1,2]

Neuhauser further explored the issue by dividing the medical staff itself into areas of high complexity and low complexity. He then examined the relationship between physician participation as voting members of the board and involvement in joint conference committee activities with the JCAH and experts' evaluations of quality. He found that in the highly complex areas of the staff the relationship between participation and quality was stronger than in the less complex areas. As noted, however, these results must be interpreted cautiously since the sample sizes involved were small, and none of the relationships were statistically significant.

Visibility of consequences was associated with greater effectiveness. Thus, greater awareness on the part of board members and administrators of where their hospital actually stood in regard to such items as autopsy rate and post-operative infection rate was related in the expected directions with the quality of care evaluations.

ENCOURAGING PHYSICIAN PARTICIPATION

In general, Neuhauser's findings tentatively suggest that greater physician participation and involvement in hospital activities may have a beneficial impact on the actual quality of care rendered in the hospital. To the extent that greater participation may lead to a greater perception and understanding of the roles of other hospital departments and employees, the results are congruent with those of Georgopoulos and Mann. At the same time, Neuhauser finds that some types of bureaucratically specified rules and procedures are also positively related to quality. This is somewhat parallel to Roemer and Friedman's general finding that highly structured medical staffs resulted in higher quality of hospital performance. It appears that a high degree of formalization of structure and participation are not necessarily incompatible, especially where physicians themselves have a strong voice in determining the rules and regulations governing their clinical activities. In addition it should be noted that Roemer and Friedman use as a prime measure of formalization of structure the percentage of physicians under contract in the hospital. And, it is exactly these physicians (full-time chiefs of staff, directors of medical education, etc.) who are more likely to take an active interest in the hospital and fill the necessary coordinative roles suggested by Georgopoulos and Mann. A summary of the principal approaches and findings of the three studies is presented in Table 1.

Table 1 essentially suggests the need to provide physicians with new types of organizational roles. The studies imply that giving physicians increased participation in the affairs of the organization through salaried employment or other means may be an effective approach to the issues of utilization—quality control and efficiency—cost control posed by the two introductory questions. Such a straightforward interpretation, however, fails to take into account the complexity of the problem by ignoring the great variety of current hospital-medical staff relationships, the personalities of individual physicians and administrators, and associated hospital idiosyncrasies. But the existing literature does suggest a common underlying theme applicable to all hospitals; namely, the need to achieve some degree of integration of administrative and clinical decision-making.

Recent developments have made inoperable the traditional distinction between administrative and clinical activities of the hospital and its doctors. Increasingly complex reimbursement schemes, legal decisions, utilization review regulations, professional standards review organizations (P.L. 92-603) and a generally more informed and demanding public (to name but a few factors) have precipitated the integration or, perhaps more accurately, confrontation of the administrative and clinical spheres of influence. Administrative activities increasingly touch upon the practice of medicine, and clinical practice, in turn, is heavily involved with issues of managerial efficiency and effectiveness.

The key concepts behind this attempt at integration would appear to be power and authority. Power is a property which generally resides in an individual not an organi-

TABLE 1
Summary of Major Studies of Medical Staff Organization

	Primary Emphasis	Principal Findings and Implications
Georgopoulos and Mann	Focused on the relationship between type and extent of physician participation and quality of coordination.	1. Those physicians more involved in hospital affairs (e.g. chief of staff) perceived greater degree of coordination. 2. Greatest amount of tension existed among doctors themselves. 3. Suggest that greater use of overlapping committee membership and coordinative roles results in less tension and better coordination of effort.
Roemer and Friedman	Focused on the relationship between degree of structure of medical staff organization (e.g. percent of physicians under contract) and scope, economy, and quality of services rendered.	1. The more highly structured the staff the greater the scope and quality of services rendered and the lower the expenses per patient day. 2. Tension and conflict highest in staffs with an intermediate degree of structure. Those highly structured have the necessary salaried physicians to provide the needed coordination and integration; in those with little structure the doctors can operate independently of administration as well as of each other.
Neuhauser	Focused on the impact of rules and regulations and visibility of consequences on quality of care.	1. Board chairmen and administrators who are more aware of their hospital's activities (visibility of consequences) have higher quality of care. 2. Rules and regulations not necessarily harmful to quality of care especially where the rules and regulations are established by the physicians themselves. 3. There is some suggestion that greater physician involvement in hospital affairs is associated with higher quality of care.

zation, while authority is generally thought of as being a property of the organization which may be bestowed upon an individual. The integration of administrative and clinical decision-making may thus be viewed as an attempt to merge the power possessed by the physician, by virtue of his technical expertise, with a legitimately defined organizational role (position of authority). The expectation is that such a merging of individual power and formal authority will result in greater accountability and control.

The particular ways in which hospitals attempt to achieve such accountability will, of course, vary widely. Examples in recent years have included appointments of full-time chiefs and/or directors of medical education, extending the length of appointment of voluntary chiefs of staff, involving physicians as voting members of the board of trustees, and mergers of medical staffs. These and related changes are aptly discussed by Johnson.[13] In addition, there have been proposals for restructuring staffs along both departmental and non-departmental lines whereby physicians would not only belong to a clinical department, but would be part of a division of community health services responsible for various aspects of emergency care, home care, nursing home services, neighborhood health services and various other satellite services.[14] Others suggest a reorganization of existing clinical departments into a division of general or primary care and a division of secondary or specialty care.[15] The primary care division would be composed of adult and pediatric generalists while the specialty care division would be organized along organ system lines. Thus, the principal tie of adult nephrologists, for example, would be with other renal specialists, rather than with specialists in other areas of adult medicine, such as cardiology and gastroenterology.

Whatever the changes, it seems clear that the ability of hospitals to adapt to their environment depends in large part on how effectively they can meet the issue of providing physicians with meaningful organizational roles. The existing research suggests some leads but, inevitably, administrators and medical staff members must work out their own solutions, taking into account their own particular set of circumstances. In any event, furthur study of the emerging patterns, involving the mutual collaboration of administrators, physicians, and social scientists, seems particularly important, given the issues faced by hospitals and their medical staffs at this point in time.

FURTHER READINGS SUGGESTED BY THE AUTHOR

(Compiled in part by the Cooperative Information Center for Hospital Management Studies of the University of Michigan.)

Ainsworth, T. H. "The Medical Staff and the Hospital." *Trustee*, April 1973, pp. 8-13.
Barr, R. "Hospital Practice: Core of Tomorrow's Medicine?" *Hospital Physician* 5 (February 1969): 77-89.
Bauerschmidt, A. "The Calculus of Hospital Administration," *Hospital Administration* 16 (Fall 1971): 50-68.
Center for Health Administration Studies. *The Impact of Changing Medical Practice on Hospital Administration.* Chicago: University of Chicago, 1963.

Emory, M. L. "Proposal for a Medical Service Corporation as a Proper Organizational Structure for Hospital Staffs." *Journal of the Louisiana State Medical Society* 122 (August 1970): 255-277.

Engel, C. "Professional Autonomy and Bureaucratic Organization." *Administrative Science Quarterly* 15 (March 1970): 12-21.

Johnson, E. "Physician Productivity and the Hospital: A Hospital Administrator's View." *Inquiry* 6 (September 1969): 59-69.

———. "Why Hospital Medical Staffs Can Do What HMO's and Foundations Can't." *Modern Hospital*, January 1973, pp. 75-79.

Levey, S. "Sources of Medical-Administrative Conflict: A Survey." *Hospitals* 35 (16 July 1962): 49.

Neuhauser, D. "The Hospital as a Matrix Organization." *Hospital Administration* 17 (Fall 1972): 8-25.

Robinson, W. M. "Medical Staffs Merge." *Hospitals* 47 (16 February 1973): 60-66.

Roemer, M., and Tennant, F. "Hospital-Physician Relations." *Hospitals* 47 (1 April 1973): 57-64.

Rothman, R. A.; Schwartzbaum, A. H.; and McGrath, J. H. "Physicians and a Hospital Merger: Patterns of Resistance to Organizational Change." *Journal of Health and Social Behavior* 12 (March 1971): 46-55.

Schulz, R. "Physicians on Boards: Survey Examines Level, Extent of Participation." *Hospitals* 46 (16 December 1972); 51-54.

Sigmond, R. M. "Changing Hospital Goals." *The Journal of the Albert Einstein Medical Center* 17 (Spring 1969): 7-16.

Toomey, R. E. "Medical Staff Organization and Administration." *Journal of the American Medical Association* 200 (12 June 1967): 964-969.

U.S., Department of Health, Education, and Welfare, Secretary's Advisory Committee on Hospital Effectiveness, *Report of the Secretary's Advisory Committee on Hospital Effectiveness: 1968.* (Washington, D.C.: Government Printing Office, 1968).

VanHouten, D. R. *Opportunity and Influences: A Study of Medical Leadership in Community Hospitals.* Pittsburgh: University of Pittsburgh Press, 1967.

Williams, K. J., "Medical Staff Issues: Past and Present," *The Hospital Medical Staff* 1 (January 1972): 2-13.

Wilson, R., "The Physician's Changing Hospital Role," *Human Organization* 18 (Winter 1960): 177-183.

FOOTNOTES

[1] O. Hall, "Research in Human Relations in the Hospital," *Hospital Administration* 1 (Fall 1956): 11.

[2] B. S. Georgopoulos and F. C. Mann, *The Community General Hospital* (New York: Macmillan Co., 1962).

[3] M. I. Roemer and J. Friedman, *Doctors in Hospitals: Medical Staff Organization and Hospital Performance* (Baltimore: Johns Hopkins Press, 1971).

[4] D. Neuhauser, *The Relationship Between Administrative Activities and Hospital Performance,* Research Series, no. 28 (Chicago: Center for Health Administration Studies, University of Chicago, 1971).

[5] It should be noted that this difference may be due to social desirability, that is, the desire of those in key positions to present a good image of the hospital thus over-emphasizing the extent of support and coordination. But it is also possible that the key medical staff members, with their greater involvement in the affairs of the hospital, have access to more information and experience

than their colleagues and, thus, may be in a better position to see how the hospital achieves coordination among the various departments.

[6] This finding is particularly significant in light of the important community relations role which a hospital's medical staff can play in interpreting the hospital to the community and vice versa.

[7] J. E. Veney and A. D. Kaluzny, "Health Administration: A Study in Role Conflict" (Paper presented at the Sixty-seventh Annual Meeting of the American Sociological Association, New Orleans, Louisiana, August 28, 1972).

[8] F. C. Mann, "Achieving an Effective Staff," *Hospital Progress,* January 1965, pp. 91-95.

[9] L. T. Berman *et al.,* "Utilization Review in Connecticut Hospitals: Three Years After Medicare," (New Haven, Conn.: Yale University School of Medicine, May 29, 1969) pp. 16-22. (Mimeographed).

[10] M. I. Roemer, A. T. Moustafa, and C. E. Hopkins, "A Proposed Hospital Quality Index: Hospital Death Rates Adjusted for Case Severity," *Health Services Research* 3 (Summer 1968): 96-118.

[11] David Starkweather, "Medical Staff Organization and Hospital Performance," *Health Services Research* 7 (Fall 1972): 254-260.

[12] B. Longest, "The Relationship Between Coordination, Efficiency, and Quality of Care in General Hospitals" (Ph.D. diss., Georgia State University, August 1972).

[13] E. Johnson, "An Emerging Medical Staff Organization," *Hospital Administration* 17 (Winter 1972): 26-38.

[14] R. Sigmond, "The Health Care Crisis and the Planning Process" (Paper presented at the Hospital Medical Staff Conference, University of Colorado, Estes Park, Colorado, September 30, 1969).

[15] E. Braunwald, "Future Shock in Academic Medicine," *New England Journal of Medicine* 286: 1031-1035.

Part II
THE MANAGEMENT OF HOSPITAL PERSONNEL

In the introduction we presented the hospital from a systems (input-output) frame of reference. Further, manpower was cited as one of its most important input resources. Consequently, serious attention should be given to the management of hospital personnel and their behavior in order to have a hospital which can accomplish its objectives. For example, Volante observes "... health care delivery systems (including hospitals) cannot reach optional effectiveness unless the 'systems' take into account the 'people' working with them. That is, the systems must be built around the realities of human behavior..."[1] Those who interact with peer employees and those who manage others need to understand why these employees behave as they do, how they can be motivated, and what approaches to take when supervising them or working with them.

In this Part we will discuss the subject of the management of hospital personnel. Included will be a presentation of motivation, leadership and supervision, and managerial approach and techniques.

EMPLOYEE MOTIVATION

To answer questions such as: why people work; why are some higher performers than others even though abilities are equal; why are some employees more satisfied and cooperative than others; why some employees have a high rate of absenteeism while others do not; and how a supervisor, department head, head of service, or administrator gets employees to do things. We must first understand the concept of motivation. It is defined as externally or self-induced behavior which seeks to satisfy needs.

NEED HIERARCHY

One of the early motivational theories seeking to explain worker behavior was presented in the 1940s by Abraham Maslow. Specifically, Maslow formulated what is called the "Need Theory of Motivation." Given that all people have needs they attempt to fulfill through behavior, Maslow identified five different levels. In summary they are:[2]

Physiological needs are those related to basic survival and human maintenance; that is, necessities of life. They include food, clothing, shelter, and the like. In most instances they are met through working behavior as it is translated into wages and the purchase of items which satisfy those needs.

2. *Safety-Security needs* are those related to maintaining one's ability to satisfy physiological needs and have physical safety. Job security (possibly through union seniority provisions) is an example.
3. *Affiliation-Affection needs* are those related to the social nature of people. The desire to be loved, have companionship, the sense of belonging fostered by work-groups, and co-worker affiliation are examples.
4. *Esteem-Status needs* are those related to the individual's self-image. Most people want others to think highly of them. Status and its signs (the physician and his stethoscope) are important. Also, prestige, reputation, attention, and a feeling of importance are needs in this category.
5. *The Self-Actualization need* is the highest in the need hierarchy. Basically it denotes the need to be what you were born to be, do your own thing, be your own person. Maslow states "A musician must make music, an artist must paint, a poet must write, if he is to be ultimately happy." Also, we could state that a dedicated physician or nurse self-actualizes when he or she heals and relieves the suffering of humanity.

Coupled with the need hierarchy are the stipulations that needs motivate and cause behavior; however, appeals to a higher order need level generally do not induce behavior if lower order needs are not already fulfilled and once a need level is satisfied, it no longer tends to be a prime motivator. For example, the granting of esteem or status, perhaps through a promotion, is not likely to motivate an individual if physiological needs are not satisfied due to an extremely low wage.[3]

Further, others (Behling and Shapiro; Bedwell) have indicated that the relative importance of needs as motivators varies with societal change. The history of the unionization movement is an example. During the 1930s industrial workers behaved in a particular manner (sought unionization) in order to satisfy physiological and security-safety needs as represented by wage increases and job security. In large part, these needs are met today and in many instances unionization is sought to satisfy the higher order needs as represented by the social functions of a union, the desire for more leisure time, and the workers' desire to humanize a job and make it more meaningful. To generalize, workers forty years ago were happy to have a job and were satisfied with one car. Today's worker wants his job to be meaningful and wants, not only two cars, but all of the other material pleasures of life by age thirty. They bring a different set of values and need expectations to the job. Simply stated, programs for health care for the needy, workman's compensation, and unemployment insurance have in part, met the security-safety needs of most people.

JOB SATISFACTION (DUAL-FACTOR THEORY)[4]

The terms "morale," "job attitude," and "job satisfaction" are often used in an interchangeable manner (Holloway). However, inherent in the concept of job satisfaction is the recognition that it is relative to the individual's needs and expectations. In turn, these are shaped by the individual's background, experiences, culture, and the like. Stated another way, job satisfaction is a function of the perceived characteristics of a job within the context of an individual's frame of reference (which can be influenced by his co-workers), and how those characteristics can satisfy his needs.

In terms of understanding employee behavior and how a supervisor can motivate employees, the Dual-Factor Theory of Motivation becomes an operational extension of the Maslow need hierarchy theory of motivation. Specifically, it translates *needs* into *job content and context variables*. The success of fulfillment is measured by the level of employee job satisfaction—the employee's overall happiness with the job.

Maintenance Dimension (Dissatisfiers)

As formulated by Herzberg et al., there are some conditions of the job *context* which operate primarily to dissatisfy employees when they are not present. However, presence (fulfillment or satisfaction) of these conditions does not necessarily lead to a high degree of motivation. Herzberg called these conditions *maintenance* or *hygiene* factors since they are necessary to maintain a reasonable level of satisfaction. He also noted that many of these factors have often been perceived by managers as motivators, but they are, in fact, more potent as dissatisfiers when they are absent. He concluded that there were a number of maintenance factors such as: organizational policy and administration, technical supervision, interpersonal relations, salary, job security, and work conditions.

Motivational Dimension (Satisfiers)

There are other job *content* conditions which, if present, tend to build high levels of motivation and job satisfaction. However, if these conditions are not present, they do not prove highly dissatisfying. Herzberg described various *motivational* factors or satisfiers such as: achievement, recognition, advancement, the work itself, the possibility of growth and responsibility.

The distinction between the two dimensions is that the absence of the maintenance factors will tend to lead to job dissatisfaction. However, the fulfillment of the maintenance factors alone will not motivate the individual or result in high job satisfaction. Should the motivational factors, however, be fulfilled, but the maintenance factors lacking, the individual will not exhibit high motivation and tend to be dissatisfied. Fulfillment of both dimensions, typically results in high employee motivation and job satisfaction. Thus, in order to promote high job satisfaction and desired employee behavior, provisions must be made to allow the individual fulfillment of both dimensions simultaneously.

When the Herzberg and Maslow motivational theories are compared it can be seen that both emphasize the same set of relationships. Both determine *what* motivates people and causes certain human behavior. Maslow identified needs of the individual while Herzberg focused on the job conditions (context and content) as they affect the individual's basic needs. In fact, one can conceptually relate the Herzberg maintenance dimension factors to the lower level Maslow needs and the Herzberg motivational dimension factors to the higher level Maslow needs.[5]

The basic advance of Herzberg's theory of motivation over the Maslow need-hierarchy is that it shows the distinction between maintenance and motivational factors. Most importantly for the application of theory in the work place, Herzberg shows that motivation tends to be derived from the *work itself,* particularly when there is satisfaction with the maintenance factors *and* the motivational factors (Myers).

LEADERSHIP AND SUPERVISION

An understanding of motivation and why people behave as they do are only two of the many ingredients necessary to successfully manage people. Once one understands the behavior of others, that knowledge must somehow be translated into a form which will result in employees performing their job responsibilities (Jacobs). The second area on which we will focus is leadership and supervision. Through each, the manager can use his understanding of motivation, establish the parameters of employee work activity, and oversee its accomplishment.

Leadership is a very complex subject and has been described in a number of different ways. Essentially it can be defined as a process of ".... influencing people to direct their efforts toward the achievement of particular goals."[6] The explicit and implicit elements of this definition are *group, goals, influence,* and *acceptance.* That is, a leader leads others who organizationally would normally be subordinates reporting to him (and in some instances other employees who may not report to him). He influences (motivates), instructs, and commands them in their work effort to accomplish some purpose such as attain organizational or personal objectives. This implies that the leader's role consists of determining what is to be accomplished, influencing (motivating) others, and overseeing their efforts. It further implies that those being led, whom we call the "followers," in turn, accept the leader in his role and accept his influence over them. In combining these elements, leadership is defined as that activity by which one person prescribes how what is to be done is determined and influences (motivates), instructs, and commands the efforts of others in order to accomplish specific purposes (objectives and/or work tasks).

The accepted manner for studying leadership is through the examination of "Leader Behavior." That is, viewing how a leader (in our case the formally appointed manager) behaves as he attempts to lead others. There are two dimensions to leader-behavior which we will examine. The first is his behavior relative to the degree of decision-making authority held by him or relinquished to the group. The second dimension is the manner in which he interacts with others and the way in which he supervises the accomplishment of specific work activities.

LEADERSHIP: DEGREE OF DECISION-MAKING AUTHORITY HELD BY THE MANAGER

In any organizational activity involving two or more people, someone must be responsible for determining what is to be accomplished, how, when, and by whom. The degree of decision-making authority dimension of leader behavior sets the overall leader-follower (manager-subordinate) relationship in terms of the determination of direction and scope of work activities along with how and when they will be performed. Various terms such as autocratic, participative, and democratic have been used as descriptors (Tannenbaum and Schmidt; Cartwright and Zander, pp. 553-572).

LEADERSHIP: MANNER OF OVERSEEING THE ACCOMPLISHMENT OF WORK ACTIVITY

The second dimension of leader behavior concerns the manner in which the leader (manager) oversees the predetermined work activity of others. Overseeing implies not only the monitoring of work but the specific assignment of tasks and the directing, instructing, and influencing of others—typically subordinates. It also carries a relationship connotation: that is, the leader's concern for workers and/or output, the way in which rules are enforced, closeness to them, and the degree to which they are represented to others in the organization. Generally, this dimension of leader behavior is called "supervision." For the sake of convention, this term will be used.

In Selection 18, "Effective Supervision Requires Leadership," the writer describes a number of supervisory styles in detail. They consist of sets of opposites such as "distant-friendly," "strict-lenient," "close-general," and "work-centered—employee-centered." It is left to the reader to review Selection 18 for the distinction between these styles. However, at this point they can be clustered in two general classifications, "work-centered and employee-centered." They embrace all other styles and characterize the directional elements inherent in each.

In Figure 1, the "work-centered" and "employee-centered" (Cartwright and Zander, pp. 554-570; Likert) descriptors characterize the basic attitude and approach of the supervisor. Specifically, in overseeing accomplishment of work, the work-centered supervisor tends to view subordinates as just another resource in the work process. Little concern is given to needs, feelings, or individual differences.

In terms of directional activity, the work-centered supervisor tends to represent and communicate downward, and employee petitions are not communicated or supported upward to the supervisor's supervisor. The rule and policy enforcement will tend to be strict; motivation will tend to be through threat or withdrawal of rewards; discipline will be negative in the sense that it is punitive rather than being constructive or used as a learning experience; and overseeing task activity is generally close with little broad delegation.

The employee-centered supervisor has the characteristics generally opposite to the work-centered supervisor. Employees are viewed as individuals with different abilities and needs and they are viewed as a primary and important resource in the work process. The directional elements presented in Figure I are basically contrasts of the work-centered elements.

LINKAGE

Within these two distinct classifications it is possible to array the supervisory style contrasts presented in Selection 18. Furthermore, it is possible to link leader decision authority styles in a general manner. For example, the employee-centered supervisor will tend to exhibit a leader decision authority style which can be characterized as one that is participative[7] while the work-centered supervisor will tend to follow a style which is more autocratic.

FACTORS AFFECTING STYLES

An overview of standard and accepted classifications of leader decision authority and supervisory styles has been presented; however, in any such presentation some have a tendency to draw the conclusions that one style is best, correct, or appropriate while another is not. In Selection 19, "A Situational Approach to Supervision," the writers present a situational model of leadership.[8] This model attempts to be predictive by suggesting the most effective leader authority and supervisory styles given the subordinate's job maturity.

Factors which affect appropriateness of leader styles and the likely resulting performance are: the nature of the work; urgency of the results; the characteristics of the workers, and the personal characteristics of the manager. If work activity must be performed immediately, perhaps under disaster or crisis conditions, the health care manager may have to adopt an autocratic decision-authority style and a close supervisory style when supervising the work activity. At other non crisis times it may be appropriate to revert to participative and general-supervision styles.

The characteristics of subordinates—their training, education, motivation, and experience—can influence the leader authority and supervisory styles adopted by the manager. This factor is closely related to the "nature of the work" since worker skills will tend to correspond closely to the type of work required. If the subordinates are skilled professionals, the manager may more readily seek their opinions (consultative or participative) relative to the determination of the work to be performed and give them fairly wide latitude when carrying it out. If they are unskilled or not necessarily dependable or experienced employees, the manager may have to make most of the the decisions himself (adopt an autocratic style) and closely supervise them.

Figure 1

Generalized Supervisory Style Classifications

Directional Elements	Work Centered (human resources are viewed as just another resource in the work process)	Employee Centered (human resources are reviewed as the primary and key resource in the work process)
1. Representation	Downward	Upward
2. Communication	Downward	Bilateral
3. Rule Enforcement	Adherence	Deviation
4. Motivation	Sanctions	Rewards
5. Discipline	Negative	Constructive
6. Task overseeing	Close	General

Finally, the personal characteristics of the manager can affect the leader authority and supervisory styles he adopts. Some individuals, by reason of their personality, traits, previous experience, values, and cultural background function better under one style than another. They may find it difficult to change even though the situation changes.

MANAGERIAL APPROACHES

One characteristic of all organizations is that they have a structured hierarchy within which all organization participants function. Linked to it is the division of the work to be performed, granting authority to individuals, and a requirement that they be accountable for the duties delegated to them. To discharge responsibilities the manager must in turn motivate, lead, and supervise certain employees and ensure that their work is performed as expected.

THEORY X AND THEORY Y

Theory X and Theory Y are part of the organizational setting just described. Each represents a managerial attitude about employees and, therefore, results in a specific exhibited approach to the management of people. Further, each makes certain assumptions about what motivates employees and each can be characterized by different leader authority and supervisory styles (Freeman; O'Donovan, 1975).

Theory X generalizes what is considered to be a "conventional" view of the way in which a manager interacts with subordinates. Basically it is characterized as the manager being responsible for directing efforts of subordinates. Further, subordinates must be *motivated* and *controlled*, their actions and their behavior *shaped*, through negative rewards if necessary, so the organization's objectives may be accomplished. Linked to this management approach are assumptions about employees (McGregor, 1960, Chapter 3).

1. Employees have an inherent dislike for work and work as little as possible.
2. They lack ambition, dislike responsibility, prefer to be led, and must be coerced, controlled, threatened, and punished in order to put forth adequate work effort.
3. They are self-centered seeking only personal need fulfillment.
4. They resist change.

This X managerial approach tends to result in leader authority and supervisory outcomes designed to force behavior and retain explicit control.

Management views its task as *force-fitting* the individual into the organization. Employees are not self-motivated or responsible and their direction and control takes on a "hard" approach. The manager feels that he must be autocratic in terms of leader decision authority and work-centered in terms of supervisory approach. If he is not, work will not get done because employees will do no more than necessary.

Theory Y embraces assumptions about employees which are opposite of the Theory X assumptions (McGregor, 1960, Chapter 4).

1. The average person does not dislike work and work can be a source of satisfaction which will be voluntarily performed.
2. External control and the use of negative sanctions are not the only means for bringing about employee work effort. Employees will exercise self-direction and self-control.
3. The employee's commitment to objectives is more a function of rewards from achievement (positive motivation) than withdrawing existing rewards (negative motivation).
4. Employees with proper direction and training will not only accept but seek responsibility particularly when it permits need-fulfillment.

Given these assumptions about employees, McGregor argues that management's approach should not be to *force fit* the individual but that of arranging "the organizational conditions and methods of operation so that people can achieve their own goals best by directing their own efforts toward organizational objectives." (McGregor, 1966, p. 15). Essentially this approach incorporates developing and using the latent potential of the organization's human resources. When linked to leader decision authority and the manner of overseeing work activity, the Theory Y approach would typically embrace the participative decision-making and employee-centered (general) supervisory styles (Rosenbaum).

Although Theories X and Y present two contrasting approaches to managing people and are based on certain assumptions, it is not possible to state Y is better than X. From an attitudinal point of view Theory Y is preferred, however. The generalized approach taken and leader authority/supervisory styles adopted will depend greatly on factors such as the nature of work, the type of employees, and the characteristics of the manager. Several things, however, are certain. First, behavioral science research has clearly demonstrated that management based on the Theory X point of view is definitely not effective over a long period of time, especially in the health care field. Workers subjected to management based upon these assumptions take little initiative, make few innovations, and enjoy little sense of achievement or job satisfaction (Levinson). Most health care employees will not function under the stringent centralized direction, control, and *force fitting* characteristics of Theory X.

Theory X and Theory Y describe the attitudes which management has toward employees. They are important concepts related to motivation because they represent a dichotomy as to how the manager approaches the task of motivating others. Also, as pointed out in Selection 16, "The Organization As A Social System," the managerial approach taken influences the manner in which employees view the organization. The manager who operates under Theory Y assumptions will see his task as that of creating an organizational climate in which the health care worker finds satisfaction and need fulfillment in work and, as a result, will be self-motivated.

PARTICIPATIVE MANAGEMENT

The term "participative management" is frequently used to denote a managerial approach which implies that subordinates participate "in an active sense" in work activity decision-making. Within the framework used here, participative management is essentially one of the leader authority styles previously presented. However, in the generic sense it means more. Some consider participative management to be use of a committee forum in making decisions. The committee is composed of individuals holding positions at the same hierarchical level in the organization (Watkins). Others consider it to be characterized by the superior and a group of subordinates interacting in decision-making (Gassett). Both of the above considerations are correct. As a managerial approach participative management has the ingredients of a participative leader authority style; most often a general supervisory style; and the mechanism by which employees (and peers) have some measure of input into the determination of work activity—its purpose, content, flow, and assignment.

From a motivational perspective, participative management can be very useful in managing hospital employees. As will be noted in Part III (Hospital Unionization), ability to have some measure of control (input into the decision-making process) of the work environment is important to employees. This not only involves day-to-day matters but also major events which result in organizational change. For example, one certainly understands the concern accounting department employees would have relative to a decision changing from manual to computerized patient-billing and accounts-payable systems. Involvement of employees and their legitimate participation in providing input (opinions, views, facts) to decisions gives them a greater feeling of control over the work situation. As a result, they are more likely to accept a decision.

Further, the motivational dimension factors can often be satisfied when a participative management approach is adopted. For example, factors such as recognition, the work itself, and responsibility can often be satisfied through this method. Participative management is a way of saying to the employees: "You have knowledge, skills, experience, and information which we want you to tell us about—your opinions, feelings, advice. Therefore, you are important and we recognize it;" in short, "you have something to contribute." By being involved, people tend to be more committed, in the broadest sense of that word. Thus, they tend to derive more satisfaction from work they are performing. Finally, participative management implies responsibility. In order to be effective, all parties must take it seriously and interact honestly. This means greater responsibility for all people involved.

Many benefits have been associated with participative management. We have mentioned involvement; motivation; satisfaction; and change implementation benefits. Watkins (p. 48) mentions commitment, which he describes as: "participation increases commitment and encourages people to feel the responsibility for the success of decisions and policies to which they have contributed—they become *their* decisions and *their* policies rather than those of the manager." Two other benefits offered by O'Donovan (1971) are that a participative management approach can enhance personal growth and development of employees and it can increase organization flexibility because of the wider experiences employees will have in the work situation.

Obviously participative management is not always a valid managerial approach. The physician often does not use it when directing the patient-care activities of subordinates. The variables which affect its appropriateness and resulting effectiveness include the type of work to be done, the skills and activities of subordinates (Crane) and the total employer-employee organizational climate. Finally, the manager's motive and sincerity play a major role in the resulting effectiveness of participative management. This is the legitimacy of the process. For example, the manager must be sincere and the subordinates must perceive this sincerity. Only going through the motions of the process, i.e., where the manager has no intention of following the recommendations of those participating, will result in employee rejection of the process and very likely the manager as well.

It should also be mentioned that there are certain risks associated with the participative management approach. In Selection 20, "Participative Management: A Valid Alternative to Traditional Organizational Behavior," the writer mentions several. The following may be added: participation is not always welcomed by all employees (some do not want the responsibility that goes with it), and one must be aware of the fact that errors can occur.

DELEGATION

When managing hospital employees effective delegation is one of the hardest things for a manager (administrator, chief of service, or supervisor). In order to *work through people* it is necessary to delegate, at least to some degree; yet, the process is given little attention. An effective manager is one who can delegate within the parameters and constraints of assigned responsibilities. Delegation is simply conferring authority and responsibility to perform certain jobs and tasks to a subordinate. All managers delegate. The executive director usually delegates in a general manner to his associate directors and heads of departments. The supervisor also delegates, but generally to a lesser degree to his or her subordinates. However, the greater the scope of delegation within the organizationally defined limits, the greater the organizational effectiveness will be.

In Selection 21, "Mastering the Managerial Skill of Delegation," the writer suggests there are negative results associated with not delegating as widely as possible. Further, it is an activity that improves with experience. Delegation has numerous benefits. It can be used to motivate subordinates. When more important tasks, duties, and assignments are delegated, the effect enables the individual to feel that his abilities are being utilized and that the supervisor has confidence in him. In addition, delegation is the primary means by which a supervisor can free more time for performing other important functions. Finally, delegation enhances organization flexibility (Haynes). If many subordinates have been delegated multiple and varied duties, personnel changes will not be as disruptive as otherwise. If one quits, is absent, or is transferred, another can do the job.

However, there are possible negative factors associated with delegating. Two important considerations are the risk of the end product, and the ability of the subordinate. Since the manager is still accountable for the actions of subordinates, caution must be exercised so that no delegation is made to those not adequately trained.

There are also multiple requirements to be met if one is to have an effective delegation process. Among these are: the duties to be delegated should be clearly thought through by the supervisor; the individual should be given appropriate authority; and a control mechanism should be established.

If an individual is responsible for performing certain duties but does not have the authority to do so, the process of delegation will be ineffective. This is often called the co-equalness of authority and responsibility. However, granting of authority does not necessarily make delegation effective. It is implicit in delegation that the supervisor remains responsible for the results even though another individual is discharging the duties. Consequently, control mechanisms ranging from simple reporting on an exception basis to detailed reporting are necessary.

BIBLIOGRAPHY

Bedwell, Raymond T., Jr. "Motivating Younger Employees." *Hospital Progress* 57(April): 60-62, 1976.

Behling, Orlando and Mitchell B. Shapiro. "Motivation Theory: Source of Solution or Part of Problem?" *Business Horizons* 17(February): 60-66, 1974.

Brannen, Ted R. "The Organization As A Social System." *Hospital Administration* 2(Spring): 19-25, 1959.

Brayfield, Arthur H., and Walter H. Crockett, "Employee Attitudes and Employee Performance." *Psychological Bulletin* 52(September): 396-424, 1955.

Bullough, Bonnie. "Is the Nurse Practitioner Role A Source of Increased Work Satisfaction?" *Nursing Research* 23(January-February): 14-19, 1974.

Cartwright, Dorwin, and Alvin Zander. *Group Dynamics.* Evanston, Illinois: Row Peterson and Company, 1960.

Crane, Donald P. "The Case for Participative Management." *Business Horizons* 2(April): 15-21, 1976.

DeVille, Jare. "Successful Leaders are Successful Motivators." *Supervisory Management* 18(July): 23-19, 1973.

Edwards, Francis G. "The Growing Need For Motivated Nurses." *Hospital Administration* 16 (Winter): 44-53, 1971.

Fielder, Fred E., and Martin E. Chemers. *Leadership and Effective Management.* Glenview, Illinois: Scott, Foresman and Company, 1974.
Freeman, Sister Roberta. "Management of People–What Is Your Philosophy?" *Hospital Administration in Canada* 16(June): 42-45, 1974.
Gassett, Hester. "Participative Planned Change." *Supervisor Nurse* 7(March): 34-40, 1976.
Goodfellow, Matthew. "Morale." *Hospital Financial Management* 28(November): 24-29, 1974.
Greiner, Larry E. "What Managers Think of Participative Leadership." *Harvard Business Review* 51(March-April): 111-117, 1973.
Gruenfeld, Leopold and Saleem Kassum. "Supervisory Style and Organizational Effectiveness In A Pediatric Hospital." *Personnel Psychology* 26(Winter): 531-544, 1973.
Haynes, Marion E. "Delegation: Key to Involvement." *Personnel Journal* 53(June): 454-456, 1974.
Hersey, Paul, Kenneth H. Blanchard, and Elaine L. LaMonica. "A Situational Approach to Supervision." *Supervisor Nurse* 7(May): 17-20, 22, 1976.
Herzberg, Frederick. "Motivation–Hygiene Profiles: Pinpointing What Ails the Organization." *Organizational Dynamics* 3(Autumn): 18-29, 1974.
Herzberg, Frederick, Barbara Mausner, and Barbara Snyderman. *The Motivation to Work.* New York: John Wiley and Sons, 1959.
Hill, Barbara Snyder. "Participative Management: A Valid Alternative to Traditional Organizational Behavior." *Supervisor Nurse* 7(March): 19-21, 1976.
Hodgetts, Richard M. *Management Theory, Process and Practice.* Philadelphia: W.B. Saunders Co., 1975.
Holloway, Robert G. "Management Can Reverse Declining Employee Work Attitudes." *Hospitals* 50(October 16): 71-77, 1976.
House, Robert J., and Lawrence A. Wigdor. "Herzberg's Dual-Factor Theory of Job Satisfaction and Motivation: A Review of the Evidence and a Criticism." *Personnel Psychology* 20(Winter): 369-388, 1967.
Jacobs, Barry J. "Leadership-Key to Management Effectiveness." *American Journal of Hospital Pharmacy* 32(December): 1287-1288, 1975.
Kerr, Steven, and Janet Schriesheim, "Let the Situation Determine Your Leadership Style." *Hospital Financial Management* 28(January):52-56, 1974.
Kaplan, Jerome. "Management by Delegation." *Journal of Long Term Care Administration* 2 (Spring): 44-60, 1974.
Krech, David, Richard S. Crutchfield, and Egerton L. Ballachey. *Individual in Soceity.* New York: McGraw-Hill Book Company, 1962.
Lawler, Edward E., and Lyman W. Porter. "The Effect of Performance on Job Satisfaction." *Industrial Relations* 7(October): 20-28, 1967.
Levinson, Harry. "Asinine Attitudes Toward Motivation." *Harvard Business Review* 51(January-February): 70-76, 1973.
Likert, Rensis. *New Patterns of Management.* New York: McGraw-Hill Book Co., 1961.
Longest, Beaufort B., Jr. "Job Satisfaction for Registered Nurses in the Hospital Setting." *Nursing Administration* 4(May-June): 46-52, 1974.
Maslow, A.H. "Theory of Human Motivation." *Psychological Review* 50(July): 370-396, 1943.
McGregor, Douglas. *The Human Side of Enterprise.* New York: McGraw-Hill Book Co., 1960.
– – –. *Leadership and Motivation.* Cambridge, Mass.: MIT Press, 1966.
Myers, M. Scott. "Who are Your Motivated Workers?" *Harvard Business Review* 42(January-February): 73-88, 1964.
Nichols, Glennadee A. "Important, Satisfying, and Dissatisfying Aspects of Nurses." *Supervisor Nurse* 5(January): 10-15, 1974.
O'Donovan, Thomas R. "Effective Supervision Requires Leadership." *Hospital Progress* 46(February): 65-67, 103, 1965.
– – –. "Can the 'Participative' Approach to Management Help Decision Makers?" *Hospital Management* 112(July): 16-17, 1971.

———. "Leadership Dynamics." *Journal of Nursing Administration* 5(September): 34-35, 1975.
Phillips, Robert I. "The Informal Organization in Your Hospital." *Radiologic Technology* 46 (September-October): 101-106, 1974.
Rakich, Jonathon S., Beaufort B. Longest, Jr., and Thomas R. O'Donovan. *Managing Health Care Organizations.* Philadelphia: W.B. Saunders Co., 1977.
Roethlesberger, F.J., and William J. Dickinson, *Management and The Worker.* Cambridge, Massachusetts: Harvard University Press, 1947.
Rosenbaum, Bernard L. "A New Approach to Changing Supervisory Behavior." *Personnel* 52 (March-April): 37-43, 1975.
Schrieber, David E., and Stanley Sloan. "An Occupational Analysis of Job Satisfaction in a Public Hospital." *Hospital Management* 108(August): 27, 30, 32, 1969.
Shore, Harvey G. "Absenteeism: How to Analyze Causes and Effects." *Supervisory Management* 20, Part 1(September): 9-17, 1975.
Slocum, John W., Jr., Gerald I. Susman, and John E. Sheridan, "An Analysis of Need Satisfaction and Job Performance Among Professional and Para-professional Hospital Employees." *Nursing Research* 21(July-August): 338-341, 1972.
Starcevich, Matt M. "Employee Organizational Attachment and Job Expectations." *Hospital Progress* 55(May): 68-73, 1974.
Tannenbaum, Robert, and Warren H. Schmidt. "How to Choose A Leadership Pattern." *Harvard Business Review* 36(March-April): 95-101, 1958.
Velghe, James C., and Gary Cockrell. "What Makes Johnny Mop?" *Personnel Journal* 54(June): 324-325, 349, 1975.
Volante, Elena M. "Mastering The Managerial Skill of Delegation." *Journal of Nursing Administration* 4(January-February):20-22, 1974.
Watkins, Brian. "Participative Management." *Nursing Mirror* (England) 7(August 16): 48, 1974.
Weiss, Alan. "Leadership Styles: Which Are Best When?" *Supervisory Management* 21(January): 2-8, 1976.
White, Catherine Harman, and Maureen Claire Maguire. "Job Satisfaction and Dissatisfaction Among Hospital Nursing Supervisors: The Applicability of Herzberg's Theory." *Nursing Research* 22(January-February): 25-30, 1973.
Wild, Ray. "Job Needs, Job Satisfaction, and Job Behavior of Women Manual Workers." *Journal of Applied Psychology* 54(April): 157-162, 1970.

FOOTNOTES
(See bibliography for full citation as necessary).

[1] Elena M. Volante, "Better Management of People Resources," *Hospital Progress*, Vol. 55, No. 6 (June, 1974), p. 64.

[2] Maslow, pp. 372-382. Also see: McGregor (1966) pp. 8-12.

[3] For an interesting study of the Maslow need theory in the hospital setting see Slocum, Susman, and Sheridan.

[4] For studies of the Herzberg Dual Factory Theory in health care organizations see: Bullough; Longest; Nichols, Schrieber and Sloan; Starcevich ; White and Maguire; and Velghe and Cockrell.

[5] Although it is beyond the scope of our presentation, the reader should be made aware of the fact that a considerable amount of controversy surrounds the hypothesis that employees having high job satisfaction are high performers. Brayfield and Crockett, in a classic review of the literature examining the relationship between morale and job performance, did not find hard evidence to support the hypothesis. Others such as House and Wigdor criticized Herzberg's dimensional construction. Further, Lawler and Porter have contended that high job satisfaction does not lead to high job performance but that job performance leads to high job satisfaction due to the re-

wards which follow from accomplished performance. Regardless of the disagreements, it has been repeatedly demonstrated that employees with low job satisfaction are more likely to exhibit absenteeism and turn-over behavior patterns.

[6] Richard M. Hodgetts, *Management Theory, Process, and Practice,* (Philadelphia: W.B. Saunders Co., 1975), p. 342.

[7] DeVille weaves into his writing both leadership dimensions without differentiating between the two. It is interesting reading in that it describes the characteristics of what we have called the "participative" and "employee centered" styles in terms of how this kind of leader leads.

[8] Fred Fiedler and his associates have developed a "Contingency Leadership Model" which is recommended to the reader. For summaries of this model, also see Gruenfeld and Kassum; Rakich, Longest, and O'Donovan (Chapter 12).

Employee Motivation

In Selection 16, "THE ORGANIZATION AS A SOCIAL SYSTEM" by Ted R. Brannen, a number of themes are developed and intertwined around the central topic—voluntary cooperation. Basically, the writer stated that the charge of the administrator is to induce voluntary cooperation among hospital employees. Linked to this hypothesis is the fact that accomplishment occurs through an understanding of motivation and an understanding of the structure and purpose of informal groups.

Multiple themes can be gleaned from this selection. First, that individual behavior is induced through attempts to satisfy needs and employee cooperation is functionally dependent upon how the individual's work effort will or will not contribute to this satisfaction. Linked to the Maslow need theory of motivation is the second theme called "organization attitude toward employees." This is analogous to the Theory X-Theory Y approach where the employee's attitude toward the organization is shaped by the organization's attitude toward the employee.

The final theme developed and linked to the first two is the understanding of the importance of the informal organization. This is significant because employee needs are partially filled by the informal organization and because the administrator's attitude toward the informal organization will shape its behavior. In order to make this distinction, a few words will be offered to characterize the informal organization.

In the text of this part we have not presented the characteristics of the informal organization or discussed its importance. The writer of this selection (16) offers information which merits elaboration and reinforcement. To characterize it, the informal organization consists of the set of emergent behavioral patterns that occur within a formal organization structure. Further, it typically does not follow formal channels of communication, departmentation—the formal grouping of activities—or the established chain of command. Finally, it consists of work groups and the loosely knit association among workers (Phillips).

The informal organization is important because it shapes attitudes of its members, especially their perception of the organization's attitude toward them. A corollary of this shaped-attitude is the group's establishment of productivity norms, an internal discipline procedure, and an informal communication system called the grapevine. The theme developed is that if the objectives of the informal organization are not congruent with those of the formal organization, voluntary cooperation will probably not occur.

Several useful benefits are derived from the informal organization. First, it is a means by which individual members can satisfy needs such as security (the group protects its members from the administration) and social (it is a means to enhance interaction among peers in a socializing sense—taking coffee breaks together). Second, it can add to the hospital's effectiveness. Often things get done through the informal organization that would not otherwise get done. Third, it offers a stability benefit provided that the formal and informal organization have common objectives (deviant behavior is internally disciplined—"Don't be absent so much or you will spoil it for us all").

The informal organization is a fact of life in every formal organization. It cannot be eliminated. Consequently, keeping in mind the need fulfillment function of the informal organization, the change process should take into consideration the importance of the informal organization as represented by employees' groups. The writer closes with the admonition that participative management, where employees have some input into the change decision-making process, should be followed. Finally, all the themes join. To obtain voluntary cooperation from employees "... the administrator must understand not only the individuals with whom he is in contact; he must also understand the informal groups into which they are organized."

Francis G. Edwards in Selection 17, "THE GROWING NEED FOR MOTIVATED NURSES," provides an interesting extension of motivation theory in the hospital. The writer begins with a definition of motivation as being human behavior instigated by needs. He next presents the Herzberg Dual-Factor approach to motivation with a discussion of the factors characteristic of the maintenance and motivational dimensions. Finally, he concludes that managers should seek to motivate employees by creating a climate where the maintenance and motivation factors can be fulfilled.

The extension of motivation theory provided in this selection builds upon the foundation of employee motivation just mentioned. That extension, called the "Domino Aspect of Motivation" is simply that the hospital's patients have physiological and psychological needs they wish to fulfill. The writer's contention, as applied to nurses, is that their technical training does not equip them with an understanding of human behavior and the importance of employee- (or patient-) need fulfillment. Consequently, when dealing with subordinates the supervisor is less likely, in the absence of natural leadership and motivation abilities, to create a working environment to enable subordinates to fulfill needs—or, in this case, satisfy the Herzberg motivational dimension factors. In these circumstances, those subordinates are not likely to truly understand the needs of patients nor, in turn, "... create an effective climate of motivation and cooperation with their patients."

16.

The Organization as a Social System

TED R. BRANNEN, PH.D.

Ted R. Brannen, Ph.D., is Dean of the School of Business at the University of Southern California, Los Angeles.

One of the most outstanding characteristics of modern society is the number and variety of tools in use. These tools fit into patterns that are combinations of interrelated parts devoted to common objectives. To operate this technological process, people are needed. Since each individual uses only a few of the tools included in the technological process, various individuals are responsible for the functioning of different parts of the process. These people must be formed into functional patterns consistent with effective co-ordination of the parts of the tool process. Patterns of technical relations between men grow out of the patterns of relations between the workers and their tools. In these patterns of relations some men must be given responsibility to co-ordinate the efforts of others.

The welfare of society, therefore, is a function not only of the availability of technology but of the efficiency with which it is used and the purposes to which it is applied. For the most part, society has delegated responsibility for the efficient use of the technological process to private and government administrators. These administrators are responsible for directing the tool complex in a manner that will achieve desired objectives.

The job of administrators is a most difficult one because, instead of performing the technical operations themselves, they must induce others to carry them out according to previously determined plans. The work of administrators will be fruitless unless the various members of their organizations are willing to contribute their efforts to the achievement of common objectives. Therefore, the primary function of administrators is to induce voluntary co-operation on the part of their subordinates and associates. It follows from this that the most important qualifications of administrators are (1) an understanding of why persons are willing to contribute their efforts and (2) skill in obtaining co-operation from the members of an organization in working toward planned objectives.

Reprinted by permission from *Hospital Administration* (currently *Hospital and Health Services Administration): Quarterly Journal of the American College of Hospital Administrators,* Chicago, Vol. 4, (Spring, 1959), pp. 19-25. Copyright 1959 by the American College of Hospital Administration. All rights reserved.

The performance of every man falls within a range of effort and efficiency. The upper limit of this range is determined by his aptitude and ability. The lower limit is determined by superiors who establish the minimum level of performance that will be accepted without provoking punishment. Men who offer conscientious voluntary co-operation perform near the upper limit of their range of productivity. Other men may do no more than is necessary to avoid punishment. The level of productivity of the individual is determined by his own desire to co-operate. In short, the attitudes of the worker toward his work, his employer, and his supervisor determine his effectiveness in the organization.

ELIMINATE PROBLEMATIC SITUATIONS

Developments in the field of psychology indicate the life-process of man is a perpetual attempt to eliminate problematic situations, that is, to satisfy needs. Each person is continually making decisions he believes will help to satisfy his needs. Employees work, follow directions, and co-operate spontaneously when doing so appears to offer a means of satisfying their needs.

Unfortunately, many administrators do not recognize the fact that the eagerness of employees to absorb training, to perform their jobs well, and to co-operate with other members of the organization can be sustained or destroyed by their relations within the organization. Administrators often interpret the energy and co-operativeness of employees as being a reflection of the inherent worthiness of the individuals. Productive employees are given credit for accepting their responsibilities because they are honorable men. Unproductive employees are often discredited as being naturally lazy, stupid, or deceitful.

Every formal organizational structure (i.e., the hierarchy of supervisors and employees) tends to be permeated with a basic attitude toward the workers in the organization. The organizational attitude toward employees is determined by the highest level of administration, and it seeps down through the entire structure. There is a causal relation between this organizational attitude and the attitudes of employees toward the organization. In turn, the attitudes of employees toward the organization strongly affect the degree of employee cooperation obtained by the organization. Employees co-operate with those from whom they receive co-operation.

THESE ARE COMMON NEEDS

Administrators must be willing to help employees satisfy their needs, and they must know what needs employees expect to satisfy through their association with the organization. There are a few needs that appear to be held in common by all employees. Although it is not always consciously recognized, the basic desire probably is for recognition of the right of every man to human dignity equal to that of every other man. All employees desire respect for their abilities, appreciation for their efforts, a sense of sharing in the control of their own destinies, and a feeling of security, that is, the absence of frightening uncertainties.

However, while we know some of the basic needs employees expect to satisfy in the organization, we know far less about what is required to satisfy these needs. What one employee thinks satisfies his needs, another employee may resent. Each man interprets the situations he encounters from his own particular point of view. The individual's perception of his environment is a conditioned reaction. It is conditioned by his own background and beliefs. Thus one employee may need careful supervision, while another may function best with a minimum of supervision. When a supervisor stops by the desk of the first worker, this may be interpreted as an expression of interest on the part of the supervisor. But the same act may be perceived by the second employee as unwarranted investigation or an expression of insufficient confidence in the ability of the worker to control his own performance.

Administrators must anticipate the reaction of employees to situations that arise. Only by an understanding of the individual, his habits, expectations, and beliefs, can the administrator know what is needed to induce his spontaneous co-operation for the benefit of the organization. The administrator must recognize the elements of satisfaction and dissatisfaction in the life of each member of the organization with whom he has direct relations. There is no short cut to sound human relations. The problems involved in meeting the needs of each employee are somewhat different from the problems presented by every other employee. Each man is unique; his situation differs in some respect from all others. Administrators must seek to understand the individual—his problems, his ambitions, the way he thinks and feels, and why he has the attitudes he has. Patience and interest are required in order to determine the peculiarities of each member of the organization.

INDUCING CO-OPERATION

It also must be recognized that expectations and interpretations are subject to change. They may be altered as a result of changes in other factors. As an employee becomes older, he may become more interested in job security and retirement benefits. He may become somewhat less concerned with opportunities for advancement.

But the problem of inducing co-operation with the formal organization is even more complex. Administrators who are familiar with the sentiments, expectations, and interpretations of individual employees may still fail to understand some of their behavior because of the influence of the "informal organization."

Most formal organizational structures are comprised of smaller groups of employees who are in frequent contact with one another. Each individual will have frequent contacts with a relatively small number of people. These individuals often form identifiable groups. Their relations become standardized, into certain patterns of acceptable behavior; each person knows what is expected of him and what he can expect of others. These groups make effective technical cooperation possible. They increase stability, provide channels of communication, and routinize many relations. Individuals derive satisfaction and a sense of security from identifying themselves with groups of this informal type. In addition, these groups have leadership positions that will be filled by one employee or another. They have certain relations with other groups, with supervisors, and with the organization as a whole. The pattern of relations and the hierarchy of status positions that grow out of these natural groupings of people are called the "informal organization."

The informal organization influences the perception of the members of a formal organization. We are all influenced by social pressures. We try to meet the expectations of people with whom we are in frequent contact. We want their good will. As members of various groups and social organizations, we encounter group values, attitudes, and sentiments that determine what is expected of the members of the group. We are subjected to considerable social pressure to conform to the group concept of acceptable behavior.

THE SYMBOLS OF RANK

The status hierarchy of the informal social organization is important to employees and is exemplified in every way possible. Each status position has associated with it certain customary symbols of rank. Everything in the work situation takes on a special meaning in terms of the social organization. Who gives directions to whom, the relation of one employee's wages to those of other employees, the size of one's desk in relation to the desks of others, and every other variable becomes associated with certain positions in the informal social organization. Administrators who do not recognize this fact and treat objects and relations solely in terms of concepts of efficiency are likely to encounter difficulty in obtaining employee co-operation.

The informal social organizations of some employee groups serve to induce co-operation with administrators, but other informal groups serve to limit co-operation. Therefore, the administrator must understand not only the individuals with whom he is in contact; he must also understand the informal groups into which they are organized. He must observe the attitudes and sentiments of these groups in order to be able to anticipate their reactions to various situations.

Once an informal pattern of relations and a hierarchy of status positions becomes established, it tends to resist change. A change resulting from action taken by administrators may be interpreted as a threat to the stability or the continuation of the informal social organization. If it is, the change will be resisted, and the members of the group will refuse to co-operate with their administrators.

ORGANIZATIONAL TREASON

Changes in methods, organization, or physical facilities that should produce substantial improvements in efficiency may result in drastically reduced efficiency if employees are suspicious or resentful of the change. The best systems cannot function properly if employees do not desire to see them succeed. This type of resistance, sometimes referred to as organizational treason, must be expected unless support is obtained from employees in advance of any change.

The most effective way to obtain prior acceptance of a change is to discuss with employees the problem that makes the change necessary. If employees are encouraged to participate in developing a solution, they will have an interest in seeing that the solution is effective. Under these conditions they will accept their responsibility to cooperate with others, and they will strive to perform their assigned tasks in order to avoid a breakdown in the chain of interrelated functions. For example, employees are always interested in receiving recognition as valuable members of an organization. If they are asked to participate in developing a cost-reduction program—and their suggestions are seriously considered—they will support the final program of action. In this way the efficiency of the organization may be substantially increased.

Unco-operative attitudes develop among employees who feel they can obtain support for their objectives only by forcing the formal organization to recognize their importance. Co-operative behavior cannot be maintained unless administrators seek to understand and satisfy the needs and expectations of individuals and informal groups of individuals.

In order to administer an organization in a manner designed to induce effective co-operation, the administrator must have a sincere interest in the needs of others. However, trying to meet needs and expectations will not produce co-operative behavior unless the administrator understands the sentiments of the individuals and groups with whom he works. The administrator must try to anticipate the reactions of others to his own actions. His directives, plans, and expressed attitudes must be viewed from the perspective of the people he is trying to influence. He must attempt to evaluate his own actions in terms of the beliefs, anxieties, and attitudes that will determine the behavior of others. To do this, he must understand the individuals and informal organizations with which he is in contact. This understanding can be gained only by observing the individuals and groups. However, it is important to remember that what the administrator sees when he tries to observe and understand the sentiments of the formal and informal organizations will be a product of his own attitudes, values, and sentiments unless he is aware of the problem and deliberately tries to view the situation from the point of view of the people and groups being observed.

17.

The Growing Need for Motivated Nurses

FRANCIS G. EDWARDS

Francis G. Edwards is a Vice President of Louis A. Allen Associates, Inc. in Palo Alto, California.

The nineteenth century angel of mercy has today been replaced by a seemingly less angelic and considerably more mercenary counterpart. With increased technical skill has come an apparent lessening of sensitivity to the sufferings of the patient. With demands for higher wages and better working conditions, the modern Florence Nightingale is undoubtedly more efficient, but somehow less comforting.

SENSITIVITY TO THE NEEDS OF THE USER

While this may seem a matter of minor moment to the hospital administrator, his management counterpart in other fields is showing growing concern with problems in motivation. He has already observed that with increased technical sophistication the product or service produced tends to become more important to the technician than the people using it. Pardonable pride in his technical accomplishments lessens his sensitivity to the needs of the user. This is particularly true when the product or service caters mainly to physical needs. Too often more subtle but equally real psychological needs are ignored or rationalized away.

In the admittedly difficult area of providing adequate nursing care for physically damaged and psychologically impaired patients, modern motivation theory gives rise to some interesting speculations and offers a strong possibility for marked improvement if seriously applied. To bring the topic into focus for the hospital administrator, he must first be aware that one of his primary functions as a professional manager is the leadership and motivation of his subordinates. Its importance, expressed in economic terms, is most readily apparent in "strained" relationships with the patients, his customers. Time-consuming, unreasonable demands and embarrassing complaints—all adding to operating costs—can be avoided if patients are properly motivated by the nursing staff. The nursing staff in turn must be motivated by their supervisors, and

---

Reprinted by permission from *Hospital Administration* (currently *Hospital and Health Services Administration*): Quarterly Journal of the American College of Hospital Administrators, Chicago, Vol. 16 (Winter, 1971), pp. 44-53. Copyright 1971 by the American College of Hospital Administrators. All rights reserved.

they in turn by their managers. To understand this fully, we must first determine exactly what motivation is and then examine the types of problems which arise when people are not motivated. Once this has been done, the experience of management in other fields can be examined to see if there are direct areas of application to hospital administration.

WHAT IS MOTIVATION?

Motivation, to behavioral scientists, is a satisfactory pattern of behavior which reaches an objective corresponding to the individual's need or needs. Since purposeful human behavior is instigated by need and directed toward objectives, reaching these objectives produces a feeling of satisfaction and a temporary disappearance of the need. This we call motivation. A motivated individual is one who accomplishes worth-while objectives related to his personal needs. In a social situation this satisfaction is greatly increased if recognition and esteem on the part of other members of the group accompanies the achievement of the objective.

Based largely on the work of Frederick Herzberg, modern motivational theory distinguishes between motivating and maintenance needs. This is particularly important in a socially structured situation such as working for a company or as part of a hospital staff. The contractual implications of employment are such that the employee feels he has a right to certain considerations. Among these considerations typically are fair policies or administration, effective supervision, adequate salary, reasonable interpersonal relations, and adequate working conditions. While precise descriptions of these conditions will vary from one type of work to another, the individual has certain standards which he feels should be met. As long as these standards are met, the individual has no reason to be dissatisfied. However, these factors, in and of themselves, do not motivate or satisfy him. For this reason they are sometimes referred to as maintenance factors, sometimes as the dissatisfiers or hygiene factors.

On the other hand, there are certain considerations to which the individual has no right in virtue of his employment contract. However, he needs them if he is going to be a completely satisified human being. These, known as motivating factors, include the work itself, achievement, recognition of this achievement, responsibility, and advancement or growth. These represent the challenge and pleasure people get out of work. They provide a basis for recognition from other members of the group and from one's supervisor. They produce a desire for advancement and a sense of continuing accomplishment.

Successful application of Herzberg's theories to various industrial situations has produced an additional observation. When people are not motivated—that is, when they are not receiving enough recognition, growth, sense of achievement, etc., they do not complain about lack of motivation or attack the motivation factors which are directly responsible. Instead, they pick on the dissatisfiers and complain about working conditions, management policies, inadequate supervision, wages, etc. Further, if the complaints are taken at their face value and salaries are increased, working conditions are improved, etc., the effect is relatively short-lived. Soon other objects or the same factors again become renewed sources of dissatisfaction and the cycle tends to repeat itself endlessly.

On the other hand, motivated workers, that is, those who are achieving a strong sense of growth, adequate recognition, a feeling of accomplishment, etc., not only do not complain about environmental factors, but tend to have a greater tolerance for substandard conditions and are quite unlikely to complain unless some major inequity develops.

IMPLICATIONS FOR MANAGEMENT

The implications of modern motivation theory for professional management are at the same time distressing and encouraging. The disquieting thought that the mini-welfare states, created by some companies, were both unnecessary and largely ineffective is in the former category. (The interesting speculation as to how many union demands might have been averted if workers had been adequately motivated must remain forever unanswered. The suspicion, however, is strong today that giving in to demands without creating better motivation simply produces more demands and a basis for further dissatisfaction.)

On the encouraging side, however, is the thought that management understanding the importance of the motivating factors, can now begin to create a climate in which workers can find personal satisfaction in everything they do. Combined with modern emphasis on management objectives, it produces a realistic climate in which the worker's need for recognition, growth, achievement, etc., can be satisfied by enlightened management handling of superior/subordinate contacts.

WORTH-WHILE OBJECTIVES

In the basic management task of securing results through others, the professional can combine an ability to effectively predetermine their courses of action with a climate that inspires and encourages each individual worker and gives him a continuing sense of his own importance so necessary to produce a continuing feeling of satisfaction. To motivate his subordinates, the modern professional must create a climate in which the individual can select and work towards worth-while objectives. He must give him necessary recognition and a sense of achievement when he accomplishes them and hold out opportunities for continuous personal growth and development.

If the manager can do this, the motivated subordinate not only produces more effective results, but can also increase both his physical and psychological capacity for useful work. Attendance records show that well-motivated, satisfied employees have fewer days off, fewer physical complaints, whether real or imaginary, and can progressively take on more difficult objectives. Of even greater significance is the observation that motivated subordinates can, in turn, create a climate in which motivation of people with whom they come in contact becomes possible. This is particularly true if they are taught to understand the important implications of motivation and its practical value, both for themselves and the company or institution they represent.

MOTIVATION IN THE HOSPITAL

Since the primary reason for a hospital's existence is to provide care for its patients and to satisfy their needs, it may be well to first examine the modern patient's needs, both physical and psychological, then to draw implications for the primary interface between the hospital administration and the patient, namely, the nursing staff. From this, we can proceed through the supervisory to the upper management levels.

In the course of the last thirty years, the needs of the average American have changed considerably in emphasis. In the era during and immediately after the depression of the 1930's primary emphasis was placed on satisfying one's bodily needs and on survival. A lot of physical and emotional energy was spent getting a job, making ends meet, and adding to or replacing one's possessions. This sense of insecurity persisted for most Americans throughout World War II. It was only in the growing affluence of the postwar period that the emphasis slowly shifted from safety and survival to a broader acknowledgment of social values, the need for status, and more recently, a strong sense of individual potential which can be actualized to an ever-increasing degree.

PROTRACTED SURVIVAL

The economic, education, and technological forces which spawned this change have also produced an extended life expectancy, superior remedies, and more sophisticated surgical techniques which have generated in modern man a stronger hope of protracted personal survival. At the same time, a growing concern and heightened dissatisfaction with ailments and physical disabilities has become apparent.

Among the par values or maintenance factors of our society today must surely be included good health and long life. For this reason the potential dissatisfaction of the individual with anything that threatens these rights is correspondingly greater. Evidence of this can be found in increasing preoccupation with health, diet, exercise, and all matters affecting one's physical well being. This is understandably heightened by the mirror-affect of mass communications, presenting health problems in highly dramatic form.

EXPECTATIONS VS. REALITIES

Concomitantly, expectations of people regarding medical services and what these can and cannot accomplish are exaggerated, and the opportunity for potential dissatisfaction greatly increased. In contrast, attitudes of patients to hospital care in less highly developed societies than ours is less demanding and considerably more permissive. In many parts of the world patients cheerfully put up with conditions that would be regarded as intolerable in any U.S. or Canadian hospital.

Seen in this light, the cool, clinical detachment of many nurses does little to provide the climate of reassurance so necessary to offset the disappointment of the individual at being confined to hospital in the first place. The proliferation of equipment, the various clinical routines and procedures to which he is required to submit, the preoccupation of the nursing staff with the mechanics of running a ward, all tend to heighten the patient's feeling of dissatisfaction with his condition.

THROUGH THE PATIENT'S EYES

Whatever his physical condition, his psychological need immediately is for adequate orientation in the new routine, a strong sense of recognition on the part of the nursing staff of his problems and their importance to him, an encouraging attitude toward the progress he makes, and an ability on the part of the nurse to see the minor objectives which he achieves through *his* eyes rather than on an absolute scale of patient achievement.

To do this adequately, minor achievements, such as eating solid food, taking a first step, sleeping through a night, etc., should all be given recognition in proportion to the patient's sense of their importance. Clearly, a nurse who is unhappy or dissatisfied with her position and is not adequately motivated will find it very difficult to develop the necessary empathy to produce this type of reaction.

THE NURSE

During the extensive period of training the nurse is required to undergo, major emphasis is placed on procedures, both diagnostic and therapeutic, knowledge of pharmacology, and other technical areas. Minor emphasis is placed on clinical psychology, with some insight into largely abnormal working of the human mind. She receives little formal training in normal human behavior, and even less in correct attitudes toward various types of patients. Supposedly, good common sense and the right type of personality will help her to improvise in the various situations which she will confront in the course of her nursing life. Even when formal training is given in this area, it unfortunately tends to take the form of a "how to be nice to patients" session and rarely explains in sufficient detail the important connection between mental attitudes and physical recuperation.

Small wonder, then, that the hardened professional tends a few years after school to classify patients into two groups: "good" patients, meaning those who make no demands outside of regular routine, and "bad" patients, meaning those who externalize psychological needs that she is not ready or equipped to satisfy. If the demands of the latter become too oppressive, a nurse will typically refer the incident to her supervisor who, depending on her type of personality, either will seek to mollify the patient through some form of verbal therapy or will reinforce the rejection which the nurse has already exhibited.

LEARNING BY PRECEPT IS RARE

Nowhere in her training is the nurse told that the role of her supervisor is to lead and motivate her so that she, in turn, can lead and motivate the patient. She is not aware of the fact that avoidance of the conflict not only does not satisfy the patient's needs, but unfortunately lessens her ability to cope with more demanding situations. If she is fortunate enough to have a supervisor with natural leadership and motivation ability, she may learn by example, but rarely will she learn by precept. Were her supervisor adequately trained in the management side of her responsibilities, she could undoubtedly anticipate a lot of the problems that nurses—particularly younger nurses and trainees—run into, and through adequate training set up a program of preventative psychological maintenance that would solve problems before they occur.

That this is not just an idle speculation was amply demonstrated in a recent two-and-a-half year study at Yale–New Haven Hospital in Connecticut, as reported in the June 20, 1969, issue of *Time* magazine. The study, under the direction of a New York psychiatrist, attempted to determine changes in attitude on the part of the nursing staff toward terminal cancer patients.

TREATING PATIENTS IN A REALISTIC MANNER

In describing the attitudes of the nurses, the article notes, "As custodians of terminal cases, nurses bear particularly heavy burdens. The girls show a tough and cold exterior—an attitude quickly acquired in hospital service." Under the psychiatrist's direction, the nurses were convinced of the importance of their task, and were asked to treat the patients in a much more realistic manner.

The success of the experiment perhaps is best summed up in the concluding works of the article: "With life rapidly slipping from her, an old Italian woman called to a nurse one day. 'It is the end, isn't it?' she asked. The nurse nodded, sat next to the old woman and held her hand. 'I don't want die alone,' the old woman said. 'You won't be alone,' the nurse replied. Ten minutes later, the old woman's labored breathing stopped, with the nurse still holding her hand."

THE NURSING SUPERVISOR

As the lowest level of hospital management, the nursing supervisor must engage in certain technical activities and provide some management functions. Among the latter, elementary planning and control and a high degree of leading and motivating skill are undoubtedly required. While new systems and procedures have placed heavy emphasis on the former, unfortunately her responsibilities in the latter area are often neglected. In order to act as an effective leader, she must know how to make logical decisions, how to communicate them effectively to her subordinates, and how to motivate her subordinates so that they in turn may obtain both personal satisfaction from their work and at the same time create an effective climate of motivation and cooperation with their patients.

This can generally be accomplished by some form of supervisory training that would adequately convey to supervisors the notion that part of their responsibility includes getting results through others. If the experience of management outside the hospital field holds true, this can prove to be one of the most valuable training investments a company or a hospital could make.

However, applying the domino aspect of motivation theory, if the supervisor is not herself adequately motivated by her immediate superior, the chances of her being able to pass this on to her subordinates is somewhat remote. It is necessary to set up an adequate instructional program throughout all levels of hospital management, so that the importance of motivation cannot only be preached, but effectively practiced.

THE HOSPITAL ADMINISTRATOR

In the evolution of modern management, as described in *Management Today,* in the spring, 1969, issue of this journal, emphasis has shifted from the autocratic to the supportive role, or from a posture of reacting to problems as they occur to an ability to anticipate problems before they arise. The change is similar from one of fighting fires by whatever means to installing a sprinkler system, so that when the fire occurs, it will automatically be extinguished.

The modern hospital administrator is called on to combine two seemingly impossible tasks. On the one hand, he must create a climate within which people can achieve their own personal objectives and, at the same time, he must also seek through them to achieve the economic objectives of the institution he manages. To accomplish the latter he must carefully predetermine what people are going to do, and have them do it in the most efficient manner possible. To accomplish the former, he must permit them enough freedom in working toward their part of the economic objectives of the institution so that they can find personal satisfaction in their work. Fortunately modern management planning systems, such as those built around management objectives permit him to overcome the apparent incompatibility.

MUST DETERMINE COMMITMENTS

As a professional manager, the hospital administrator must determine the economic, functional, service, and patient commitments of the hospital. He must communicate them effectively to all levels of supervision, and, through them, to the nursing staff. At the same time, he must create the necessary motivational climate so that all levels, depending as they do on the level above, and ultimately on him, can find the necessary freedom and self-determination to obtain maximum satisfaction from the work that they perform.

If all employees understand the intimate connection between profitability and patient satisfaction, the hospital will not only survive, but will have an opportunity to grow and expand its services to satisfy both the needs of patients today and the more demanding and complex needs of patients tomorrow.

FURTHER READINGS SUGGESTED BY THE AUTHOR

Argyris, Chris. *Personality and Organization.* (New York: Harper & Rowe, 1957).

Gellerman, Saul W. *Motivation and Productivity.* (New York: American Management Association, 1963).

Herzberg, Frederick, Bernard Mauser, and Barbara Synderman. *The Motivation to Work.* (New York: John Wiley & Sons, Inc., 1960).

Katz, Daniel. "The Motivational Basis of Organizational Behavior," *Behavioral Science,* April, 1964

Leadership and Supervision

In the next two selections the subject of leadership is presented. The first is descriptive while the second offers a model that seeks to indicate the leader behavior pattern most likely to be successful as the situational variable of employee "job maturity" changes. Selection 18, "EFFECTIVE SUPERVISION REQUIRES LEADERSHIP" by Thomas R. O'Donovan, examines the subject of leadership utilizing the broad category scheme that was previously presented. The writer does not make a clear distinction between the two leader-behavior dimensions we have identified; namely leader decision-making authority and the manner in which the leader oversees (supervises) the work activity, but the distinction is implied.

This selection begins with a discussion of the benefits of effective leadership. Next, it offers various contrasts such as "close versus general" characterizing supervisory styles and then clusters those styles with a description of the "person-centered—work-centered" supervisory styles. The latter corresponds to our previous presentation of the "employee-centered—work-centered" dichotomy. Finally, this selection closes a presentation of three leader decision-making authority styles labeled democratic, mature autocratic, and bureaucratic. Essentially, these three leader authority styles are analogous to those previously mentioned. Some of the insights offered by the writer relative to these styles make this selection informative.

In the text, it was noted that a number of factors affect the leader's decision-authority and supervisory styles. Among them are: the nature of the job, the urgency of the results, the characteristics of the subordinates, and the personality of the manager. In a few words these factors can be summarized as, "the situation." Selection 19, "A SITUATIONAL APPROACH TO SUPERVISION" by Hersey, Blanchard, and La Monica, offers an analysis with the aim of predicting leader behavior patterns most appropriate and effective given different situations.

This selection is rather complex, however, its attempt to be predictive makes it informative. That is, guidelines are offered whereby a situational variable (the job maturity of the subordinate) can be identified by the leader. Leader behavior can then be modified to correspond to the type most likely to be effective.

18.
Effective Supervision Requires Leadership

THOMAS R. O'DONOVAN

Thomas R. O'Donovan, Ph.D., is Administrator of Mount Carmel Mercy Hospital in Detroit, Michigan.

The concept of leadership refers to a process in which an individual is able to obtain voluntary cooperation in a goal or activity from another person or group of persons. Managers and supervisors who possess formal delegated authority in an organization become more effective when their style of leadership brings forth willful cooperation from their subordinates. This article will discuss some of the ways the supervisor can obtain the full support of his team. A major goal of any hospital is to provide a high level of patient care. Such care is administered by people. Therefore, supervision of these people is vitally important to the achievement of hospital goals. Without leadership, the supervisor's ability to obtain willful cooperation from his subordinates is impossible.

KINDS OF LEADERSHIP

The style of leadership that a supervisor should adopt depends upon a great many factors. His own personal goals and values, the character and goals of the organization, the type of subordinates involved, and the particular situation all will influence the choice of a particular leadership style. Each situation has to be considered on its own merit; however, some general statements can be made that are highly useful. Principles of leadership, like vitamins, are useful only when they are used correctly, and adaptation must be made to the individual situation. What is correct in one case may not be correct in another. A "correct" leadership style is important because of its effects on employe morale and productivity.

An improper leadership style may result in:

    a. A lowering of employe morale and motivation because of oversupervision (sometimes referred to as "snoopervision"), overly strict or distant supervision, etc. Management is interested in employe morale not only because of a humanistic concern for the employe's wellbeing but also because of its effects on employe productivity.

Reprinted by permission from *Hospital Progress: Journal of the Catholic Hospital Association,* St. Louis, Vol. 46 (February, 1965), 65-67, 103. Copyright 1965 by the Catholic Hospital Association. All rights reserved.

b. A lowering of employe productivity. This may be a decrease in either quantity or quality of employe work output per given unit of input. In a hospital for example, lower employe productivity would be reflected in a lower quality of patient care, increasing expenses, and waste.
  c. Increased employe absenteeism and turnover.
  d. Employe resistance to change.
  e. A decrease in the individual development of employes.

We shall identify six major question areas and give the implications for each area: 1. Shall I supervise my subordinates very closely by keeping tabs on every detail or shall I supervise them only in a general way? 2. As a supervisor, should I attempt to identify with my subordinates or with my superiors? 3. In the management of subordinates, should I tend to be distant toward them or friendly? 4. Should I be strict or lenient in supervision? 5. Should I tend to be "person-centered" in my leadership style or "work-centered?" 6. Which of the following specific leadership styles works best and under what conditions: the mature autocratic, the democratic, or the bureaucratic?

CLOSE VERSUS GENERAL SUPERVISION

Whether or not we should supervise subordinates very closely or in a general way depends upon a large number of variables. Unskilled or clerical jobs tend to require closer supervision than professional or managerial jobs. For example, maids and porters generally need closer supervision than medical secretaries and nurses. Supervision of unskilled or clerical jobs is typically related to actual job performance while supervision of the professional or managerial employe is related more to the checking of results. If an employe has been trusted in the past to do a good job, a supervisor would be grossly unfair if he did not demonstrate his trust appropriately.

New employes may require closer supervision than employes who have been on the job for a long period of time. This point may seem self-evident, but we must be quite careful not to give the impression that this temporary closeness of supervision is merely a "taste" of what is to come.

Close supervision is important in emergency situations. In a highly critical situation, it may be neccessary to give very specific instructions and follow every detail very closely. For example, in our orbital flights, the top officials of the National Aeronautics and Space Administration watch details very closely because small errors can cause complete disaster. The surgeon-nurse supervisory relationship during an operation is another example.

In general, people who have an optimistic view of how well their subordinates will perform tend to supervise in a general way, while the more pessimistic supervisors who feel that they cannot trust their employes to do an honest or accurate job will tend to watch things in closer detail. Obviously, if supervision is *too* general, control over results is reduced and serious error may creep in before it is possible to determine the problem. In most organizations, however, there is a tendency to supervise too closely rather than not close enough. The problem for the supervisor is one of striking a happy medium.

Several studies are available in the research literature that provide useful information regarding the second question. The Prudential Insurance Company Study[1] of office employes examined the productivity of work groups under supervisors who had different patterns of identification. The first group of supervisors tended to identify more with subordinates than with higher management. The results of the study showed that productivity was higher in the group in which the supervisors tended to identify more with the subordinates than with upper management. A similar study of foremen was performed at General Electric Company.[2] Here the findings were quite similar. The foremen in high-producing areas tended to identify more with their subordinates than with upper management.

Certain people, in interpreting these findings, point out that it is not a question of *which* group one should identify with, but *how* much identification should be made with each group. In other words, it is important to identify with both groups. The workers who report to a superior must trust him and respect his willingness to support them. At the same time, management must depend upon the supervisor to carry out established policies. Obviously, this situation can create conflict in the supervisory role. The superior is literally the "man-in-the-middle." It is up to him to determine the best course of action for his particular situation. The most that can be said is that there is no firm answer as to which group should be identified with the most. It depends upon the individual situation.

Nonetheless, the supervisor must occupy a different role than the worker, although a lack of organizational resources may make this impossible in certain temporary situations. The supervisor who plays a different role does not perform the same functions as rank and file workers, but assumes more of the functions traditionally associated with leadership. Research studies of clerical workers, railroad workers, and workers in heavy industry point out that supervisors with the better production records gave a larger proportion of their time to supervisory functions, especially to the interpersonal aspect of their jobs. The supervisors of the lower producing sections were more likely to spend their time in tasks which the men themselves were performing or in the paperwork aspect of their jobs.

DISTANT SUPERVISION?
FRIENDLY SUPERVISION?

Whether or not a supervisor should be distant or friendly with his subordinates is another question which cannot be answered easily one way or the other. One should be distant enough to retain the respect of his subordinates, yet friendly enough so that he can work well with them as a team. In the military service, officers are instructed not to become too involved in the personal lives of their troops. This is especially true in war time. In corporate management a military type of organization is seldom needed, but there is much to be learned from the military experience. If one is too friendly with subordinates, it may prevent him from disciplining an employe when discipline is warranted, or from organizing and structuring work activity. On the other hand, a too distant attitude may be interpreted by the employe as a lack of interest in him as an individual, with resultant lower employe morale. The supervisor again has to draw a happy medium, depending upon the particular situation.

STRICT SUPERVISION?
LENIENT SUPERVISION?

Douglas McGregor[3] provides us with a solid analysis of the role of supervision with regard to strictness versus leniency. He suggests that there are two major parts in the leadership process. The supervisor must have a warm, genuine human concern for the well-being of his subordinates and at the *same* time, he must require and maintain a high standard of performance. He suggests that the supervisor must be fair with his subordinates but at the same time he must be firm. If the supervisor does not require a strict standard of performance, then both performance and respect will tend to degenerate. If the supervisor is too wishy-washy, he cannot command the respect that is needed. The important thing is that these two behavior patterns must co-exist. If we are firm but not fair, we tend to lose the cooperation of the group. If we are fair but not firm enough, we lose control of the group.

PERSON-CENTERED?
WORK-CENTERED?

The issue of being "person-centered" rather than being "work-centered" refers to the following: the "person-centered" supervisor tends to look toward the individual human being as the center of the productivity wheel. He interprets his job as one of increasing employe motivation. A supervisor who is "work-centered" tends to ignore the human factor and concentrates on the production and technical aspects of the job. The "work-centered" supervisor thinks of his employes as cogs in the wheel of production.

Many studies have shown that the "person-centered" supervisor is far more effective than the "work-centered" supervisor.[4] Employe productivity and morale tend to be much higher when the supervisor is "person-centered." Many supervisors are work-oriented because their experiences have been heavily weighted this way. They have been trained to make things or to perform things. They were trained to accomplish the work that they are now delegating. For this reason, when confronted with a work problem, some supervisors who have this tendency will look around the problem involved to the work itself in searching for the cause. If the problem is with the people involved, it may be completely overlooked.

Several years ago, the Survey Research Center of the University of Michigan[5] studied the leadership and production aspects of a large number of clerical departments of the Prudential Life Insurance Company. Many sections of this company had comparable working conditions. The clerical work output was measurable and it was possible to relate production records to various kinds of supervisory practices. One finding of the study was that approximately 85 per cent of the supervisors in the high-producing groups were "employe-centered" whereas only 30 per cent of the supervisors in the low-producing groups were "employe-centered."

This last section will describe three different leadership styles and discuss briefly their implications. These approaches were adapted from the writings of Eugene E. Jennings.[6]

THE DEMOCRATIC APPROACH

The democratic supervisor looks to the group for direction. He values the group above himself and above the organization. He caters to the group's wishes and desires. He tends to knit his group into a harmonious team, so that the resultant cohesion disguises who is actually running things. Rather than making himself indispensable, his primary goal is to develop subordinates so that he becomes almost unnecessary. The democratic supervisor seeks, therefore, to involve every member in determining group activities and objectives. He is more interested in group competency than in his individual competency.

In its extreme form, this is the description of the "democratic" supervisor. Perhaps no supervisor is this way all the time. Most will vary their pattern to fit the situation and they must do this to be effective. The majority of supervisors agree that they should be democratic and seek the participation of subordinates. What if time and circumstances do not permit? Some subordinates do not wish to share in many decisions. People change, both as supervisors and as subordinates.

One can appraise himself and fellow supervisors, but will be unable to classify each supervisor as democratic, mature autocratic, or bureaucratic. Most supervisors attempt to adjust their behavior pattern as needed. The better supervisors know how to adjust to the needs of their subordinates. However, we do tend to lean toward one model more than to any other and constant shifting of gears is no easy task.

THE MATURE AUTOCRAT

The mature autocrat is not the ruthless autocrat that existed in the "captains of industry" era. Reference is not had here to the complete "one-man show" style of leadership although this is one of the styles available to supervisors. The mature autocrat is the supervisor who wants to run with the ball but, at the same time, wants to make the team feel needed. The mature autocrat is a highly competent individual and an excellent decision-maker. He controls individually and uses personal influence. He is a decision-maker but he works through and with people. The mature autocrat is highly polished while the typical stereotype of the autocrat tends to be very crude.

The most important quality that the mature autocrat should possess is sincerity. This means that the mature autocrat makes up his mind and then works with the group in such a way that they come up with the same decision. Thus, when the decision is implemented, group members feel they have played a significant role. If, however, a supervisor attempted to use this leadership style and was insincere, then the entire model and perhaps the entire work group organization would likely split wide open. Mature autocracy and insincerity are incompatible. If at any time, the group does *not* come up with the same decision as the mature autocratic supervisor, he must either successfully show why the group's decision cannot be implemented (i.e., due to top management policy), or he must accept the group's decision. Thus, the mature autocrat doesn't "get his way" all the time and does not expect to. His major skill is in his ability to predict the group's reactions.

THE BUREAUCRAT

The bureaucrat does not recognize the individual or the group as much as the organization. He is a system-builder and places his faith in the ultimate perfectability of that system. This supervisor allows no violation of rules and procedures under any circumstances. If violation occurs, disciplinary action follows immediately. He wants every potential situation covered in a procedures manual so that individual judgment becomes unnecessary. This is a brief description of the bureaucratic model of leadership as viewed in its extreme form.

Managers today are tending more toward the bureaucratic leadership style than toward the mature autocratic or the democratic style. The aggressive attitude of the autocrat assures the enterprise of periodic rejuvenation and is largely the reason why our business system in the past has maintained its healthy vigor. As businesses increase in complexity, the importance of a bureaucratic structure becomes increasingly important. However, at the same time that bureaucrats replace autocrats, the essential creativity of our business system may be subjected to considerable dilution. The organization cannot become too engulfed in excessive rules and regulations. What the organization requires is a style of supervisory leadership that is a balance of the bureaucratic, the autocratic, and the democratic approaches—the *multicrat*.

CONCLUSION

As can be readily seen, most of the major areas discussed overlap closely.[7] A supervisor who is distant may also be strict. A supervisor who identifies with superiors may be somewhat distant. Each of these major subject areas that have been examined should be integrated with the others in order to establish the kind of leadership style that each supervisor would look forward to shaping for himself. These things have to follow in a natural way. A leadership role cannot be turned off and on like a faucet. The integration of a leadership style depends on individual philosophy and values, individual opinions, and individual attitudes toward people. A successful supervisor is a product of his team.

The choice of a leadership pattern is usually quite limited because of the factors listed at the beginning of this article. Certainly one limiting factor is the style of leadership exhibited by the supervisor's supervisor. The supervisor can, however, look ahead months or years to strategically determine at which point on the continuum he will act. This point will vary with the objectives he wishes to accomplish, his own personality and values, the characteristics of the situation.

There is no *one* leadership style correct for all supervisors at all times and in all places. This does not mean, however, that leadership cannot be scientifically examined. When the *total* situation has been carefully examined, a correct and satisfying pattern of leadership can be developed. Leadership is an art built upon scientific inquiry. We must be ourselves but at the same time, we must understand and watch ourselves. Supervision requires "super-vision."

REFERENCES

[1] Morse, Nancy C., *Satisfactions in White Collar Jobs.* Ann Arbor, Survey Research Centers, University of Michigan, 1953.

[2] Ponder, Quentin D., "The Effective Manufacturing Foreman," in *Proceedings of the Tenth Annual Meeting.* Madison, Wis., Industrial Relations Research Association, 1957, pp. 51-54; General Electric Company, Public and Employee Relations Research Service, *The Effective Manufacturing Foreman* (processed 1957).

[3] McGregor, Douglas, *The Human Side of Enterprise.* New York, McGraw-Hill Book Co., Inc., 1959.

[4] Cartwright, Dorwin and Zander, Alvin. eds., *Group Dynamics,* Evanston, Ill., Row, Peterson, 1953.

[5] Kahn, Robert L. and Katz, Daniel, "Leadership Practices in Relationship to Productivity and Morale," *Group Dynamics.* Dorwin Cartwright and Alvin Zander, eds., Evanston, Ill., Row, Peterson, 1953, pp. 612-628.

[6] Jennings, Eugene E., *The Executive.* New York, Harper, 1962.

[7] Jennings, Eugene E., *An Anatomy of Leadership,* New York, Harper, 1960.

19.
A Situational Approach to Supervision: Leadership Theory and the Supervising Nurse

PAUL HERSEY, KENNETH H. BLANCHARD, and ELAINE L. LaMONICA

Paul Hersey, Ph.D., is Professor of Organizational Behavior and Management and Director, Center for Leadership Studies, Ohio University.

Kenneth H. Blanchard, Ph.D., is Professor of Leadership and Organizational Behavior and Director, Center for Curriculum and Organizational Development, School of Education, University of Massachusetts.

Elaine L. LaMonica, R.N., Ed.D., is Associate Professor, Department of Nursing Education, Columbia University

Recognition that nurses need to become effective managers, supervisors, and administrators had pervaded the writings of nursing theorists[1] over the years. The methods for providing nursing care have moved from case to functional, followed by establishment of the team concept, and then primary nursing. Styles of leadership have varied in each: autocratic, democratic, or laissez faire behavior of the leader in any given situation.

The variety of environments in nursing practice have expanded concurrently with the various preparations provided by educational institutions for prospective nurses. It has become increasingly apparent that nurse leaders must broaden their views, their knowledge, and their experience of leader behavior to accommodate the added responsibility placed on them by their organizational administration, by the specific goals of the facility, and by the individual experiences, backgrounds and needs of their nurses.

The purpose of this article is to provide the nurse supervisor with a leadership theory which may be helpful in determining the situational demands which she may confront. This theory is intended to provide a conceptual framework that may enable nursing leaders to increase their effectiveness in working with individual nurses and their individual environments.

A "BEST" STYLE OF LEADERSHIP?

The quest for an ideal type of leadership has appeared in management literature ever since the apparent conflict between the Scientific Management and the Human

---

Reprinted by permission of *Supervisor Nurse*, Vol. 7, No. 5 (May, 1976), pp. 17-20, 22. Copyright 1976 by *Supervisor Nurse*. All rights reserved.

Relations schools of thought. The scientific management school emphasized a concern for task (production), while the human relations movement stressed concern for relationships (people).

The recognition of task and relationship as two different styles of leader behavior has pervaded the works of management theorists[2] over the past several decades. These styles have been defined as:

Task Behavior:

The extent to which a leader organizes and defines the roles of individuals and members of her group by explaining what activities each is to do as well as when, where and how tasks are to be accomplished. It is further characterized by the extent to which a leader defines patterns of organization, formalizes channels of communication, and specifies ways of getting jobs accomplished.

Relationship Behavior:

The extent to which a leader engages in personal relationships with individuals or members of her group; the amount of socio-emotional support and psychological strokes provided by the leader as well as the extent to which the leader engages in interpersonal communications and facilitating behaviors.[3]

These two styles have been variously labeled, including such popular terminology as autocratic vs. democratic, employee-oriented or production-oriented, and goal achievement or group maintenance.

For some time, it was believed that task and relationship were *either/or* styles of leader behavior and, therefore, could be depicted on a single dimension, a continuum, moving from very authoritarian (Task) leader behavior at one end to very democratic (Relationship) leader behavior at the other.[4]

In more recent years, the feeling that task and relationship were *either/or* leadership styles has been dispelled. In particular, the leadership studies initiated in 1945 by the Bureau of Business Research at Ohio State University questioned this assumption.[5]

Observing the actual behavior of leaders in a wide variety of situations, the Ohio State staff found that leadership styles tended to vary considerably from leader to leader. The behavior of some was characterized mainly by structuring activities of followers in terms of task accomplishments, while others concentrated on providing socio-emotional support in terms of personal relationships among themselves and their followers. Other leaders had styles characterized by both task and relationship behavior. There were even some individuals in leadership positions whose behavior tended to provide little structure or consideration.

No dominant style appeared. Instead, various combinations were evident. Thus, it was determined that task and relationship are not *either/or* leadership styles as an authoritarian-democratic continuum suggests. Instead, these patterns of leader behavior can be plotted on two separate axes as shown in Figure 1.

The Basic Leader Behavior Styles

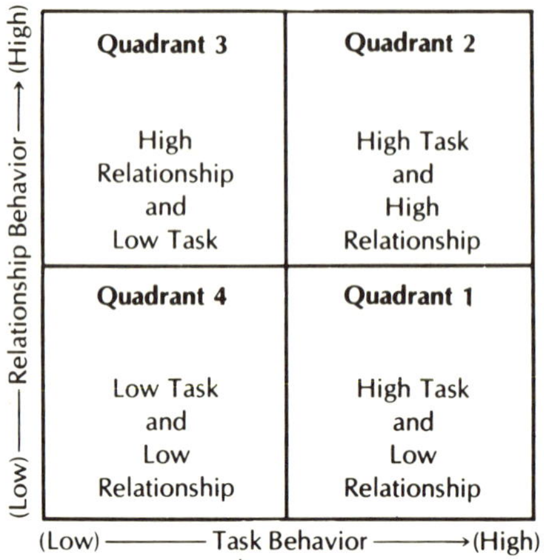

(High)	**Quadrant 3** High Relationship and Low Task	**Quadrant 2** High Task and High Relationship
(Low) ← Relationship Behavior →	**Quadrant 4** Low Task and Low Relationship	**Quadrant 1** High Task and Low Relationship

(Low) ——— Task Behavior ——→ (High)

Figure 1.

Tri-Dimensional Model:

After identifying task and relationship as the two central aspects of leader behavior, numerous practitioners and writers tried to determine which of the four basic styles depicted was the "best" style of leadership, that is, the one which would be successful in most situations. At one point, high task/high relationship (quadrant 2) was considered the "worst" style.[6]

Yet, evidence from research in the last decade clearly indicates that there is no single all-purpose leadership style.[7] Successful leaders are those who can adapt their behavior to meet the demands of their own unique environment.

If the effectiveness of a leader behavior style depends on the situation in which it is used, it follows that any of the four basic styles in Figure 1 may be effective or ineffective depending on the situation. The difference between the effective and the ineffective styles is often not the actual behavior of the leader, but the appropriateness of this behavior to the situation in which it is used. In an attempt to illustrate this concept and build on previous work in leadership, an effectiveness dimension was added to the task and relationship dimensions of earlier leadership models to create the Tri-Dimensional Leader Effectiveness Model[8] presented in Figure 2.

**The tri-dimensional
leader effectiveness model**

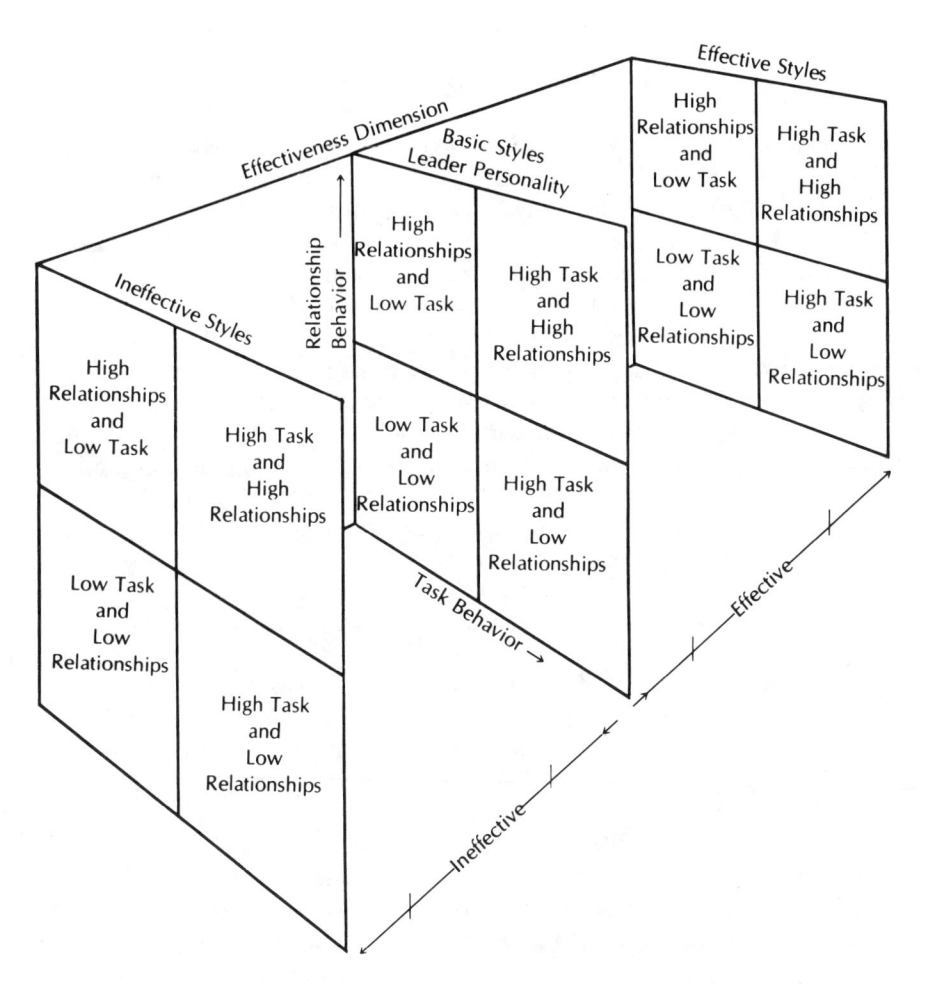

Figure 2.

The middle quadrants represent the four basic leader behavior styles; the left quadrants illustrate the four basic styles when they are ineffective (used in an inappropriate situation); and the right quadrants illustrate the four basic styles when they are effective (used in an appropriate situation).

The Tri-Dimensional Leader Effectiveness Model is distinctive because it does not depict a single ideal leader behavior style which is suggested to be appropriate in all situations. In essence, an effective leader must be able to *diagnose* the demands of the environment, and then *adapt* her leader style to fit these demands, or develop the means to change some of the other variables or all of them.

SITUATIONAL LEADERSHIP THEORY

Even nursing supervisors who realize that they must adapt their style of leadership to meet the demands of their environment are frustrated by the conclusion that the type of leader behavior needed "depends on the situation." They find little practical value in theory unless they can begin to see HOW leadership depends on the situation and, therefore, WHAT style tends to be effective with particular individuals and groups in changing environments. Yet, few theoretical frameworks have been developed to help supervisors diagnose the demands of their situation. This scarcity of practical situational leadership theories was one of the forces which motivated Hersey and Blanchard to develop *Life Cycle Theory of Leadership*.[9] This situational theory is based on a relationship among the amount of direction (Task Behavior) a leader gives; the amount of socio-emotional support (Relationship Behavior) a leader provides; and the "maturity" of her followers or group. Followers in any situation are vital, not only because individually they accept or reject the leader, but also because as a group they actually determine whatever personal power she may have. Maturity is defined in Life Cycle Theory as the capacity to set high but attainable goals (achievement-motivation),[10] willingness and ability to take responsibility, and the education and the experience of an individual or a group. These variables of maturity should be considered in relation to a specific task to be performed. That is to say, an individual or a group is not mature or immature in any global sense, but is mature or immature only in terms of a specific task. Thus a new graduate may be very responsible in providing care for three or four individual patients, but not experienced in leading a team who care for sixteen patients.

According to Life Cycle Theory, as the level of maturity of one's followers continues to increase in terms of accomplishing a specific task, leaders should begin to *reduce* their task behavior and *increase* relationship behavior until the individual or group is sufficiently mature for the leaders to decrease their relationship styles according to the level of maturity of the followers. This cycle can be illustrated by the bell-shaped curve going through the four leadership quadrants as shown in Figure 3.

As can be seen in Figure 3, the curvilinear function of the cycle would be portrayed on the effective side of the Tri-Dimensional Leader Effectiveness Model. To determine what style is appropriate with what individual or group, some benchmarks of maturity have been provided for determining appropriate leadership style by dividing the maturity continuum into three categories—low, moderate, and high.

This theory of leadership states that when working with people who are low in maturity in terms of accomplishing a specific task, a high task style (quadrant 1) has the highest probability of success; whereas in dealing with people who are of average

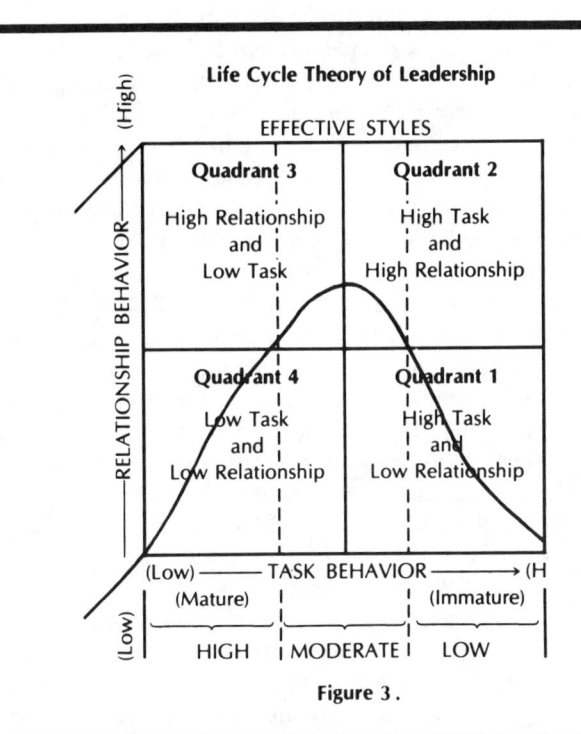

Life Cycle Theory of Leadership

EFFECTIVE STYLES

Quadrant 3 High Relationship and Low Task	**Quadrant 2** High Task and High Relationship
Quadrant 4 Low Task and Low Relationship	**Quadrant 1** High Task and Low Relationship

RELATIONSHIP BEHAVIOR (Low to High) — TASK BEHAVIOR (Low to High)

(Mature) — HIGH | MODERATE | LOW — (Immature)

Figure 3.

maturity on a task, moderate structure and moderate-to-high socio-emotional style (quadrants 2 and 3) appear to be most appropriate; and a low task and low relationship style (quadrant 4) has the highest probability of success working with people of high task maturity.

Modifying Levels of Maturity:

In attempting to help a staff nurse or a group to mature, *i.e.*, to get them to take more and more responsibility for performing a specific task, a nursing leader must be careful not to delegate responsibility or to increase socio-emotional support too rapidly. If the leader does this, the individual nurse or group may take advantage and view the leader as a "soft-touch." Thus the leader must develop the maturity of followers slowly on each task that they must perform, using less task behavior and more relationship behavior as they mature and become more willing and able to take responsibility. When a staff nurse's performance is low on a specific task, one cannot expect drastic changes overnight. For a desirable behavior to be obtained, a supervisor must reward as soon as possible the slightest behavior exhibited by the nurse in the desired direction and continue this process as the individual's behavior comes closer and closer to the nursing leader's expectations of good performance. This is a behavior modification concept called *positively reinforcing successive approximations*[11] *of a desired behavior*. For example, a head nurse might want to move a new graduate through the cycle so that she would assume significantly more responsibility as a team member. If the new graduate is normally dependent on her head nurse for clarification and direction regarding the care of her four assigned patients, the head nurse can reduce the close supervision by asking the new graduate what she thinks needs to be done and adding to this only when quality care will not be provided for the patient. This will allow the staff nurse to begin to trust her own experience and knowledge. If the responsibility is well-handled, the head nurse should reinforce this behavior with increases in socio-emotional support or relationship behavior. This is a two-step process: first, a reduction in structure, and second, if adequate performance follows, an increase in socio-emotional support as reinforcement. This process should continue until the new graduate is carrying out all phases of patient care as a mature individual. This does not mean that the nurse's work will have less structure, but rather that the structure now will be internally provided by the individual instead of being externally imposed by the head nurse. When this happens, the cycle as depicted by Life Cycle Theory of leadership in Figure 3 begins to become a backward bending curve and to move toward Quadrant 4 (low task behavior and low relationship behavior). The staff nurses are able not only to structure many of the activities in which they engage while working on a specific task, but also are able to provide their own satisfaction for interpersonal and emotional needs. At this stage of maturity staff nurses are positively reinforced for their accomplishments by the supervisor not looking over their shoulders on a specific task and by the supervisor leaving them more and more on their own. It is not that there is less mutual trust and friendship but rather that less overt behavior is needed to prove it.

Although this theory suggests a basic style for different levels of task maturity, it is not a one-way street. When people begin to behave less maturely for whatever reason, *i.e.*, crisis at home, change in unit assignment, etc., it becomes appropriate for the supervisor to adjust behavior backward through the curve to meet the present maturity level of her group. For example, take the staff nurse who is presently working well on her own. Suppose, suddenly, the nurse faces a family crisis which begins to affect her performance on the job. In this situation, it may be appropriate for the supervisor moderately to increase structure and socio-emotional support until the individual regains his or her composure.

In summary, it is important for nursing supervisors to be aware of any progress of their subordinates so that they are in a position to appropriately reinforce improved performance. It must be remembered that change through the cycle from Quadrant 1 to Quadrant 2, 3 and 4 must be gradual. This process by its very nature cannot be revolutionary but must be evolutionary—it requires gradual developmental changes, a result of planned growth and the creation of mutual trust and respect.

FOOTNOTES

[1] As examples see the following: L. Douglass. *Review of Team Nursing.* St. Louis: C.V. Mosby Co., 1973; L. Douglass and E. Bevis. *Team Leadership in Action: Principles and Application to Staff Nursing Situations.* St. Louis: C.V. Mosby Co., 1970; Grace Eckelberry. *Administration of Comprehensive Nursing Care.* New York: Appleton-Century-Crofts, 1971; T. Kron. *The Management of Patient Care.* Phila.: W.B. Saunders Co., 1971.

[2] As examples see the following: Robert F. Bales, "Task Roles and Social Roles in Problem-Solving Groups," in *Readings in Social Psychology,* E.E. Maccoby, T.M. Newcomb and E.L. Hartley (eds.) New York: Holt, Rinehart and Winston, 1958; Chester I. Bernard, *The Functions of the Executive.* Cambridge, Massachusetts: Harvard University Press, 1938; Dorwin Cartwright and Alvin Zander (eds.). *Group Dynamics: Research and Theory,* second edition. Evanston, Illinois: Row, Peterson and Company, 1960; D. Katz, N. Maccoby, and Nancy C. Morse. *Productivity, Supervision, and Morale in an Office Situation.* Detroit, Michigan: The Darel Press, Inc., 1950; Talcott Parsons. *The Social System.* Glencoe, Illinois: The Free Press, 1951.

[3] These definitions have been adapted from The Ohio State definitions of "Initiating Structure" and "Consideration," Andrew W. Halpin, *The Leadership Behavior of School Superintendents.* Chicago: Midwest Administration Center, The University of Chicago, 1959, p. 4; and Roger M. Stogdill and Alvin E. Coons (ed.), *Leader Behavior: Its Description and Measurement,* Research Monograph No. 88. Columbus, Ohio: Bureau of Business Research, The Ohio State University, 1957.

[4] Robert Tannenbaum and Warren H. Schmidt, "How to Choose a Leadership Pattern," *Harvard Business Review,* March-April, 1957, pp. 95-101.

[5] Stogdill and Coons, *op. cit.,* note 3.

[6] See Andrew W. Halpin, *op. cit.,* note 3. Robert R. Blake and Jane S. Mouton. *The Managerial Grid.* Houston, Texas: Gulf Publishing, 1964; and Rensis Likert. *New Patterns of Management.* New York: McGraw-Hill Book Company, 1961.

[7] As examples see A. K. Korman, " 'Consideration,' 'Initiating Structure,' and Organization Criteria–A Review," *Personnel Psychology: A Journal of Applied Research,* XIX, No. 4, Winter 1966, pp. 349-61; and Fred E. Fiedler. *A Theory of Leadership Effectiveness,* New York: McGraw-Hill Book Company, 1967.

[8] Paul Hersey and Kenneth Blanchard. *Management of Organizational Behavior: Utilizing Human Resources.* Englewood Cliffs, New Jersey: Prentice Hall, Inc., pp. 81-87. For a discussion of an early attempt to add an effectiveness dimension to the task and relationships dimensions see William J. Reddin, "The 3-D Management Style Theory," *Training and Development Journal,* April 1967, pp. 8-17; see also Reddin, *Management Effectiveness.* New York: McGraw-Hill Book Company, 1970.

[9] This theory was first published in Paul Hersey and Kenneth H. Blanchard, "Life Cycle Theory of Leadership," *Training and Development Journal,* May, 1969, and was further refined in Hersey and Blanchard, *Management of Organizational Behavior, op. cit.,* note 8.

[10] David C. McClelland, J. W. Atkinson, R. A. Clark, and E. L. Lowell. *The Achievement Motive.* New York: Appleton-Century-Crofts, Inc., 1953, and *The Achieving Society.* Princeton, New Jersey: D. Van Nostrand Co., 1961.

[11] The most classic discussions of behavior modification, or operant conditioning, have been done by B. F. Skinner. See Skinner. *Science and Human Behavior.* New York: The Macmillan Company, 1953.

Managerial Approaches

The last two selections in this part elaborate on the managerial approaches of participative management and delegation. In Selection 20, "PARTICIPATIVE MANAGEMENT: A VALID ALTERNATIVE TO TRADITIONAL ORGANIZATIONAL BEHAVIOR" by Barbara Snyder Hill, the subject of participation is presented. Viewing the manager as a change agent, a primary role is involving subordinates. The writer suggests that participative management is a healthy, viable approach useful in managing hospital employees. Benefits, as well as risks involved, are presented.

The final selection in this part (21), "MASTERING THE MANAGERIAL SKILL OF DELEGATION" by Elena M. Volante, focuses on the importance of delegation for supervisory nurses. Although it focuses on one particular employee classification, the principles apply to all who manage other people. Building on the contention that delegation is a difficult skill to learn, the writer identifies numerous costs or disadvantages that occur from ineffective delegation. Following that, supervisory attitudes toward delegation and the steps involved, with guidelines, are presented.

20.
Participative Management: A Valid Alternative to Traditional Organizational Behavior

BARBARA SNYDER HILL

Barbara Snyder Hill, R.N., M.S., is Assistant Professor, Department of Nursing, Indiana University - Purdue University.

Traditionally, organizational management has been practiced through superior-subordinate relationships. These relationships have resulted in high productivity, but not without many psychological and sociological consequences. In recent years the humanization of organizations within society has received much study. Participation of subordinate members in the management of an organization can be rewarding for both the individual and the organization. Major benefits of management through participation have been revealed in business and nursing literature. Its acceptance as a preferred method should be a careful consideration for all organizations.

The exercise of authoritarian management appeared at the time of the Industrial Revolution and was founded in the philosophy of the basic evilness of man. Inherent in this philosophy was the belief that the subordinate man would work only when chided and monetarily rewarded because he had little initiatory or motivational drive. Believing this, the superior man controlled his subordinates' lives so that the organizational goals were met. Production was at an all time high at the expense of low morale. The evidence of low morale—absenteeism and high turnover—was usually ignored or ill-handled.

Research has shown that the behavior of the subordinate members can be improved when consideration of their humanness is a factor in achieving organizational goals. Theorists including Tannenbaum and Blake have consistently shown that high productivity and high consideration can occur simultaneously.[1] It appears that many behaviorists are urging the move toward participation of all group members as the potential panacea for organization.

Group decision-making as the *alpha* of participative management in health organizations would more surely meet the needs of our present society than traditional methods. This concept was advanced by Pellegrino when he wrote that for the good of the patient, decision-making must be restructured to meet the demands of a demo-

---

Reprinted by permission of *Supervisor Nurse*, Vol. 7, No. 3 (March, 1976), pp. 19-21. Copyright 1976 by *Supervisor Nurse*. All rights reserved.

cratic society and a highly organized system of health care delivery.[2] The patient has a right to expect his needs to be dealt with effectively. This right can only be achieved if the patient is involved with the decision as it relates to his illness and its outcome.

The process of social exchange, lacking in authoritarian management, is a prime ingredient in participative management. Knowles wrote that these relationships are "characterized by attitudes of cooperation based on feelings of mutual trust and openness."[3] He stated that this process provides a stark contrast to traditional "patterns of competitiveness and impersonality which are frequently destructive and negative in dimension."[4] Huse and Bowditch have stated that leadership is the effort to influence or change the behavior of others in order to accomplish both organizational and personal goals.[5] He added, however, that the ultimate control in the influence and change process rests with the changee. It is important for the follower to understand the problem and the reasons for the proposed change, because he perceives the problem on his own terms. Both the leader and the follower must be adept in the sharing of ideas and the assumption of responsibility for change.

PREPARATION

Effective participative management can become a reality only after a great deal of prior planning relative to climate and to leader and member preparation. The development of a favorable climate of relationships is essential. This climate can be accomplished through the reinforcement of certain attitudes of the leader and the group members. Leadership style is a product of individual development over time and cannot be easily changed.[6] Therefore, training for leaders that will concentrate on enhancing an optimistic view of the nature of man must be instituted. When a leader employs this outlook he will be more accepting of himself and more responsive to others' needs. The successful leader of a synergistic group represents a consistency of values which leads to the development of professionalism on the part of the members. The leader actually encourages in members the growth of attributes and attitudes associated with life itself. Together, the synergistic group achieves self-discipline, self-control, and simultaneously more effectively meets both organizational and personal goals.

Members of a group look for the most articulate and powerful person among them and expect him to represent their interests. The leader performs a service to the members and should be selected for the extent to which he can represent the members' interests.[7]

A dynamic leader is one who functions as a change agent. Knowles states that the leadership role is really a value carrier to be emulated by the organizational members. In other words, the leader should be able to crystallize the organizational values so that they will coincide with both group and individual goals.[8]

The preparation of the group members' attitudes is also inherent in the effectiveness of all organizations. Educators are beginning to respond to the plea for participation from employees and students. The teacher's relationship with the principal was found to be a much more important satisfier than the teacher's relationship with other teachers.[9] This finding implies that communication to the subordinate and understanding by him of the group's objectives are essential. The causative factors in low morale and job dissatisfaction were policy and administration. Recognition, responsibility, achievement, advancement and a voice in management are job satisfiers.[10] Teachers (as group members) must be prepared for participative decision-making by being informed and willing to make suggestions. It must be communicated that their position will not be jeopardized by the expression of those suggestions. Teachers must also assume an active role in gaining information about present and future trends. Involvement of all group members is the key to making the good decision better.

Participative organizational behavior must include a plan for student involvement if it is to be effective in today's educational society. Involved nursing students become graduates who are self-directive and creatively responsive to patients.[11] Mauksch contended that involvement in group decision-making is better than a traditional classroom experience. In addition more learning would take place in a classroom if the learning experience decisions were the result of shared ideas. When the student has assumed the role of constructive dissent (ability to examine critically and objectively positions held by others) then education has become a mind-liberating force.

The leader-member preparation for group participation promotes a climate in which the clarification of individual expectations and ideologies merge with organization goals. Synergistic clinical decision-making in hospitals can be achieved only after analysis and resolution of role incongruities, conflicts, and expectations.[12] The resultant rational delivery of health care would begin to close the gap between the expectations of the consumer and those of the providers.

Summarizing, participative management requires careful planning prior to the implementation of the theory. The leader selection and preparation will not provide successful implementation unless preparation of the group members is also instituted. The careful preparation of the leader and members will encourage that climate which fosters participative decision-making.

EFFECTS

What can organizations expect if implementation of participative management occurs? Some of Likert's research findings relative to the effects of participative management implementation demand our close attention:

- Freedom to set one's own work pace is directly related to productivity.
- An effective interaction-influence system is required for high performance.
- Participative methods of management enhance human resources for longer gains.
- In a favorable organizational climate, participative management methods reduce resistance to change and increase productivity.[13]

These findings, though business-oriented, hold implications for nursing education and nursing practice. For example, Pellegrino reported that larger community understanding and agreement on goals for health personnel was an incentive-producing process.[14]

Because of conflict in hierarchical control in large hospitals, Starkweather has developed a model for "troika" management of complete and separate hospital divisions.[15] The "troika" composition for each "mini-hospital" would include an administrative assistant, a physician, and a chief clinical nurse. Authority would be delegated to this group, skilled in communication, to make important decisions regarding their "mini-hospital." Integration of goals nearer to the consumer level would be a beneficial result.

Mackie, a nurse educator, developed and tested a model using two different teaching approaches to compare student satisfaction.[16] One group had a traditional classroom situation. The second group participated in defining their own goals and activities within broad limits. Students also selected specific content, resource material and the methods of presentation. The instructor participated as a group member and offered suggestions and guidance. Both satisfaction and concrete learning ability improved under the latter plan.

It was found that the practice of participative management in the university setting has become a limited reality.[17] The process by which decisions are made was almost uniform in nature. Those who were interviewed neither stated nor implied that "orders" were given or received; rather consultation and coordination were the words used to describe the interaction of the faculty with the department chairman. The five institutions studied appeared to have administrators who conducted themselves as equals, not superiors of their colleagues. However, a distortion of the participative decision-making process occurred when a member's salary increment was dependent on decision-making agreement with the department chairman. The need for change of evaluation procedures was noted.

Thus, the method for evaluation becomes of prime importance to successful implementation of participatory decision-making. Peter Drucker's *Management by Objectives* is a widely used plan for evaluation of participative management. This approach is based on the clarification of goals at the outset.[18] It should link the goals of the manager and his unit to the total objectives and success of the enterprise, and also to the needs and objectives of the individual group members. Management by objectives motivates and develops managers and ensures three outcomes in addition: the work gets done better; the overall objectives are met; and the organizational objectives more closely fit the individual objectives, in turn motivating the individual member. The process is one in which the leader and the members share equally in defining the goals for the organization; the group and the individual. Together they also decide the major areas of responsibility for each in terms of what each is expected to do. These measures then serve as guides for determining the contribution of each member as well as the unit as a whole. There must be agreement on the standard of performance and positive reinforcement of the desired behaviors.

Greater involvement in goal setting results in better communications, increased productivity, and increased motivation and agreement for both the leader and the group members. Management by objectives needs to be a continuous process to meet the changing needs of the organization and its members.

THE RISKS

Participative management is not without fault, and may involve a certain amount of risk. Tannenbaum wrote that some unfavorable by-products have been suggested by Strauss.[19] These include:

1. Individuals whose opinions have been rejected by the group may become alienated from it.
2. Participation may lead to greater cohesion but it may be cohesion against management.
3. Participation may set up expectations of continued participation which management may not be able to satisfy.
4. Participation often takes a great deal of time, can be frustrating to those involved, and frequently results in watered-down solutions.

However, participative management *is* a valid alternative to traditional organizational behavior. The incorporation of member consideration in accomplishing high productivity is an effective motivator. Even though there are some disadvantages to this method of operation, careful planning and evaluation will effect a successful implementation. Through participation in decision-making leaders and members can achieve a higher sense of self-esteem while becoming sensitive to others' needs. Health organizations and the society of which they are a part would reap an abundant harvest of understanding and achievement from the implementation of participative management.

FOOTNOTES

[1] Huse, Edgar, and James L. Bowditch. *Behavior in Organizations: A Systems Approach to Managing.* Reading, Massachusetts: Addison-Wesley, 1973.

[2] Pellegrino, Edmund D., "The Changing Matrix of Clinical Decision-Making in the Hospital," in *Organizational Research on Health Institutions,* pp. 301-327, edited by Basil Georgopoulos, Institute for Social Research, The University of Michigan, Ann Arbor, Michigan, 1972.

[3] Knowles, Henry, and Boye O. Saxberg. *Personality and Leadership Behavior.* Reading, Massachusetts: Addison-Wesley, 1971, 164 pp.

[4] *Ibid.,* p. 145.

[5] *Op. cit.* Huse and Bowditch.

[6] *Op. cit.,* Knowles.

[7] Hobbs, Walter, and G. Lester Anderson, "The Operation of Academic Departments," in *Readings in Organizations,* pp. 106-119, edited by James L. Gibson, *et al.* Dallas: Business Publications, 1973.

[8] *Op. cit.,* Knowles.

[9] Ellenberg, F. C., "Factors Affecting Teacher Morale, Meaning for Principals," *NASSP Bulletin,* 37-45, December, 1970.

[10] Howard, Alvin, "Junior High and Middle School-Teachers' Involvement on the Management Team," *NASSP Bulletin,* 110-117, May, 1973.

[11] Mauksch, Ingeborg G., "Let's Listen to the Student," *Nursing Outlook,* 20:103-107, February, 1972.

[12] *Op. cit.,* Pellegrino.

[13] Pigors, Paul, and Charles A. Myers, *Personnel Administration, A Point of View and A Method.* New York: McGraw-Hill, 1973, 588 pp.

[14] *Op. cit.,* Pellegrino.

[15] Starkweather, David B., "The Rationale for Decentralization in Large Hospitals," in *Readings in Organizations.* See Note 7.

[16] Mackie, Joan Barcy, "Comparison of Student Satisfaction with Educational Experiences in Two Teaching Process Models," *Nursing Research,* 22:262-266, May-June, 1973.

[17] *Op. cit.,* Hobbs and Anderson.

[18] *Op. cit..,* Huse and Bowditch.

[19] Tannenbaum, Arnold S. *Social Psychology of the Work Organization.* Belmont, California: Wadsworth Publishing Company, 1966, 136 pp.

21.
Mastering the Managerial Skill of Delegation

ELENA M. VOLANTE

Elena M. Volante, B.A., is Director of Public Relations for the McLean Hospital in Belmont, Massachusetts.

Delegation is a key managerial function. It is a means, or process, if you will, through which a supervisor (or manager) gets the necessary work done through other personnel or sources.

The question for every RN who supervises others is not whether she delegates. In fact, the nature of her role requires that she assign work to those who report to her. Rather, the question is how much and how effectively she delegates. A second question is whether she is content to delegate, as best she can, acting by trial and error as she goes along; or whether she improves her skill in delegating as she would any other by conscious analysis of what is involved and concentrated effort to master the skill.

The ability to delegate skillfully is a major issue concerning all kinds of supervisory positions in hospitals. There was a time when what is inelegantly but accurately referred to as "seat of the pants" management was enough. But today, our organizations are becoming increasingly complex and require more sophisticated managerial techniques than ever before. These skills do not come easily, but many can be acquired through conscious effort.

Delegation is a major skill that must be mastered by the RN in a supervisory role. Failure to delegate effectively has the potential for many negative results:

1. It results in higher management costs. If tasks that could be done by those who report to a supervisor are, in fact, done by the supervisor herself, they are more costly. Obviously, she is paid more than those who work for her. This is one of the biggest hidden costs in management, i.e., work done at the wrong level by the wrong person.

2. If a supervisor is busy doing things that those who report to her could well do, she has little time left to plan and do those things only she has the skill, knowledge, and authority to handle. This is a second hidden cost for all kinds of institutions;

Reprinted by permission of the *Journal of Nursing Administration,* Vol. 4, No. 1 (January-February, 1974), pp. 20-22. Copyright 1974 by *Journal of Nursing Administration.* All rights reserved.

namely, professional personnel are not finding time to do the work they have been hired and paid to do. They are too busy doing work others are paid to do.

3. Still another major cost of ineffective delegation is engendered by the supervisor who cannot bring herself to delegate and thus does not enable her staff to grow. Most developmental theorists believe that employees best develop by doing, by being given challenging opportunities to increase their skills and abilities on the job. The supervisor who is reluctant to "let go" deprives those who work for her of the opportunity to develop as individuals. And she deprives her organization of potentially higher employee contributions.

ATTITUDES THAT LEAD TO UNDERDELEGATING

There are many attitudes on the part of supervisors that lead to their not delegating as much as they should. Some are valid and some are not. Time and risk factors as well as feelings about subordinates and the self underlie some of the attitudes commonly expressed by supervisors to explain or rationalize why they do not delegate more.

Time Factors

1. Initially, it takes more time to explain what's needed than for me to do the job myself.
2. I'm constantly interrupted to answer questions and give guidance while the work is in progress.
3. Finally, at some point, I have to check that it's been done and done right—something I could avoid if I did it myself.
4. If the task involves other departments, I can usually get decisions and cooperation from them more easily and quickly than the people who work for me can.

Risk Factors

1. If my people make a mistake, I'll be blamed.
2. If they make more than a couple of mistakes while they're learning, their performance may be unfairly judged.

Feelings About Subordinates

1. My people are not experienced enough.
2. They are already too busy.
3. They have less knowledge than I about the total situation and are more likely to overlook something.
4. If I ask them to do more, they will expect higher salaries.
5. I can't depend on them to keep me informed about developing problems before they reach a crisis stage.

Personal Feelings

1. I like doing some of this work myself.
2. I get less personal recognition for work I get done through others than for work I do myself.
3. By sharing responsibility and knowledge, I lose control, power, and prestige.
4. Delegating to others involves planning for and with them—if you're action-oriented like I am, the real satisfaction comes from doing something rather than planning for someone else to do it.

Do you see anything of yourself in these kinds of comments? If you do, you probably should take another look at the attitudes expressed and ask yourself whether in your situation and in your unit those attitudes are valid and justifiable.

STEPS TOWARD BETTER DELEGATION

Whenever you ask someone in your unit to do something, you are engaged in delegation. What are some steps to follow to insure that you delegate as wisely as possible? Some of the important ones follow:

Define the Task to be Done

Determine in your own mind just what it is you wish to have done. That is, define the task. So often, supervisors go to someone who works for them with a fuzzy concept of precisely what is needed. Without careful conceptualization, without a clear understanding of what you want done and why, you cannot possibly communicate effectively with someone else. If you really want to work at delegating, you should not hesitate at this stage of the game to put in writing—for your own use—a few sentences describing the task. This is a simple technique whose chief value is that it forces you to recognize whether or not your thinking has crystalized. If you cannot put the key facts down on paper, the chances are that trying to "wing it" orally will not be fully effective.

Relay Your Definition of the Task

Tell the person you have selected to perform the task precisely *what* you want done, as you have defined it in your own mind. Go on to explain the reasons behind the task, the purpose it is to serve, etc. Ask for and take time to answer questions. If people have an understanding of why something is needed, chances are they can bring a great deal more thought of their own to the project and help both themselves and you.

Notice that we have said define "what" you want done. This means the end results you expect, including when you wish it done and what standards or yardsticks you will use to determine whether it is adequate. In delegating, whether or not you should prescribe "how" to do the task depends very much on the subordinate involved. For example, if the subordinate is an experienced, fairly knowledgeable person, it is best for that person's own self-development that the step-by-step means to achieve the results you have requested not be mapped. If you define only the "what's" and leave room for them to develop the "how's," they will have greater opportunity to relate to the task and feel a sense of responsibility. Obviously, however, you can invite such persons to come back and talk with you after they have thought through how they are going to go about it, what approaches they plan to use, etc. And you can make it clear that you are there as a resource person for support and interest.

Other employees may be relatively inexperienced, afraid of responsibility, or otherwise uncomfortable about your not indicating how to go about producing the results you have defined. In such cases, direction and guidance on step-by-step possibilities for achieving assignments will need to be greater on your part. This is a large area of judgment for the supervisor and it requires her to familiarize herself with the different skills, abilities, and personal characteristics of those who work for her.

Establish Controls and Checkpoints

Another important step in delegating is the establishing of controls and checkpoints to insure feedback. Since you remain accountable for work you delegate, it is essential that you follow through here. Lawrence Appley, former president of the American Management Association, once said, "Employees respect what the manager inspects." Very often supervisors delegate a task, assume it will be done, and then go on to something else. Obviously, a supervisor does not have to check every piece of work. On the other hand, she should have some means of periodically assessing the work going on. This may be done by informal meetings, by formal meetings, through written reports, or by just walking out onto the nursing floor periodically and actually observing what is going on. If employees sense that you are interested in following through, chances are they will do likewise.

Establish Dialogue

Finally, open dialogue between the supervisor and each of the individuals who report to her will help. How do they feel about what is being delegated to them? What is her judgment about how they are handling delegated tasks? Can some joint goals be worked out to enable them to develop more as individuals and release time for the supervisor for tasks which only she can tackle?

SUMMARY

While many management practices are open to debate due to different philosophies and styles of managing, there is substantial agreement on the need to delegate effectively. The purpose of this article has been to help the supervisor examine how well she delegates and how she might go about improving this managerial skill. The pay-offs from effective delegation are important for the supervisor herself, for those she supervises, and for her institution. The supervisor wins time to plan and do important work that requires her special knowledge and skills. This is often work which could help her unit become more effective, but which she has had to put off or let slide for lack of time. Those she supervises have increased opportunities for responsibility and growth. The institution benefits from the broadened activities of both the supervisor and her people.

Part III
HOSPITAL UNIONIZATION

In this part, HOSPITAL UNIONIZATION, we will examine a relatively recent phenomenon. Included will be a description of the union movement in the health care industry, labor legislation, and a discussion of unionization issues and procedures.

THE UNION MOVEMENT

Unionization in the health care industry grew slowly through the late 1950s, increased in the 1960s, and was given further impetus in the 1970s by the 1974 Taft-Hartley Amendments. This, however, was not the case in other industries. From the turn of the century to the 1930s union membership in the United States rose gradually. It increased during prosperity and decreased during recession. In 1925, unions represented 4 million employees, constituting 3.5 percent of the nonagricultural work force.[1]

One factor which fostered the growth of unionization after 1930 was the maturation of our industrialized economy. Another, and perhaps more important factor, was a changed attitude on the part of the federal government. Prior to the 1930s, the federal government was essentially anti-union. However, with the Depression, Congress recognized a responsibility to blue-collar workers. That change of attitude was expressed in 1932 with the passage of the Norris-LaGuardia Act and again in 1935 with the passage of the Wagner Act. Finally, in 1947, Congress enacted another major piece of labor legislation, the Taft-Hartley Act.

Sketching the rise of unionization in hospitals, Metzger and Pointer report that the earliest instance of unionization occurred in 1919.[2] However, through the 1950's most unionization activity was directed not toward hospitals, but basic industries such as steel, chemicals, plastics, automobiles, and manufacturing organizations. Some of the reasons why large, established labor organizations did not focus attention on hospitals are offered by Davis and Foner (1975):

1. Hospital employees were among the lowest paid in the country and their organization would not swell union treasuries.
2. Hospitals are widely dispersed, making organization difficult.

3. Exclusion of not-for-profit hospitals from federal labor law (pre-1974) meant that recognition often required a strike.
4. The nature of the hospital's humanitarian service fostered society's attitude which was anti-union and anti-strike.
5. A large number of the workers were minorities, thus, organization of these workers required a "crusading spirit" and societal attitude change.

In the late 1950s, unions focused some attention on health care organizations, particularly hospitals. Among the various unions and associations currently representing employees are: the "1199" locals of the National Hospital and Health Care Employees' Union; Teamsters; American Federation of State, County, Municipal Employees Union; American Nurses' Association; various state nurses' associations; the American Society for Medical Technology; and American Federation of Physicians and Dentists. Although there were unionization efforts in the 1950s, it was not significant. The decade of the 1960s was quite different.

Some of the reasons for the upward thrust of the union movement in hospitals in the 1960s can be attributed to the civil rights movement which focused attention on unskilled and semi-skilled employees (many of whom were employed in lower level positions). In addition, societal values changed; professional employees such as teachers, nurses, and most recently physicians were no longer adverse to joining a union (Stanton).[3] Finally, the enactment of the Medicare and Medicaid programs in 1965 created a fundamental shift in the financing of health care and, in part, diminished the validity of the "we are not-for-profit and cannot pay higher wages" argument.

Reporting on an American Hospital Association study of unionization in the nation's hospitals, Match et al., indicated that 3.0 percent of the nation's registered hospitals had at least one union in 1961. By 1967 the percentage had risen to 7.7 percent, and in 1970 it had almost doubled to 14.5 percent. In 1973, it was estimated that 17.0 percent of the nation's hospitals had at least one collective bargaining agreement (Phillips, 1974a), and this is expected to increase in the future.

Nineteen hundred seventy-four was a year in which the environmental setting changed vis-à-vis hospitals and unions. Not-for-profit health care organizations had been specifically excluded from the provisions of the 1947 Taft-Hartley Act (Pointer, 1970b). However, the 1974 amendments to the act eliminated this exclusion. Thus, unions and employees now seeking to unionize have the benefit of coverage by federal labor law. Observers (Phillips, 1974a; Pointer, 1974), predicted that a new era of aggressive unionization of health care organizations would begin in 1974 with that environmental change. This is demonstrated by recent activity reported by Rosmann. In the first year after enactment, 1,600 representation petitions were filed with the National Labor Relations Board (NLRB).

In 1932, congressional changed attitude toward labor was expressed with the passage of the Norris-LaGuardia Act, officially known as the Anti-Injunction Act. It was a landmark piece of legislation. The intent of the Act was to place restraints upon employers and courts when dealing with employees and their efforts to unionize.

WAGNER ACT OF 1935 AND EMPLOYER UNFAIR LABOR PRACTICES

The second and more important piece of labor legislation was the Wagner Act of 1935, officially entitled the National Labor Relations Act (NLRA). The intent of the NLRA was to rectify the existing employer-employee power imbalance by restraining various forms of employer unfair labor practices and creating environmental conditions which would enable unionization to spread throughout all sectors of the economy.[4] Specifically enumerated in the 1935 NLRA was a set of employer unfair labor practices. In summary, it is an unfair labor practice for an employer to:[5]

1. Interfere with the employees' right to join a union.
2. Dominate or interfere with the affairs of a union.
3. Discriminate in regard to hiring or any other condition of employment which would encourage or discourage union membership.
4. Discriminate or discharge an employee who gave testimony or filed charges under the Act.
5. Refuse to bargain in good faith.

TAFT-HARTLEY ACT OF 1947 AND UNION UNFAIR LABOR PRACTICES

In passing the Wagner Act (NLRA) Congress enabled unions to grow in size and strength. The power imbalance previously favoring employees had been substantially equalized. However, by 1946 it had shifted too far toward the employee, to the detriment of the employer. Consequently, Congress amended the NLRA with the Taft-Hartley Act of 1947, officially called the Labor-Management Relations Act (LMRA). One of its provisions was the delineation of union unfair labor practices. Summarized, they are to:[6]

1. Interfere or restrain employees in the exercise to their right to join or not join a union.
2. Cause an employer to discriminate against employees on the basis of union membership.
3. Refuse to bargain in good faith with an employer.
4. Engage, induce, or threaten strikes or refuse to work when the purpose is to force an employer to force another employer to recognize a union (secondary boycott).
5. Charge discriminatory membership fees.

EFFECT OF THE NLRA AND TAFT-HARTLEY ACTS

The net effect of these two acts was that constraints were imposed on employers, employees, and unions. Certain specified recognition and negotiation procedures were established and the administrative agency for overseeing labor recognition and disputes, the National Labor Relations Board (NLRB), was created (1935) and strengthened (1947).

Although both acts set behavior parameters for employers and employees, under the provisions of the 1947 Taft-Hartley Act, not-for-profit hospitals were specifically excluded. Thus, employees did not have the benefit of federal labor law (such as unfair labor practices) when attempting to organize, although state labor laws did apply.

Prior to the 1974 amendment many argued for and against retaining the 1947 exclusion. The arguments against retention of the exclusion generally centered on the fact that some states had labor legislation applying to not-for-profit hospitals, others did not. As a result, there was inconsistency (Metzger, 1970). Further, it was argued that most hospital strikes were for the purpose of recognition and deletion of the exclusion would eliminate need for this form of strike (Pointer, 1973). Those arguing for the exclusion contended that elimination would result in a significant rise in unionization, increase costs appreciably (Lewis, 1974), and cause supervisory conflicts of interest (Emanuel, 1971). Additional reasons described by Pointer (1973) were that not-for-profit hospitals were humanitarian and would deal fairly with employees since they are semi-public in nature.

1974 AMENDMENTS TO TAFT-HARTLEY

The 1974 not-for-profit hospital amendments to the Taft-Hartley Act broadly defined a health care organization as:

> any hospital, convalescent hospital, health maintenance organization, health clinic, nursing home, extended care facility, or any other institution devoted to the care of sick, infirm or aged persons. [7]

The 1974 amendments also recognized the role of those organizations. Because of this, special provisions were developed. Among them were longer notices for the modification or termination of a contract, specific strike notices, a procedure for the conciliation of labor disputes, and exemption of individuals with religious convictions from paying dues to a union (Rakich, 1974).

Contract Notices

Realizing that hospitals provide unique and essential services to patients, section 8(d) of the Act was amended to require a 90-day (versus a 60-day) notification to the other party to modify an existing contract. A 60-day notice to the Federal Mediation and Conciliation Service (FMCS) and applicable state agency was also required. When a breakdown in bargaining occurs during initial contract negotiations following certification and recognition, a 30-day notice must be given to the FMCS and appropriate state agency. These provisions allow for longer periods for parties to reach agreement, plan for work stoppage, and to enable the FMCS to provide assistance.

Strike Notice

Another unique provision is the strike notice. Specifically, the union must give at least 10 days notice to the employer and FMCS preceding a work stoppage and that stoppage cannot occur before the end of the 90-day notice of a desire to change an existing contract. When bargaining for an initial contract after recognition, that 10-day notice cannot be given until the end of the 30-day notice of an impasse. The strike notice enables hospitals to discharge, transfer, or otherwise plan for the care of patients.

Conciliation of Labor Disputes

The 1974 amendments also provide that if, in the opinion of the Director of the FMCS "... a threatened strike or lockout affecting a health care institution will ... substantially interrupt the delivery of health care in the locality concerned ... " he can appoint an impartial board of inquiry to help resolve the issue. The act specifies various time constraints for appointment of the board, investigation, and reporting during which the employer and union must maintain the status quo, unless they both concur to a change. This enables the FMCS to enter into discussions and help resolve issues involving health care organizations before total breakdown.

Individuals With Religious Convictions

Public Law 93-360 also exempts hospital employees from paying dues to a union, even if there is a union-shop agreement, when the individual ... "is a member of and adheres to established and traditional tenents or teachings of a *bona fide* religion, body, or sect which has historically held religious conscientious objections to joining or financially supporting labor organizations...." The individual must, however, donate an equivalent amount to a charitable fund. The purpose of this provision was to recognize the unique position of the employees of many of the nation's religiously affiliated hospitals.

Even with the unique provisions many issues remain for administration. For example, the definition of common and appropriate bargaining units is presented as a major concern in Selection 22, "Recognition and Negotiation under Taft-Hartley" (also see Amundson). In Selection 25, "The Nurse as a Professional and Unionist," the writers describe instances in which hospital support of a professional nurses' association, which later takes on the role of a union, can be considered an employer unfair labor practice. Further, attention must be given to what actually constitutes a strike notice, and what is a *bona fide* religion. Finally, the importance of solicitation and distribution activities and the hospital's policies related to them are discussed in Selection 26, "Solicitation Rules Will Need Revision" (also see Epstein, 1975a). These and other issues will be resolved by the NLRB.

National Labor Relations Board (NLRB)

The NLRB has responsibility for overseeing recognitional, jurisdictional, and other labor relations matters in the United States. It is an administrative body with the power to promulgate regulations having the force of law. As with many administrative bodies, the NLRB actually performs three functions; it investigates the need for regulation (executive function), promulgates rules and regulations based on investigated needs (legislative function), and enforces these regulations (judicial function).

Even though appeals by the employer or union can be made to the courts if either party is not satisfied with an NLRB decision, the courts tend to practice a form of judicial restraint—unless the NLRB is clearly in error the decision will not be modified by the judicial system. Therefore, when conflicts exist and where reasonable minds may differ on the ultimate outcome of the conflict, the NLRB decision is generally not disturbed. As a result, hospitals now have to cope with the NLRB administrative procedures, rules, and also its rulings (Lewis, 1975; M. Miller). Among the activities of the NLRB are:

1. To supervise union recognition elections and certify their outcome.
2. To designate collective bargaining units within health care organizations[8] and designate who is a supervisor.[9]
3. To resolve findings of facts in conflicts.
4. To interpret labor/management agreements.
5. To determine what constitutes an unfair labor practice.

Now that not-for-profit hospitals are covered by the Taft-Hartley Act they have to function within the constraints of statutory and administrative law. As stated by Epstein (1975a); "...a new set of rights and responsibilities for managers (administrators and their representatives) and for employees has been imposed on a traditional relationship." Since hospitals, as a rule, have not had the experience unions have had with the law, recognition/negotiation procedures, and the NLRB, retention of competent counsel is strongly urged (Emanuel, 1974). At the minimum, the administration should be very precise and cautious so that it does not commit an unfair labor practice. At the same time it must be aware of employer rights (NLRB Layman's Guide; Pointer, 1974b; Singleton).

UNIONIZATION ISSUES AND PROCEDURES

After an orientation to the union movement and federal labor law, the remainder of this section will describe and discuss some of the reasons why employees join unions. It will also examine administrative philosophies relative to unionization, and suggest various constructive responsive steps which can be taken to minimize the likelihood that a hospital's employees will attempt unionization.

WHY EMPLOYEES UNIONIZE[10]

One might ask: "What causes employees to want to join a union?" Previously, it was reported that one of the primary causes has been lack of a clearly defined and operational personnel administration/labor relations department (Osterhaus, selection 24; Pointer, 1974b). Implicit is the presumption that an operational department would implement orderly policies and procedures related to staffing, utilizing, compensating, and training the hospital's human resources. Although there was merit to this charge, it can be stated that today personnel administration/labor relations activities of hospitals have matured. In part this is because of environmentally imposed laws, executive orders, and regulations, e.g., the 1964 Civil Rights Act and affirmative action programs. It has also been reported that pay is a primary reason why hospital employees unionize (M. Miller; Match et al.). However, in recent years hospital employee compensation has increased substantially and is no longer below other sectors of the economy.

Although these two previously cited factors are material to the issue, they do not fully answer the questions, "What does an employee expect from a union and what promises can be made by unions to employees which the administration does not or has not made?" There are a multitude of interrelated factors including unfulfilled needs and dissatisfaction with one and/or all of the three following areas: (1) the conditions of employment, (2) democracy in the work setting, and (3) the content of employment.

As indicated in Part II, THE MANAGEMENT OF HOSPITAL PERSONNEL, today's hospital employees seek more from their employment than just a pay check. Certainly conditions of employment including pay, consistency among pay grades, fringe benefits (health insurance, holidays, and vacation time), and physical and nonphysical working conditions (work breaks, cleanup time, safety conditions, parking, hours of employment, employee schedules, and assignment to specific duties) are important. Dissatisfaction can motivate employees to seek unionization as a way to rectify problems. However, it can be argued that maturation of hospital personnel administration/labor relation activities in recent years has remedied many of the previously existing deficiencies.

Democracy in the work setting represents another group of factors which can cause employees to unionize. This specifically refers to established procedures which restrain unfair, unwarranted, or inconsistent administrative action. Matters of concern are layoffs on the basis of seniority, freedom from arbitrary administrative action, fair employee appraisal, compensation increases, and procedures for promotion and discipline. Inconsistency and the absence of legitimacy in the eyes of the employees generally results in deterioration of morale and job satisfaction. One function of a union and one of its attractions is that it generally establishes, through the negotiation and contract activities, criteria and procedures which lead to democracy in the work setting.

Perhaps one of the most important group of factors which can cause employees to unionize is the content of employment, particularly for professional employees (Robinson). This generally refers to the total atmosphere of employment. Inherent elements are: the desire on the part of employees to be treated as individuals rather than just as another input resource, and knowing that supervisors have a sincere concern for their welfare. The ability to expand one's job responsibility, particularly for professional employees, to engage in valid and legitimate participative decision-making and have some control over the parameters of one's job (M. Miller; Phillips, 1974b), and to seek and derive job satisfaction from their employment, are important to employees. Further, the ability to communicate freely upward and the dissemination of information downward are important to employees (A. Imberman, Stanton) and are considered part of the content of employment.

The hospital manager should be aware of the many factors which cause employee dissatisfaction. The answer to the question, "Why do employees unionize?" is not simple, nor can a standard answer be offered. On the contrary, the answer is very complex and the causes vary according to hospital. However, one point is certain. If employees perceive that their needs are not being met in regard to the conditions of work, democracy in the work setting, and content of employment, they will probably seek a vehicle (union) which can correct them.

Concerted administrative attention and action in these areas can do much to strengthen the employee-employer relationship. However, one overall perspective is often lost—the employee's wants and desires sometimes escape the hospital administrator. It must be remembered that employees typically are not administration-oriented in an all encompassing perspective. They react to their immediate supervisor and the treatment displayed by the supervisor is generally extrapolated by the employee as representing the total management attitude (Emanuel, 1974).

ADMINISTRATIVE PHILOSOPHY

Though hospital union recognition and bargaining activities are covered by federal labor law, the issue of "administrative philosophy" toward unionism has not yet been addressed. Specifically, how should the administration respond to the current unionization phenomenon? In Selection 24, "The Effects of Unions on Hospital Management," two administrative philosophies at opposite ends of the conservative-liberal spectrum are discussed.

This selection was written prior to 1974, but it raises valid considerations. The conservative administrative philosophy encompasses the standard arguments as to why hospitals should not be unionized. Among them are since hospitals are predominately not-for-profit, it is not in the public interest; by nature of the life-and-death situation the interruption of service cannot occur; and hospitals do not have money to distribute in the form of higher wages. The liberal philosophy, on the other hand, notes the attitude that times are changing and the administration should adopt progressive internal personnel procedures and policies. By implication, if a hospital's employees seek a union, the administration should work constructively with it to reduce animosity and promote harmony (Shershin and Boxx).[11]

Regardless of the administration's philosophical approach to the issue, four fears worthy of further consideration and reflection are raised in this selection. They are: strike, unionization will cost money, loss of control, and organized labor will complicate hospital administration.

Strike Fear

Hospitals provide unique services which set them apart from other types of organizations. Because of this, concern about a strike is valid. The strike issue could be explosive. Simply defined, it is the mechanism by which a union, certified by the NLRB to represent employees, can seek to force the administration to meet its demands. Although strikes will continue to occur they are costly for the administration in terms of time, loss of revenue (Brody and London), and legal expenses. They are also costly for employees in lost wages, and potentially for the patient's well-being.

The strike fear is a fact of life and the administration must learn to cope with it. However, two points need to be mentioned. First, if employees gain union recognition, the administration should be reasonable in the negotiation process in order to minimize the likelihood of a strike and foster a positive labor relations attitude after a contract is signed. Second, employees and their representatives have a duty to be reasonable in their requests so that the administration and union together can discharge their responsibility to the patient without resorting to work stoppages.

This posture is superbly described by one writer as follows:

> The health care industry, in all its diversity, exists for the benefit of patients; patients do not exist for the benefit of either health care industry management or labor. Collective bargaining in this field, and even the right to strike, will be acceptable as long as they do not claim too great a price from the sick, do not cause needless deaths or suffering, and do not make conventional hospital care economically impossible. This past decade, the data suggest, there has been a kind of informal conspiracy between hospital managements and hospital workers to raise wages, improve working conditions, and otherwise increase the competitive power of hospitals to attract workers in the labor market. Now there is increasing pressure to keep health care costs from rising further. If either or both sides exploit the new situation with less than a full sense of the responsibility they owe the public, especially the sick, such misconduct will boomerang.[12]

Cost Fear

A union will certainly affect costs through wage and benefit levels as well as through the need to allocate resources (time and money) in the recognition and negotiation processes (W. Imberman). Payroll already accounts for more than two-thirds of all hospital expenditures. However, should the administration attempt to keep the hospital union free, it will have to make concerted attempts to ensure that wage rates and fringe benefits are competitive. Should a union become established, the administration will be required to make its employees' renumeration competitive (Coleman and Sperling). Thus, the fear of higher costs will probably occur, not as much through wages, but costs affected by employee utilization.

Complicated Administration and Control Fears

A discussion of the last two fears can be combined. Without question a union contract would complicate personnel administration because of the need to negotiate and resolve impasses and later to follow grievance procedure steps once a contract is ratified. Further, specific personnel activities ranging from wage and salary compensation to transfers and terminations will be formalized (Krinsky).

The final fear, loss of control, is in our view the most important one. The administration's prerogative of managing the institution and its personnel is critical. Thus, flexibility in personnel utilization (manpower input resources) is directly related to the issue of costs. Because hospitals are labor intensive, and with the rising labor intensity and changing technologies requiring more personnel with greater skills, administrative flexibility in the utilization of personnel is crucial to cost containment. Thus, a union's effect on the administration's control prerogative is of major importance (R. Miller).

STRATEGY

If the administration wishes to prevent unionization, action must be taken early, not during an organization attempt (Rakich, 1973). The best strategy to follow is creation of a work environment where the majority of employees will feel no need to organize (Stanton). In virtually every instance, the administration's lack of perception and response to the legitimate needs and grievances of its employees gives rise to an organization drive. In such an environment the institution is the loser, whether or not the election is won.

The best posture for promoting an environment where employees will not seek a union is to be progressive and constructive with consideration given to balancing many competing constraints—responsibility to patients, employees, and the administrator's accountability for costs and effectiveness. This posture requires not only a meaningful commitment on the part of the administration, but also the need to work through the supervisor from whom most employees generally form their opinion of the administration. The supervisor is a major link in the whole chain (V. Cleland; Emanuel, 1974; Shershin and Boxx).

BIBLIOGRAPHY

American Hospital Association. "Statement on Employee Relations for Health Care Institutions." Chicago, Illinois, 1975.
Amundson, Norman. "Alternatives to the Strike in Collective Bargaining." *Journal of Nursing Administration* 5(January): 11-12, 1975.
Brody, Paul E. and Jordan London. "How Costly is a Strike?" *Hospitals* 49(September 16): 53-56, 1975.
Chamot, Dennis. "Professional Employees Turn to Unions." *Harvard Business Review* 54(May-June): 119-127, 1976.
Clelland, Rod. "Grievance Procedures: Outlet for Employee, Insight for Management." *Hospitals* 41, Part I(August 1): 58-60, 1967.
Cleland, Virginia S. "The Supervisor in Collective Bargaining." *Nursing Administration* 5(September-October): 33-35, 1974.
Coleman, Francis T. and Louis Sperling. "NLRB Unit Determinations Expanding." *Hospital Progress* 57(August): 43-46, 66, 1976.
Cunningham, Robert M., Jr. "Strike." *Modern Health Care* 5(February): 41-48.
Davis Leon J. and Moe Foner. "Organization and Unionization of Health in the United States: The Trade Union Perspective." *International Journal of Health Services* 5:1: 19-26, 1975.
Denton, John A. "Attitudes Toward Alternative Models of Unions and Professional Associations." *Nursing Research* 25(May-June): 178-180, 1976.
Elkin, Randyl D. "Recognition and Negotiation Under Taft-Hartley." *Hospital Progress* 55(December): 50-53, 63, 1974.
―――. "Negotiating and Administering A Union Contract." *Hospital Progress* 56(January): 41-43., 1975.
Emanuel, William J. "Taft-Hartley Exemption." *Hospitals* 45(April 16): 66-68, 1971.
―――. "Nonprofit Hospitals and the NLRA Exemption." *Hospital Progress* 54(January): 69-70, 76, 1973.
―――. "Coping with the NLRA." *Hospital Forum* 17(November): 15-16, 1974.
―――. "Hospital Policy: Professional Associations as Unions." *Hospital Progress* 57(January): 51-55, 1976.
Emanuel, William and Alfred Klein, "Solicitation Rules Will Need Revision." *Hospitals* 49(August 16): 47-51, 1975.

Epstein, Richard L. "Employee Relations." *Hospitals* 49(April 1): 75-77, 1975a.
———. "The NLRB Bargaining Unit Decisions." *Trustee* 28(July): 7-9, 1975b.
———. "Guide to NLRB Rules on Solicitation and Distribution." *Hospitals* 49(August 16): 43-47, 1975c.
Holloway, Robert G. "Management Can Reverse Declining Employee Work Attitudes." *Hospitals* 50(October 16): 71-77, 1976.
"How to Win the Labor Tug of War." *Modern Healthcare* 2(September): 56-61, 1974.
Imberman, A. A. "Communication, an Effective Weapon Against Unionization." *Hospital Progress* 54(December): 54-57, 1973.
Imberman, Woodruff. "How Expensive is an NLRB Election?" *MSU Business Topics* 23(Summer): 13-18, 1975.
Kralewski, John E. "Collective Bargaining Among Professional Employees." *Hospital Administration* 19(Summer): 30-41, 1974.
Krinsky, Edward B. "Problems of Discipline and Discharge." *Hospitals* 48(May 16): 48-50, 1974.
Lewis, Howard L. "Wave of Union Organizing will Follow Break in the Taft-Hartley Dam." *Modern Healthcare* 1(May): 25-32, 1974.
———. "Separate Collective Bargaining." *Modern Healthcare* 4(July): 51-54, 1975.
Marcus, Sanford A. "The Purposes of Unionization in the Medical Profession: The Unionized Profession's Perspective in the United States." *International Journal of Health Services* 5:1:37-42, 1975.
Match, Robert K., Arnold H. Goldstein, and Harold L. Light. "Unionization, Strikes, Threatened Strikes, and Hospitals—A View from Hospital Management." *International Journal of Health Services* 5:1:27-36, 1975.
Matlack, David R. "Goals and Trends in the Unionization of Health Professionals." *Hospital Progress* 53(February): 40-43, 1972.
Metzger, Norman. "Labor Relations." *Hospitals* 44(March): 80-4, 1970.
———. "The Arbitration Procedure." *Hospitals* 48(April 16): 47-49, 1974.
———. "NLRA Boards of Inquiry Have Been Used Sparingly." *Hospitals* 50(July 1): 55-57, 1976.
———. *Personnel Administration in the Health Services Industry.* New York: Spectrum Publications, Inc., 1975.
Metzger, Norman and Dennis D. Pointer. *Labor Management Relations in the Health Services Industry.* Washington, D.C.: Science and Health Publications, 1972.
Miller, Michael. "Nurses Right to Strike." *Journal of Nursing Administration* 5(February): 35-39, 1975.
Miller, Ronald L. "Collective Bargaining: A New Frontier for Hospitals." *Hospital Progress* 56(February): 58-60, 65, 1975.
Nash, Al. "The Hospital's Value System and the Union." *Hospital Administration* 19(Fall): 49-64, 1974.
National Labor Relations Board. *A Layman's Guide to Basic Law Under the National Labor Relations Act.* Washington, D.C.: U.S. Government Printing Office, 1971.
NLRB General Council. "Guidelines of the National Labor Relations Board to the 1974 Nonprofit Amendments to the Taft-Hartley Act." *Labor Relations Report* 86:33:88 LRR 371-393, 1974.
Osterhaus, Leo B. "The Effects of Unions on Hospital Management." *Hospital Progress* 48(June-July): 68-72, 78,79, 1967.
Pepe, Stephen and Robert L. Murphy. "The NLRB Decisions on Appropriate Bargaining Units." *Hospital Progress* 56(August): 43-46, 69, 1975.
Phillips, Donald F. "Taft-Hartley: What To Expect?" *Hospitals* 48(July): 18a-18d, 1974a.
———. "New Demands of Nurses-Part 2." *Hospitals* 48(September): 41-44, 1974b.
Pointer, Dennis D. "The Labor Law Status of Health Care Facilities: Part 1 The Wagner Act." *Hospital Progress* 51(September): 44-47, 1970a.
———. "The Labor Law Status of Health Care Facilities: Part 2: The Taft-Hartley and Landrum-

Griffin Acts." *Hospital Progress* 51(October): 83-86, 1970b.
———. "The Labor Law Status of Health Care Facilities: Part 3: Proprietary Hospitals, Nursing Homes, and State and Federal Government Hospitals." *Hospital Progress* 51 (November): 72-75, 1970c.
———. "Hospital Labor Relations Legislation: An Examination and Critique of Public Policy." *Hospital Progress* 54(January): 71-75, 1973.
———. "How the 1974 Taft-Hartley Amendments Will Affect Health Care Facilities (Part 1)." *Hospital Progress* 55(October): 68-70, 1974a.
———. "How the 1974 Taft-Hartley Amendments Will Affect Health Care Facilities (Part 2)." *Hospital Progress* 55(November): 58-61, 1974b.
———. "Hospitals and Professionals—A Changing Relationship." *Hospitals* 50(April): 117-121, 1976.
Pointer, Dennis D. and Norman Metzger. *The National Labor Relations Act: A Guidebook for Health Care Facility Administrators.* New York: Spectrum Publications, Inc., 1975.
Public Law 93-360. "Amendments to the National Labor Relations Act." 93rd Congress. S. 3203. (July 26), 1974.
Rakich, Jonathon S. "Hospital Unionization: Causes and Effects." *Hospital Administration* 15 (Winter): 7-18, 1973.
———. "The Impact of the 1974 Taft-Hartley Amendments on Health Care Facilities." *Business Law Review* 7(December): 1-7, 1974.
Rakich, Jonathon S., Beaufort B. Longest, Jr., and Thomas R. O'Donovan. *Managing Health Care Organizations.* Philadelphia: W.B. Saunders Co., 1977.
Reynolds, Lloyd G. *Labor Economics and Labor Relations.* Englewood Cliffs, New Jersey: Prentice Hall, 1970.
Robinson, A. Selden. "Collective Bargaining in the Technical and Professional Fields." *Personnel Journal* 55(June): 278-281, 1976.
Rosasco, Louise C. "Collective Bargaining: What's a Director of Nursing to Do?" *Hospitals* 48 (September 16): 79-82, 113, 1974.
Rosmann, Joseph. "One Year Under Taft-Hartley." *Hospitals* 49(December 16): 64-68, 1975.
Schwartz, Harry. "Public Will Not Tolerate Disruptive Strikes." *Hospitals* 49(November 16): 43-46, 1975.
Sellentin, Jerry L. "Labor's Concerns Face Management." *Hospitals* 50(April 1): 65-67, 1976.
Shershin, Michael J., and W. Randy Boxx. "Building Positive Union-Management Relations." *Personnel Journal* 54(June): 326-331, 1975.
Singleton, Barry W. "Negotiating A Collective Bargaining Agreement." *Hospital Progress* 56(October): 57-59, 80, 1975.
Sloane, Arthur A., and Fred Witney. *Labor Relations.* Englewood Cliffs, New Jersey: Prentice Hall, 1972.
Stanton, Erwin S. "Unions and the Professional Employee." *Hospital Progress* 55(January): 58-59, 68, 1974.
Sweeney, Sr. Margaret, and Edith H. Belsjoe. "Employee Communications During and After a Union Campaign." *Hospital Progress* 48(April): 52-55, 60, 1974.
Zimmerman, Anne. "Taft-Hartley Amended: Implications." *Nursing* 75(February): 284-296, 1975.

FOOTNOTES
(See bibliography for full citation as necessary)

[1] U. S. Bureau of Labor Statistics, *Handbook for Labor Statistics* (Washington, D.C.: Government Printing Office, 1950), p. 139.

[2] See Metzger and Pointer (1972, Chapter 2) for a history of the labor movement in the health services industry.

[3] For discussions of unionization of professionals
  (a) in general see: Chamot; within hospitals, Pointer (1976).
  (b) for nurses see Denton; Kralewski; Matlack; R. Miller.
  (c) for physicians see Cunningham; Marcus.

[4] Lloyd G. Reynolds, *Labor Economics and Labor Relations* (Englewood Cliffs, New Jersey: Prentice Hall, 1970), pp. 462-463.

[5] See: National Labor Relations Board, *Layman's Guide to the NLRA* (pp. 19-29); Pointer and Metzger (Chapter VI).

[6] See: National Labor Relations Board, *Layman's Guide to the NLRA* (pp. 29-44); Pointer and Metzger (Chapter VII).

[7] For a copy of the 1974 amendments see PL 93-360, 93rd Congress, S. 3203, July 26, 1974 or Pointer and Metzger (pp. 235-237).

[8] This is probably one of the most significant areas of NLRB responsibility. Rulings on bargaining unit configuration will have a long run impact on hospitals. A major concern is that the proliferation of many and varied bargaining units will complicate the administration's task in dealing with unions and possibly result in the use of union whipsaw tactics. For discussions on bargaining units, criteria for classification, and concern for large numbers of units see: Coleman and Sperling; Epstein (1975b); Lewis (1975); R. Miller; Pepe and Murphy; Pointer (1974b); and Pointer and Metzger (Chapter V).

[9] The role of the RN as a professional nurse and a supervisor can create a conflict of interest. For a definition of a "supervisor" under the NLRA see Rosasco; Zimmerman.

[10] See Rosmann for an American Hospital Association survey giving reasons why employees unionize and "How to Win The Labor Tug of War" (1974). For further details on these three areas see: Rakich, Longest, and O'Donovan (Chapter 10).

[11] For a case history of such a philosophy see Nash.

[12] Harry Schwartz, "Public Will Not Tolerate Disruptive Strikes," *Hospitals*, Vol. 49 (November 16, 1975), p. 46.

The 1974 Taft-Hartley Amendments

The subjects of recognition, negotiation, and administration of union contracts under the 1974 Taft-Hartley Amendments have not been addressed. Presuming an election occurs and the NLRB certifies a union as the sole bargaining agent for a group of employees, the next step in the process is negotiation. Selection 22, "RECOGNITION AND NEGOTIATION UNDER TAFT-HARTLEY" by Randyl D. Elkin, describes those activities. After providing the reader information about the 1974 Taft-Hartley Act Amendments, this selection presents the next step, recognition and its requirements. Further, emphasis is placed on the importance of bargaining unit determination and the criteria used by the NLRB in establishing units.

Selection 23, "NEGOTIATING AND ADMINISTERING A UNION CONTRACT" by Randyl D. Elkin, provides a sequel. Once a union has been certified by the NLRB as the exclusive bargaining agent for a group of employees, the next step is negotiation of a contract. This does not imply, however, that there must be an agreement. In negotiation there are three classes of bargainable issues; those that are mandatory, permissible, and those that are illegal per se. Mandatory issues consist of conditions of employment including wages, fringe benefits, hours of employment, and criteria for promotion and transfers. Failure to bargain "in good faith" about these issues is an unfair labor practice. Permissible or nonmandatory issues include establishing a grievance procedure, discipline practices, and union security. The latter normally encompasses the establishment of a union shop (a newly hired employee must join the union after a specific period of time) and the check off (collection of union dues by the administration through payroll deduction). Failure to bargain about these issues is not an unfair labor practice. The final category of issues consists of those that neither party can negotiate about and have binding because they are illegal. Examples are a union shop (where an employee must be a union member before being hired), the inclusion of supervisors in a bargaining unit with their subordinates, or that the hospital pressure a sub-contractor to recognize a union.

Once a contract is negotiated and ratified, it is a private law between the two parties. Elkin points out that a contract can contain management rights clauses which delineate those prerogatives exclusively reserved for the administration. Another provision in most contracts is a grievance procedure which is defined as the internal jurisprudence system for handling employee grievances. Finally, the arbitration procedure, which can be specified in the grievance procedure, is described (also see Metzger, 1974).

22.
Recognition and Negotiation Under Taft-Hartley

RANDYL D. ELKIN

Randyl D. Elkin, Ph.D., is the Director of the Graduate Program in Industrial Relations, West Virginia University.

Nonprofit hospitals once again are covered under the rubric of national labor law. In July, the passage of an amended Senate Bill 3203 removed the section 2 (2) exemption for nonprofit hospitals from coverage under the Labor Management Relations Act (LMRA or, more commonly, Taft-Hartley).[1] In addition to striking the exemption, the new bill added several sub-sections to the LMRA in recognition of the special nature of the services delivered by nonprofit hospitals.

The extended coverage will no doubt stimulate collective bargaining in health care institutions. New faces will appear in hospital labor relations. The actions of hospital administrators and their employees will be tempered by the new freedoms and restrictions of the LMRA. This article discusses the expected impact of the removal of the exemption upon the recognition and negotiation processes of collective bargaining. A subsequent article will examine the new legislation's impact on hospital management and employees once a collective bargaining agreement has been reached.

Much information about the effect of the new legislation can be gleaned from the experiences of those already covered by the LMRA or similar laws. Proprietary hospitals with gross revenues exceeding $250,000 have been covered under the LMRA since 1967. Federal hospitals have been covered since Executive Order 10988 became effective in January, 1962. State and local government hospitals are covered by state bargaining laws in about 19 states. Bargaining is not new to nonprofit hospitals either. An estimated 18 percent of the 3,565 nonprofit hospitals had collective bargaining agreements as of December, 1973.[2]

RECOGNITION

Selection or rejection of an employee representative exclusively for the purpose of collective bargaining is very closely regulated under the LMRA. The Wagner Act was

---

Reprinted by permission from *Hospital Progress: Journal of the Catholic Hospital Association*, St. Louis, Vol. 55 (December, 1974), pp. 50-53, 63. Copyright 1974 by the Catholic Hospital Association. All rights reserved.

passed to eliminate the causes of industrial strife or unrest which obstructed the free flow of commerce. Recognition strikes were then and still are a major source of work stoppages in unregulated employment. Often, the only way employee representatives can gain recognition from intransigent employers is through economic force in the absence of a legal procedure. The LMRA institutionalizes the conflict over recognition by providing a recognition procedure and outlawing employee strikes and employer lockouts over recognition. Administrators operating under the LMRA should avail themselves of competent legal counsel.

The LMRA establishes an employee bill of rights in section 7:

> Employees shall have the right to self-organization, to form, join, or assist labor organizations, to bargain collectively through representatives of their own choosing, and to engage in other concerted activities for the purpose of collective bargaining or other mutual aid or protection, and also shall have the right to refrain from any or all of such activities except to the extent that such right may be affected by an agreement requiring membership in a labor organization as a condition of employment as authorized in section 8(a) (3).

The process of organizing for recognition may begin spontaneously within the employee group or may be stimulated by organizers from various employee health organizations. In either case, at some point the administrator will be confronted by an employee or organizational representative who claims that he represents the majority of a group of employees and wishes to begin bargaining on the group's behalf. This individual usually claims to have cards signed by a majority of the employees authorizing a particular labor organization to bargain in their behalf.

The response of most employers is to refuse recognition (or to refuse an audience in the first place) without looking at the authorization cards. The employer, one or more of his employees, or the labor organization may petition the National Labor Relations Board (NLRB) to begin election proceedings. The NLRB investigates informally to determine if there is "reasonable cause to believe a question of representation exists." The NLRB requires that any organization claiming representation status must prove that it has representation interest from at least 30 percent of the employees. Interest is usually proven via authorization cards. Once interest is established, a formal hearing is set up to determine:

1. Whether the NLRB has jurisdiction;
2. Whether there is veritable question of representation; and
3. The existence of an "appropriate bargaining unit."

If the first two conditions are met and an appropriate unit has been determined, a date is set for a secret ballot. If the election is won by a bargaining representative, he is certified by the NLRB as the "exclusive bargaining representative" for all employees in the "appropriate bargaining unit."

APPROPRIATE BARGAINING UNIT

The "appropriate bargaining unit" is determined by the NLRB. All employees in the unit, and only those employees, are eligible to vote in the election. The election, which is supervised by the NLRB or its agent, is decided by a majority of those voting. The ballot will list the organization or organizations claiming representation status and a "no union" choice. If none of these receives a majority, there is a runoff between the top two vote-getters. For example, if Union A received 40 percent of the vote, Union B 20 percent, and "no union" 40 percent, the runoff balloting would pit Union A against "no union." If the majority of those voting select Union A in the second ballot, Union A is the exclusive bargaining representative and must bargain for *all* of the employees in the appropriate bargaining unit. If the "no union" choice receives a majority, no exclusive bargaining agent would be permitted. Either outcome sets an "election bar" against further organizational effort or challenge of exclusive representative status for a period of 12 months from the election date. If the labor organization wins the election and within that 12 months enters into a collective bargaining agreement with the hospital, then there is a "contract bar" against challenging the organization's representation status for the duration of the contract.

The determination of the appropriate bargaining unit is extremely important to the hospital's industrial relations and health service delivery. Fragmentation of units is the chief pitfall of unit determination. Many small units cause nonuniform benefits, whipsawing, multiple strike threats, added management overhead to administer contracts, and budget coordination problems. The public sector has experienced the difficulties inherent in too many units.[3] The NLRB is mindful of these difficulties and weighs such considerations during the hearing to determine the appropriate unit. The hospital administrator should present a detailed analysis supporting his own judgment about the appropriate unit during the hearing.

The NLRB uses the following criteria to establish the unit: (1) "community of interests" in wages, hours, and working conditions; (2) "geography and physical proximity" of employer operations; (3) "employer's administrative or territorial divisions;" (4) the degree of "functional integration" of the employer's operations; (5) the "interchange of employees" between various locations; (6) "bargaining history" in the industry and/or area; (7) "employee desires;" and (8) "extent of organization" of the employees.[4]

By far, the most important factor in unit determination has been community of interests. By law, supervisory personnel are excluded from the unit. Payment from the same salary schedule, interchangeability of employees between job classifications, common educational and training requirements, method of hire, common supervision, and a host of other considerations are scrutinized to determine the extent of this interest. Structural considerations are far from settled for hospitals, but a number of organizations tend to become exclusive bargaining agents. Registered nurses are usually represented by the state affiliate of the American Nurses' Association in a unit separate from licensed practical nurses and nurses' aides. LPNs may form a separate unit represented by their state affiliate of the National Federation of Licensed Practical Nurses. Or LPNs and nurses' aides may be found to have a community interest with technicians and blue-collar workers. Because of the community of interest doctrine, nonprofessionals and blue-collar workers often are grouped together in a large unit represented by either the Service Employees International Union or the American Federation of State, County, and Municipal Employees. The structural precedents are still being set for the health care field through the case-by-case investigations of the NLRB.

If it is opposed to bargaining, the hospital management has a relatively free hand in making its opposition known. It may set up a counterorganizational drive. However, once the hospital has been notified that it is being organized, it becomes subject to the unfair labor practices section of the LMRA. The counterorganizational drive shall in no way "interfere with, restrain, or coerce employees in the exercise of the rights guaranteed in sec. 7." Legal counsel should be obtained to ensure that no employer actions become unfair practices. Hospital administrators can cite relevant facts about unions, union leaders, and their activities only if these actions do not threaten, coerce, or mislead the employees about unionization. The employer may review his past record of wage and salary payments but may neither give nor promise to give a nonregular pay increase during the organizational campaign.

Overstepping legal boundaries may cause the NLRB to set the election aside. A new election would be held. Frequent and flagrant violation of section 7 rights may cause the NLRB to mandate bargaining between the hospital and labor organization. It is important to keep in mind that the tenor of future labor-management relations will be affected by employer actions during an organizational drive. A bitter organizational drive often yields a bitter, conflict-ridden postorganizational negotiation and contract administration relationship.

Just as there are legal constraints on management behavior during organizational drives, there are also restraints upon union actions. Employees have the section 7 right to refrain from any or all organizational activities as well as freedom from union coercion. A labor organization violation of section 7 employee freedoms is cause for an election rerun.

UNFAIR LABOR PRACTICES

The other major portion of the LMRA concerns unfair labor practices. Unfair labor practices initially, with the passage of the Wagner Act in 1935, applied only to employers. Taft-Hartley applied unfair labor practices to unions in 1947. Briefly, under section 8(a) employers are guilty of unfair labor practice if they:

1. Interfere with, restrain or coerce employees, in the exercise of their rights of self-organization and collective bargaining through representatives of the workers' own choosing;
2. Establish and maintain company-dominated labor organizations by financial assistance or in other ways;
3. Discharge or otherwise discriminate against employees for joining a union or for being active in support of a labor organization;
4. Discharge or otherwise discriminate against employees for testifying in an NLRB case;
5. Refuse to bargain collectively with a union designated by a majority of employees in a unit appropriate for collective bargaining purposes to represent said employees in collective bargaining.[5]

The labor organization shall not:

1. Restrain or coerce employees in the exercise of their section 7 rights or an employer in the selection of his bargaining representative;
2. Cause or attempt to cause an employer to discriminate against an employee on the basis of union membership;
3. Refuse to bargain in good faith with an employer as representative of his employees;
4. Engage in a secondary boycott;
5. Charge excessive or discriminatory membership fees;
6. Cause an employer to pay, in the nature of an exaction, for services not rendered; and
7. Picket to gain recognition where an exclusive representative already exists.

Although it is a major NLRB responsibility to prevent these unfair labor practices, the Board does not act unless an unfair labor practice charge is filed. The process begins when the complaining party files an unfair labor practice charge on the NLRB form. These forms are obtained from and must be returned to the appropriate NLRB regional office. Once again, competent legal advice should be sought the first time such a charge is contemplated.

If the unfair practice involves picketing, a boycott, or work stoppage, investigation of the charge will be expedited. The complaining party must document the alleged unfair practice incident as fully as possible during an interview with the NLRB field examiner (investigator), who subsequently will interview the other party. During the investigation, the field examiner will try to obtain an informal settlement.

If no settlement is achieved, and if the evidence supports the existence of an unfair practice, a complaint will be issued and a hearing on the complaint will be scheduled. After a complaint has been issued, the Board may petition the federal district court for a temporary injunction to stop the unfair practice. A hearing on the complaint will be held before a trial examiner; the case is prosecuted for the board by an attorney from the regional office. The trial examiner then must file an intermediate report citing the findings in the case and recommending disposition. If an exception is filed by either party, the NLRB will review the case and, although rare, may allow further oral arguments from the parties. The vast majority of cases, however, are settled informally before they reach the NLRB. The Board may either dismiss the complaint or issue a cease and desist order enforceable by the U.S. Court of Appeals.

NEGOTIATION

If recognition is obtained by the labor organization, the labor-management relationship enters a new phase. The National Labor Relations Act does not require the bargainers to come to an agreement. It requires only "good faith" bargaining. The duty to bargain in good faith requires the parties "to meet at reasonable times and confer in good faith with respect to wages, hours, and other terms and conditions of employment...." It also requires notification of the other party and the Federal Mediation and Conciliation Service (FMCS) if a contract is to be modified or terminated.

Recognizing the special impact any work stoppage will have on the health services delivered by hospitals, Congress extended the notification procedure as follows. When a contract is already in effect, the party desiring to modify or terminate the contract must:

1. Notify the other party to the contract in writing 90 days prior to contract expiration;
2. Meet and confer with the other party about the contract changes;
3. Notify the FMCS and any state mediation agency 60 days prior to termination; and
4. Continue the existing contract for 90 days or until termination, whichever is later.

Good faith bargaining for an initial agreement following recognition or certification requires 30-days' notice to the FMCS. Congress also added a subsection (g) to section 8 requiring a labor organization to give 10 days written notice to the health care institution and the FMCS prior to engaging in any strike, picketing, or other concerted refusal to work. When the agreement is an initial one, the 10 days must come after the 30-days' notice to the FMCS.

A further amendment to Title II of the Taft-Hartley Act adds a special clause concerning conciliation of health care industry disputes. It empowers the director of the FMCS to determine if a threatened or actual strike or lockout will substantially interrupt the delivery of health care. If the director thinks it will, he may establish an impartial board of inquiry. The director must do so within the first 30-days' notification of the 60 days required when a contract already exists, or within 10 days after notice when an initial contract is concerned.

A board of inquiry must make written findings of fact with recommendations for settlement within 15 days. The parties must maintain the status quo during the 15 days of the board-of-inquiry operations and for 15 days after the board has rendered its findings of fact and recommendations. Therefore, when a board of inquiry is established, the requirement of maintenance of the status quo will expire at the same time the notice requirements have been fulfilled. This is an oddity in impasse procedures. The usual sequence places a fact-finding board after the notice requirements have been met.

The threat of a strike or lockout has long been recognized as the prime force for settlement in both the private and public sectors. Mediation often occurs as the 11th hour approaches. Fact finding is rarely used in the private sector, and usually it is used in the public sector only after contract expiration or impasse. Outlawing a strike and adding another step such as fact-finding only extends the dispute. The weaker party waits to see if the recommendations will lend support to its side. It is doubtful that serious bargaining will occur prior to the last 15 days, particularly when low paying hospital jobs are involved. The position of the labor organization may be substantially strengthened by waiting for the fact finders' recommendations.

SUMMARY

The removal of the Taft-Hartley exemption for nonprofit hospitals confers new legal rights and restrictions on nonprofit hospital management. This article has discussed the basics of the Taft-Hartley provisions concerning recognition and negotiation.

At this time, hospital management needs information. To that end, the following actions should be taken:

1. Widen the information base from which labor-management decisions are made. There is a myriad of literature on collective bargaining. A few hours reading time will save legal fees and decrease confusion. Some references are suggested below.

2. Obtain access to the services of a competent, current *labor* lawyer.

3. Adopt a "do-it-yourself" approach to labor-management relations. The law establishes procedure and precedent; it does not make management decisions.

REFERENCES

Beal, Edwin F., et al., *The Practice of Collective Bargaining,* Richard D. Irwin, Inc., Homewood, Ill., 1972.
Davey, Harold W., *Contemporary Collective Bargaining,* Prentice-Hall, Inc., Englewood Cliffs, N.J., 1972.
Hepner, James O., et al., *Personnel Administration in Health Care Facilities,* C.V. Mosby Co., St. Louis, 1969.

FOOTNOTES

[1] Nonprofit hospitals were covered under the National Labor Relations Act (Wagner Act) of 1935. The Labor Management Relations Act (Taft-Hartley) of 1947 amended section 2(2) of the

Wagner act to exclude nonprofit hospitals. The new bill strikes the section 2(2) exemption from Taft-Hartley; so hospitals are once again under national labor law.

[2] A. A. Imberman, "Communications: An Effective Weapon Against Unionization," *Hospital Progress,* December, 1973, p. 54.

[3] See Eli Rock, "The Appropriate Unit Problem in the Public Service: The Problem of Proliferation," *Michigan Law Review,* March, 1969, pp. 1001-16; and William J. Emanuel, "Nonprofit Hospitals and the NLRA Exemption," *Hospital Progress,* January, 1973, pp. 69 ff.

[4] A discussion of the history and application of each factor is presented in John E. Abodeely, *The NLRB and the Appropriate Bargaining Unit,* University of Pennsylvania Press, Philadelphia, 1971.

[5] Harold W. Davey, *Contemporary Collective Bargaining,* Prentice-Hall, Inc., Englewood Cliffs, N.J., 1972, p. 60.

23.
Negotiating and Administering a Union Contract

RANDYL D. ELKIN

Randyl D. Elkin, Ph.D., is Director of the Graduate Program in Industrial Relations, West Virginia University.

When PL 93-360 became effective Aug. 25, 1974, nonprofit hospitals were no longer exempt from the National Labor Relations Act. Therefore, many administrators will soon be engaged in the three basic processes of collective bargaining: recognition, negotiation, and contract administration.

If a labor organization achieves exclusive representative status and meets the procedural requirements for recognized negotiation,[1] the hospital administrator must be concerned with the scope of those negotiations. If negotiations culminate in a collective bargaining agreement, hospital management must administer the contract. This article emphasizes labor-management relations rather than legal aspects of contract negotiation and administration.

Analyses of contract negotiation processes vary from purely theoretical treatises to practical, how-to-do-it manuals.[2] A list of frequently mentioned suggestions follows:

1. Both the union and management negotiating committees should be reasonably small. If the union or company committee is too large and everyone insists on participating, much time will be consumed, tempers will become frayed, and much irrelevant material may be introduced.

2. One person must be in charge of conducting the negotiations for each side. Division of authority in negotiation is fatal to orderly procedure and usually impedes the agreement-making process.

3. The parties should agree in advance on the time of day and desired length of bargaining sessions. Each side can then make its plans accordingly.

4. Careful preparation for negotiations should include exchange of demands or proposals for study before actual bargaining begins. A frequent source of trouble is the springing of a complicated new proposal during negotiations.

5. Advance agreement on procedures will eliminate such unnecessary arguments as whether subject X is "in order at this time."

Reprinted by permission from *Hospital Progress: Journal of the Catholic Hospital Association*, St. Louis, Vol. 56 (January, 1975), pp. 40-43. Copyright 1975 by the Catholic Hospital Association. All rights reserved.

6. Negotiators should have authority to make decisive commitments in the course of negotiations. Company negotiators generally have the power to bind their principals. In most unions the negotiated terms are subject to ratification or rejection by the membership. Membership rejection can be a serious problem.

7. Negotiations should begin with well-planned agenda that include a complete statement of all disputed issues together with a listing of proposals and counter proposals on the disputed points.

8. If possible, an agreed statement of relevant economic data should be employed. This can be done when the parties have made effective use of a prenegotiation conference.

9. The negotiators should first resolve the less controversial issues and reduce their agreement to writing before proceeding to the tougher issues.

10. The difficult issues can be divided into those that involve money outlays and noneconomic demands.

11. Many noneconomic issues can be negotiated individually in terms of their intrinsic merit rather than in terms of the bargaining strength of the principals. This generalization would clearly not apply, however, to union demands relating to such "noneconomic" matters as union security or seniority.

12. Finally, and of critical importance in most negotiations, a decision must be made as to whether to bargain out the demands involving money outlays one by one or to negotiate on an economic package basis.[3]

Hospital administrators confronted with the uncertainties of negotiating their first labor contract may be tempted to hire a labor lawyer to act as chief management negotiator. Such action usually is not necessary. A labor lawyer should be present on the management negotiating team for reference and for purposes of drawing up formal contract language, but he need not and probably should not be chief negotiator.

BARGAINING SCOPE

As the exclusive bargaining representative certified by the National Labor Relations Board (NLRB), the labor organization has a 12-month period during which to persuade management to enter into a written agreement. Limitations are placed on what subjects may be included in the agreement. However, the recency of the removal of the Taft-Hartley exemption and the peculiarities of the health industry will require that the legal scope of negotiations be determined on a case-by-case basis.

The law vaguely states that the scope of negotiations be restricted to "wages, hours, and other terms and conditions of employment." The NLRB and the courts have established three categories to delineate bargaining scope. The first category consists of "mandatory" items such as wage rates, pensions, seniority accumulation, and subcontracting. These are bargainable to the extent of strikes or lockouts. The second category consists of "permissible" issues about which the parties may bargain by mutual consent. However, since such issues are either too remote from the employment relationship or are prerogatives of one of the parties, neither side may insist on bargaining on these issues. Such permissible items include performance bonds, change of a party negotiator, and the rehiring of replaced economic strikers.[4] The final category includes items outside the scope of negotiations. Requiring that an employee be a union member prior to being hired is an example of such an illegal demand because it violates section 8(a) (3) of the Taft-Hartley Act.

MANAGEMENT RIGHTS CLAUSES

The test of a contract derived from collective bargaining is whether the parties can live reasonably well under these newly established formal rules of the shop. Once an agreement has been signed, the bargaining relationship enters the executive phase of contract administration.

Contrary to the convictions of many administrators, labor organizations do not want to manage the hospital. They perceive a dividing line between those functions that are solely management's and those that are jointly labor's and management's. Frequently, this line is very broadly drawn and subject to shifts, but nevertheless it is there.

Hospital management may protect its prerogatives in at least two fashions. Explicit management rights clauses similar to those regularly appearing in industry contracts may be included. Some are very explicit and lengthy listings of management functions. Others are brief and state in effect that anything not explicitly stated in the contract is the sole and exclusive province of management. The other major approach adopts the attitude that anything in the contract is fair game for future union bargaining pressure. Rather than list and possibly lose prerogatives, those taking this second approach prefer to waive the contractual management rights clause, therefore assuming that anything not explicitly listed in the contract is management's right.

Management rights clause provisions frequently address residual rights, flexibility in operations, and discipline. One example of such a clause is:

> The management of the plants and the direction of the working forces and the operations of the plants, including the hiring, promoting and retiring of employees, the suspending, discharging or otherwise disciplining of employees for just cause, the laying off and calling to work of employees in connection with any reduction or increase in the working forces, the scheduling of work and the control and regulations of the use of all equipment and other property of the company, are the exclusive functions of the management; provided, however, that in the exercise of such functions the management shall observe the provisions of this agreement and shall not discriminate against any employee or applicant for employment because of his membership in or lawful activity on behalf of the union.[5]

Some contracts also add a section to the grievance clause stating that the management rights clause is not subject to interpretation or application by an arbitrator.

Hospital management rights clauses will vary in content according to the type of labor organization, i.e., professional, blue-collar, or white-collar membership. The content of management rights clauses contained in contracts with the latter groups probably will be similar to those discussed above. However, contracts with professional employees are likely to address responsibility for patient care. Such clauses are common in contracts with registered nurses for two reasons. First, nurses have identified greater control over patient care as a bargaining goal. Second, appropriate bargaining unit determination demands that nurses with largely supervisory functions be distinguished from those without these functions.

INDUSTRIAL JURISPRUDENCE

Employees do not organize solely to gain economic benefits.[6] They also organize to establish a system of industrial jurisprudence, which is addressed in those aspects of the contract that give employees freedom from arbitrary management decision-making. Employees want decisions to be made on the basis of known criteria applied consistently according to established procedure. It is management's right to determine how many individuals must be laid off, but the specific individuals may be contractually determined by seniority and ability. Management may have the right to decide to fill a nurses' aid vacancy, but it may be required by contract to exhaust internal sources of labor supply before going to external sources.

A good grievance procedure is the epitome of industrial jurisprudence. There are two ways to gain freedom from arbitrary management decision-making. One is to usurp that function (or gain a say in management decision-making similar to that achieved by the codetermination model in West Germany). The other method, used in the United States, is to effectively challenge any management decisions that appear to be arbitrary.

Prior to grievance procedures that in addition require final and binding arbitration, economic force was the effective challenge. Since World War II grievance procedures (95 percent of which end in arbitration) have institutionalized this conflict. They are *quid pro quo* for a no-strike clause in the contract. In the absence of negotiators with perfect foresight, the day-to-day decisions of contract administration will cause grievances. Whether the employee is right or wrong under the contract makes no difference; a grievance exists any time an employee questions the interpretation and application of the contract.

An effective grievance procedure will dispose of the problem quickly and equitably. A poor or nonfunctioning procedure may cause, at worst, a wildcat strike. Arbitrator Harold W. Davey suggests four principles which should govern the handling and adjustment of grievances.

1. Grievances should be settled promptly, preferably at the first step of the procedure, and on their merits.
2. The procedure and forms must be easy to use and clearly understood by both employees and supervisors. According to the Taft-Hartley Act, an employee has the right to attempt to adjust his grievance directly without appealing to the formal grievance procedure. Yet the employee's grievance should not be settled contrary to

the agreement, and a union representative has the right to be present during the adjustment sessions.

3. Grievance procedures should provide a timed avenue of appeal that progresses through a higher level of management and labor organization power at each step.

4. The procedure should end in arbitration which is final and binding upon all concerned parties.[7]

ARBITRATION

Hospital management is obligated to administer the contract fairly and to resort to discipline only for just cause. The labor organization has a parallel responsibility to reject grievances without contractual merit. Nevertheless, in a well-functioning grievance procedure a small percentage of grievances will proceed to arbitration.[8]

Arbitration may be performed on an *ad hoc* basis or by a permanent arbitrator. Lists of arbitrators are provided on request by the Federal Mediation and Conciliation Service (FMCS) free of charge and by the American Arbitration Association (AAA) for a small service fee. An arbitrator may be chosen from the list by several methods, but requesting an odd number of arbitrators from AAA or FMCS is a common solution. Each side involved in bargaining then proceeds to alternately eliminate a single name. The remaining arbitrator is then contacted to set a hearing date. He probably will suggest several possible hearing dates a month or more off, and he may request a brief statement of the grievance, a copy of the contract revealing the disputed language, and any other materials the two parties may jointly decide to send. The parties do not have to keep the hearing date if the grievance or grievances are settled before the hearing. But if the settlement occurs near the hearing date, the arbitrator may charge a service fee for preventing him from scheduling another hearing on that date. The hearing is held on neutral turf—frequently in a nearby motel or hotel room. It is conducted by the arbitrator in a fashion akin to the rules of evidence.

If the parties have not decided upon a statement of the grievance, the arbitrator's first task is to get the parties to phrase the grievance in a one-sentence, yes or no question. The hearing will open with both sides explaining what it is they intend to prove. The labor organization will present its opening statement first unless the case involves disciplinary action, wherein the burden of proof lies with management. Management must show that the disciplinary action was for "good and just cause" and that the penalty was in keeping with the infraction.

The majority of the hearing is devoted to the second phase wherein each side presents its case. Witnesses may be called for direct examination and are subject to cross examination, redirect, etc. The arbitrator has a duty to the record. He may ask questions about things that are unclear to him or about things that he believes have been omitted from the record. These procedures are followed by closing comments by both sides.

The parties may have a court reporter prepare a transcript of the hearing (done about 10 percent of the time) and may submit posthearing briefs. The arbitrator will study these documents, his notes, and the contract, and make an award sometime after the hearing.

The arbitrator is bound by the contract; he can neither add to nor delete from it. His duty is to interpret and apply it. The award will state the agreed upon facts, the contentions of the two sides, and the arbitrator's reasoning. The final page will contain the arbitrator's award: grievance sustained or denied. Occasionally, the arbitrator will modify the penalty imposed by management if he believes the "punishment" is too harsh for the "crime."

Unfortunately, grievance arbitration is expensive (but much less expensive than a work stoppage) and can involve considerable delay. In 1972, the FMCS alone had requests for 13,005 panels. A review of cases for 1972 indicates that $590 was an average total charge per case for the arbitrator alone.[9] A partial accounting of management arbitration cost in 1965 found that arbitrator fees (shared equally with the labor organization) were about 20 percent of the fee cost of a one-day hearing.[10] In 1972, a sampling of FMCS cases revealed the following average time trend for grievances requiring arbitration.[11]

Number of days between:

Filing of grievance and request for panel	75.2
Request and sending of list	15.1
Date list is sent and appointment	43.8
Appointment and hearing	61.1
Hearing and award	46.4
Total time between panel request and arbitration award	166.4
Total time between grievance filing and award	241.5

Currently, there is considerable experimentation designed to cut the costs and delays in arbitration. Certainly, the newly organizing health care industry provides an excellent opportunity for innovation in grievance arbitration.

SECURITY CLAUSES

The recent amendment to Taft-Hartley added a union security clause (section 19) to the NLRA. Such a clause provides that the employer aid the labor organization in enrolling employees and in keeping them enrolled. There are at least half a dozen varieties of union security clauses, each providing the labor organization with varying degrees of security.

The clause offering the greatest security is the "closed shop," which requires union membership prior to hiring. Such a clause is illegal under Taft-Hartley. The "union shop" clause is the most security a union can legally have under national law. Under this clause, after a certain number of days, often 30, the employee must either join and maintain membership in the labor organization or seek employment elsewhere. However, under section 14 (b) of Taft-Hartley, states can outlaw the union shop. Eighteen "right-to-work law" states have done so. In these states and others, unions frequently obtain "agency shop" clauses whereby the employee need not join the labor organizations. But because he receives all the benefits and services of having a labor organization, he must pay a service fee equal to the membership fee. Under a "maintenance of membership" clause, employees have the option of joining the union or staying nonunion after a specific number of days. If they join, they must maintain their membership as a condition of employment. Under the modern meaning of "open shop," there is no security clause other than NLRB exclusive recognition. Any of these types of security clauses may be coupled with a form of union security called the "checkoff," whereby the employer automatically deducts the membership fee from the pay of all employees who voluntarily sign the checkoff authorization form. The money then is remitted to the labor organization.

When a security clause requires membership as a condition of employment, the employer shall not terminate the employee for lack of membership so long as that person pays an amount to the union equal to union fees. The addition of section 19 to Taft-Hartley allows an employee of a health care institution to pay an amount equal to the initiation fees and dues of the organization to a tax-exempt nonreligious charitable fund chosen by the employee. Yet such an arrangement can be made only if the employee is a member of and adheres to the teachings of a religion, body, or sect which has historically held conscientious objection to joining or financially supporting a labor organization.

Collective bargaining is a continuous labor-management relationship of recognition, negotiation, and contract administration. The removal of the exemption from Taft-Hartley affords nonprofit hospital management and employees an opportunity to select the best aspects of current collective bargaining and to innovate to create more viable forms that will more readily benefit both parties.

FOOTNOTES

[1] See Randyl D. Elkin, "Recognition and Negotiation Under Taft-Hartley," *Hospital Progress*, December, 1974, pp. 50ff.

[2] The following books can be helpful when preparing for negotiations: Leland B. Cross, *A Collective Bargaining Agreement Checklist for Employers*, Indiana State Chamber of Commerce, Indianapolis, 1968; James O. Hepner, *et al., Personnel Administration and Labor Relations in Health Care Facilities*, The C. V. Mosby Company, St. Louis, 1969; and Meyer S. Ryder, *et al., Management Preparation for Collective Bargaining*, Dow-Jones-Irwin, Inc., Homewood, Ill, 1966.

[3] Harold W. Davey, *Contemporary Collective Bargaining*, 3rd ed., Prentice-Hall, Inc., Englewood Cliffs, N.J., 1972, p. 129.

[4] These items and a synopsis of important cases outlining the board and court rationale can be found in Russell A. Smith, *et al., Labor Relations Law*, 4th ed., The Bobbs-Merrill Company, Inc., New York City, 1968, pp. 741-61.

[5] *Agreement Between Bethlehem Steel Corporation and United Steelworkers of America,* Aug. 1, 1974, p. 91.

[6] See Sr. Margaret Sweeney and Edith H. Belsjoe, "Employee Communications During and After a Union Campaign," *Hospital Progress,* April, 1974, pp. 52ff.

[7] Davey, pp. 146-48.

[8] See Norman Metzger, "The Arbitration Procedure," *Hospitals,* April 16, 1974, pp. 47-49 and May 1, 1974, pp. 45-47.

[9] James F. Power, "Improving Arbitration: Roles of the Parties and Agencies," *Monthly Labor Review,* November, 1972, pp. 20-21.

[10] R. W. Fleming, *The Labor Arbitration Process,* University of Illinois Press, Chicago, 1965, p. 50.

[11] Power, p. 21.

Unionization Issues and Procedures

In Selection 24, "THE EFFECT OF UNIONS ON HOSPITAL MANAGEMENT" by Leo B. Osterhaus, the "conservative-liberal" administrative philosophy spectrum toward unionization is presented. The writer goes on to identify the factors which stimulate and inhibit unionization. Finally, the four fears of unionization—strike, cost, loss of control, and administrative complication—are presented.

An event of the past ten years, slow at first but lately becoming a cascade, is professional unionization. Many in the public sector—such as teachers and policemen—have formed unions or quasi-unions. The vanguard in the health care area have been nurses' associations. Because of their major role in the delivery of health care and their numbers, the nurse as unionist is an important issue. In Selection 25, "THE NURSE AS A PROFESSIONAL AND AS A UNIONIST" by Richard L. Epstein and K. Bruce Stickler, the basic conflicts between professional and union member, the roles of nurses' associations and the administration, and federal labor law are presented.

The writers outline distinctions between a professional and labor organization. The basic message of this selection is that when a professional association, such as a national, state, or local nurses' association becomes concerned with pay, hours of work, or any other conditions of employment, it is defined as a labor organization under the Taft-Hartley Act. Consequently, the nurse who is an active professional association member and a supervisor, is placed in a paradoxical position.

To resolve the inconsistencies the reciprocal theory is offered, i.e., the administration's response to nurses' organizations, or any other professional association should be based on its momentary function or activity. The test is: "Is it functioning as a professional or labor organization for that activity at that point in time?"

In our discussion of the 1974 Taft-Hartley Amendments, a number of matters of concern to the administration were discussed. One of them was its policy on solicitation and distribution by union organization representatives and/or the hospital's employees. In Selection 26, "SOLICITATION RULES WILL NEED REVISION" by William J. Emanuel and Alfred Klein, the reader is provided with a complex, yet well written and informative treatment of this subject. The primary point is that a hospital's policies on solicitation and distribution must be enforceable and there must be "consistency of application in a non-discriminatory manner" for outside organizers as well as inside organizers (employees). Should these conditions not be met, the

NLRB can declare them illegal. Further, to be non-discriminatory, they must be formulated prior to an organization attempt. The writers also trace through typical situations of concern and offer a sample policy for the reader's consideration.

Selection 27, "GRIEVANCE PROCEDURE: OUTLET FOR EMPLOYEE, INSIGHT FOR MANAGEMENT" by Rod Clelland, is the last in this part. It serves to point out the function of a grievance procedure, whether implemented on the administration's initiative or as part of a labor agreement. Drawing on the motivational foundation which was presented in Part II, THE MANAGEMENT OF HOSPITAL PERSONNEL, the writer presents the grievance procedure as a safety valve for constructively dissipating employee frustration, satisfying human needs, and, simply, solving problems that might otherwise be ignored.

24.
The Effect of Unions on Hospital Management

LEO B. OSTERHAUS, PH.D.

Leo B. Osterhaus, Ph.D., is the Director of the Center of Business Administration at St. Edwards University in Austin, Texas.

As organized labor has increased in numbers and scope, not only has it affected every individual in the United States, but the ramifications of its influence are evident in organizations and institutions that have traditionally been isolated or specialized in their functions, if not in their activities. Such an institution is the hospital.

In spite of deeply rooted traditions which surround hospitals with an almost religious-like aura, significant trends in public opinion and acceptance of unions as democratic institutions lend validity to the doubts of some and wishes of others that hospitals are prime targets for accelerated union activities.

Attracting organized labor to the hospital field are 7,123 hospitals employing almost two million people.[1] Related activities such as nursing homes, clinics and other medical treatment facilities swell this total.

It is generally conceded that working conditions and wages in the hospital have not kept pace with industry, even for the same skills; rather a reliance has been placed on appeals to the "will to serve humanity." Although this has been successful to a limited degree, these conditions beckon the unions. Sloan, in describing hospital labor problems, stated that although hospitals have paid low in the past, they must pay more and must eliminate possible causes for demands or unions will make them do it.[2]

Much of the organization of labor in the hospitals has occurred since World War II. A few hospital employes like engineers were organized loosely in the thirties, but the major drives have been in the past 10 years. One of the reasons for the delay in unionization in the hospital is probably the fact that the Labor Management Relations Act of 1947, usually referred to as the Taft-Hartley Act, specifically excludes nonprofit hospitals from its provisions which protect or encourage collective bargaining. Voluntary hospitals are also generally excluded from the provisions of state laws.

---
[1] Statistics were obtained from *Hospitals,* Part II, Guide Issue, Aug. 1, 1966, p. 428.
[2] Raymond Sloan, *This Hospital Business of Ours,* New York, G. P. Putnam's Sons, 1952, p. 216.

Reprinted by permission from *Hospital Progress: Journal of the Catholic Hospital Association,* St. Louis. Excerpts from two parts, Vol. 48 (June 1967), 68-72; (July, 1967), 78-79. Copyright 1967 by The Catholic Hospital Association. All rights reserved.

It would be a mistake to attribute the existence of unions today to any single cause; they resulted from a combination of many historical circumstances which existed in the hospital environment. In general, hospitals have lagged far behind industry in recognizing the need and providing for the industrial relations staff function. Hospital administrators have handled grievances poorly. They have failed to provide comparable wages and salaries, and the training in communication and supervision has failed to be effective in many cases.

SCOPE OF THE STUDY

It is generally stated that hospital costs are closely related to many of the labor-management problems. Costs in nonfederal short-term general and special hospitals have been increasing faster than the costs of any other segment of the medical care area. The proportion of the total cost represented by payroll expenses has increased from 50 per cent in 1946, to 70 per cent in 1964. Two-thirds of the increase in total expense per patient day between 1946 and 1964 can be accounted for by the increase in payroll expenses.[3]

With the increasing influence of labor unions on hospitals, and the pressures being placed upon hospitals to improve their manpower practices, the hospital is being forced to meet industrial employment conditions by increasing hospital wages and fringe benefits and shortening the workweek. Industrial employers have been able to meet some of their increasing labor costs through increased productivity; therefore, the author studied the potential of productivity increases in hospitals to see if they can compensate for higher labor costs.

The type of labor hospitals employ is a function of their employment conditions and creates certain manpower problems such as high turnover, absenteeism and high supervisor-employe ratios. Although the type of labor employed may result in low labor costs, it is necessary to include the effects of these problems in an evaluation of total actual cost and to estimate whether changed employment practices allowing for improved labor standards might not lead to an actual reduction in labor costs.

CONSISTENT DATA LACKING

Because of the critical relationship of manpower problems, labor unions and hospital costs, and the growing impact of these problems on hospital operation, research leading toward possible solutions and the development of effective policies is urgently needed. Data on which the research would be based, however, is not available. Studies have been made of specific manpower problems in individual institutions or small groups of institutions. But no comprehensive, consistent data has been collected from enough institutions over a wide area to provide the researcher with a base of correlated and verified information on patterns and trends of hospital personnel practices, policies and problems. After the author collected and organized these descriptive data, he then evaluated the effects of current practices on hospital efficiency and costs.

[3] *Hospitals,* Part II, Guide Issue, Aug. 1, 1965, p. 438.

While manpower and industrial relations problems in hospitals fall directly within the purview of the applied disciplines of personnel administration and labor relations, the techniques of labor economics, cost accounting, and industrial management have also been used to analyze the significance of hospital operations on specific policies and practices. The most productive approach to hospital manpower and industrial relations problems seemed to be an interdisciplinary approach capable of using the relevant information and techniques of both basic and applied disciplines and of the medical care field.

PHILOSOPHY OF LABOR RELATIONS

Although most industries have probably thought at one time or another that "they were different," and organized labor "did not have a place" in their establishments, hospitals do seem to present other than routine labor-management problems.

The basic labor relations philosophy of the hospital field is shaped by hospital management, hospital associations, and other professional groups closely allied to the hospital and medical care field.

Hospital management is a diffused and varied group without a unified, concise stance on common problems. It is difficult to determine anything specific concerning hospital management. Not only is the ownership of hospitals diverse, but hospitals themselves are identified so closely with the general public that it is difficult to isolate public opinion from hospital management opinion. The direct public influence is immediately experienced.

The American Hospital Association, the unofficial voice of most hospitals, states as a policy: "It is for the hospital governing board to decide the hospital policy toward union recognition and collective bargaining."[4] The same organization states further: "It is hoped that such a hospital will approach the problem with due regard for: 1. the law, 2. sound personnel policies, 3. proper management principles, and 4. accepted community practices."[5]

As indicated from a review of recorded statements from leaders and other individuals in the field, attitudes toward unions vary from: 1. Violent opposition,[6] 2. toleration as long as individual union members do not interfere in any way with hospital operations and management,[7] 3. acceptance as bargaining equals to management,[8] and 4. acceptance because the ownership of the hospital or union represents a sizable portion of the clientele.[9] The majority opinion seems to cluster around the second attitude which may possibly be explained by the size and location of hospitals in this country. Undoubtedly, this attitude toward unions has been

---

[4] American Hospital Association, *Hospitals and Employe Groups*, Personnel Relations Series No. 2, Chicago, American Hospital Association, p. 5.

[5] *Ibid.*, p. iv.

[6] Grandville L. Jones, "Unions in Hospitals Are Wrong and Unnecessary," *Mental Hospitals*, September, 1957, p. 27.

[7] E. D. Barnett, "Satisfied Employes Promote Good Hospital Care," *Hospital Council Bulletin*, June, 1949, p. 19.

[8] San Francisco Bay Area.

[9] Hospitals owned by unions and hospitals furnishing hospital services to union groups.

influenced by the fact that most hospitals have less than 100 beds and are located in small communities where organized labor is weak.

The management philosophy of these rather conservative administrators is based on the following factors:

1. The granting of control of employes and/or activities in a hospital to a union which knows little about the problems of the care of the sick is incompatible with safe patient care.

2. Hospital operation is a continuous one, and to interpose any force that would tend to destroy its continuity would be harmful.

3. Hospital activity, unlike industry, must strive for 100 per cent efficiency in its professional elements and cannot accept any interference that might appear if seniority, tenure, etc., were used primarily as a basis for selection of employes in the nursing units and treatment and diagnostic areas.

4. Because hospitals are nonprofit organizations, no profits are available to share, or with which to bargain.

5. Unions divide the loyalty of employes between management and unions.

6. Hospital employes enjoy a high status in the community without union aid.

7. Unions are powerless if the weapons of strikes, work stoppages and slowdowns are removed. As these weapons cannot be tolerated in hospitals without endangering life, unions would be unnecessary appendages.

8. The right of employes to organize is secondary to the right of human beings to receive adequate attention when ill or injured.

9. The Taft-Hartley Act is the law of the land—a public mandate, and since hospitals were specifically exempted from this law, unions should not attempt to organize in hospitals.

10. Unionization in hospitals is not in the public interest.

11. As it is assumed that with unionization comes additional labor costs, some leaders point out that this additional cost would have to be borne directly by the patients. The vital difference in the purchasing of hospital services is that the patient does not have a real choice of whether to purchase or not to purchase—he must buy hospitalization.

FOUR FEARS

The above theories (or expositions) are based on four fears:

1. Strikes. Management realizes that hospitals are helpless against strikes if desired health care standards are to be maintained. Endangering lives and/or delaying the relief of suffering is unthinkable. Past records of strikes, in spite of their paucity, have magnified this fear.

2. Unionization will cost money. A study of the wage rates confirms this fear. As hospital costs are reaching alarming proportions, administrators appear to be condoning, currently at least, a lower hospital charge at the expense of hospital employes' wages.

3. Control will be lost. Management has a fear that unions will assume an unnecessary number of management's prerogatives. A divided control would be disastrous in a hospital if exhibited to any degree.

4. Organized labor will complicate administration and require that a central control be established to insure that personnel administration is consistent. Detail procedures will have to be given the supervisors on how to handle simple disciplinary problems and complaints. All actions will have to be documented completely so that the case can be supported if it goes to arbitration.

A MORE LIBERAL VIEW IS EMERGING

Enlightened writers have been warning for years that hospital management should re-evaluate the philosophy of purchasing labor, and vitalize hospital personnel policies. These warnings, stripped of their more highly theoretical (but probably more important) discussions, are based on hard reality that can be ascertained by even the most recalcitrant. These are:

1. Unionization is now generally accepted as a way of life, and this trend may affect the favorable public reaction enjoyed by the hospital in the past in hospital-labor disputes.

2. Noneconomic incentives accruing to hospital employes are currently over-rated. Gordon in commenting on this states:

> There appeared to be a general acceptance of the proposition that nonmonetary incentives have sometimes been over exploited and are not a substitute for a fair wage scale that is equitable within the hospital and that provides a necessary standard of living for the worker and his dependents.[10]

3. A social revolution has taken place that should be considered in the over-all operation and relationships of hospitals. This change is best illustrated by the following comment:

> In the fields of wages and salary administration, many new concepts have been introduced. In this field, as in the field of relations with organized labor, we are dealing with group pressures, and we have as yet not resolved the dilemma of conflicts between individual and group aspirations.[11]

4. Sound personnel policies and a modern personnel department are needed with or without a union; they are not a luxury or a frill but a necessity in these enlightened times. Hospitals must quit vacillating and establish these departments or this will be just another defenseless weakness. Everett W. Jones states:

> The constant upgrading of administrative abilities and leadership and the development of sound personnel and public relation practices may well determine the ultimate fate of our voluntary hospital system.[12]

Many people connected with the hospital field complain that the worker today is more interested in the monetary return than in service to the sick. These and similar

---

[10] Paul J. Gordon, "Why Anyone Works in a Hospital," *The Modern Hospital,* June, 1954, pp. 76-78.

[11] B. A. Lindberg, "Looking in on Hospital Personnel Administration," *Hospitals,* May, 1953, p. 65.

[12] Everett W. Jones, Hospital Consultant at the National Board of Methodist Hospitals and Homes Convention, Indianapolis, Ind., 1945.

statements are emanating from both the conservative and the liberal side of the question as evidenced by the following:

1. Hospitals are competing with industry for personnel in the face of a diminishing labor pool, particularly since the change in status of women workers after World War II. To meet competition, wages and other benefits must approach parity with industry.

2. Hospitals must present an attractive career program for the three-quarter million new workers entering the labor market every year, or fall heir to the castoffs from industry.

3. Hospitals should recognize that they have a basic obligation to both their employes and the public in their employe relations.

The above facts, reinforced with a new philosophy, have resulted in enlightened efforts to accept unions,[13] and writings such as those of the AHA, Stevens,[14] Freeman,[15] and Metzger[16] have furthered the cause.

A very limited number of administrators have advanced the theory that unions actually benefit hospital operations. This attitude, as limited in converts as it may be, is found in the mental hospital field,[17] but it is not entirely limited to this area.[18] The limitation of the scope of this attitude is emphasized since one of the two major problems that contribute to limited unionization in mental hospitals is the fact that hospital administrators are slow to recognize unions. Today, for an administrator to advocate that unions do benefit hospital operations is an undertaking of some trepidity.

In summary, the majority of hospitals are conservative in their thought and action toward unions, but a trend to a more liberal view is indicated.

FACTORS STIMULATING UNIONIZATION

The magnitude of the nonunion labor force in the hospital industry apparently has been one of the factors attracting the eyes of union organizers during recent years. In 1964, there were 7,127 hospitals in the United States employing a total of 1,886,839 fulltime personnel with an annual payroll of $7,974,623,000.00.[19] Of all the hospitals this vast industry, only 435 hospitals in 1965 had contracts with labor organizations.[20] This fact certainly provides an incentive to the labor organizer, especially in light of recent declines in over-all labor union membership.

[13] Ray Bruner, "Toledo Plan' Supported by Hospitals and Labor," *The Modern Hospital,* July, 1959, pp. 76-77.

[14] R. D. Stevens, "How Administrators Can Negotiate with a Union," *Southern Hospitals,* December, 1956, p. 26.

[15] John R. Freeman, "You Can Too Learn to Live with Unions." *The Modern Hospital,* November, 1964, pp. 95-98.

[16] Norman Metzger, "Living with a Collective Bargaining Agreement for the First 100 Days," *Hospital Management,* October, 1964, pp. 49-52.

[17] Pamphlet entitled *Mental Health Story,* published by the American Federation of State, County and Municipal Employes, AFL-CIO; Jack R. Ewolt, "Employes Union: Pro and Con; Unions Can Benefit Hospital Administration," *Mental Hospitals,* September, 1957, pp. 26-27.

[18] Arthur Hare, "Hospitals and Union in Harmony." *The Modern Hospital,* February, 1948, p. 74.

[19] *Hospitals,* Guide Issue, Aug. 1, 1965, Part II, pp. 431-451.

[20] Interview with Edward W. Weimer, director, Administrative Services, AHA, Aug. 2, 1965.

Poor labor relations practices are thought to be one of the major factors contributing to the general labor movement. This condition has apparently provided a major boost in the unionization of employes in the hospital industry.

> In general, hospitals have lagged far behind industry in recognizing the need for, and providing, the industrial relations staff function. In many hospitals of several hundred employes, the personnel function is performed as "the other hat" of an already harried administrator, or his assistant.[21]

Inadequacies in personnel or industrial relations have been especially noticeable in the area of grievance procedures in hospitals. "In some hospitals, there is little provision made for the settlement of grievances, an oversight that stimulates interest in unions."[22] In recognition of this shortcoming, concerted efforts of the American Hospital Assn. have been directed toward personnel relations during the past several years. These efforts have taken the form of numerous workshops and institutes conducted for hospital administrators and their assistants on the subjects of labor relations, as well as publications aimed at improving personnel policies of member hospitals, especially in the areas of employe handbooks and grievance procedures.[23]

Another factor which would seem to contribute to the encouragement of labor unions in hospitals is the matter of wages.

> A disproportionate chunk of the charity of too many hospitals has been involuntarily carried by underpaid employes who supply the hospital with essential services.[24]

The Bureau of Labor Statistics' survey of hospital wages conducted during 1963 showed a number of hospital employes receiving less than what is usually considered to be the minimum wage. Almost 130,000 of the one million workers covered by the survey were receiving less than $1.25 per hour.[25] Another factor to keep in mind is that this survey was limited to hospitals in metropolitan areas with populations in excess of 250,000. A much larger percentage of low-paid employes can normally be expected in hospitals in smaller cities and in rural areas.

Even though the wage issue is usually not the greatest motivating factor for union membership, it would seem to rank high in importance for workers in the hospital industry. The difference between the wages of hospital workers and those employed in work outside the hospital industry is such that hospitals sometimes have been accused of "exploitation."[26] The mere mention of this word, of course, strikes at the very heart of the labor union movement, and it provides additional impetus for the drive to unionize hospital employes.

---

[21] James L. Centner, "Hospitals and Collective Bargaining," *Personnel Journal,* November, 1959, p. 203.

[22] Walter L. Daykin, "The Hospital and Employe Organizations," *Hospital Administration,* Fall, 1958, p. 7.

[23] For example, see the following pamphlets published and distributed by the AHA. *Suggested Employe Dissatisfaction Procedure, Preparing an Employe Handbook,* and *Hospitals and Employe Groups.*

[24] Carl I. Flath, "Hospitals and the Labor Movement," *Southern Hospitals,* July, 1960, p. 26.

[25] U.S. Department of Labor, Bureau of Labor Statistics, *Industry Wage Survey: Hospitals,* June, 1964, p. 12.

[26] George Kirstein, "Why Hospitals Exploit Labor," *The Nation,* July 4, 1959, pp. 3-6.

FACTORS INHIBITING UNIONIZATION

Although many hospitals have long had a small number of employes who belonged to unions, the unions have been slow to develop in hospitals for a variety of reasons. Foremost among them is that unions were preoccupied with more lucrative fields and thus delayed their action in this particular field. Some of the other more important reasons which prevented unionization of hospital employes are discussed below.

Dispersion and size of hospitals are factors which inhibit unionization. Of the 7,127 hospitals registered by the AHA in 1964, 4,009 had less than 100 beds. The average institution had approximately 260 fulltime employes.[27] These hospitals were dispersed throughout the United States, and the majority of the small hospitals were located in small communities. This fact made unionization difficult except where employes could be included with other organized groups from other industries in the community.

The nature of the hospital force itself has been a major inhibiting factor.

> Many hospital employes are women whose work is a temporary interlude between school, marriage and the rearing of a family. In other words, these female employes lack permanency, and it is a well-established principle that it takes permanent employes to form a strong labor movement. Employes of this type customarily lack labor-consciousness and are inclined to view problems that arise as temporary. In addition, a sizable proportion of the employes in hospital work are older workers who are unfamiliar with union operations; many are pleased merely to have employment. Consequently, they often are reluctant to engage in any activity which might jeopardize their job status.[28]

The hospital also has a multiplicity of professional and semiprofessional employes. Tead, in addressing the American College of Hospital Administrators, stated that among the factors that highlight and complicate the jobs of administrators is the critical function of utilizing a wide variety of specialized vocational groups within the organization as well as by the organization itself, and the difficulty of keeping the primary social objective of the institution foremost in mind.[29] This problem would apply with equal force to the union officials as well as the hospital executive.

Hospitals, proportionally, have a greater number of varieties of professional, semiprofessional, skilled, and semiskilled personnel than any other organization. This factor, combined with the reluctance of many of these personnel to be identified with unions, has impeded progress of unions.

Both national and state labor legislation has been a major deterrent for hospital unionism. Although these laws generally do not prohibit hospital employes, neither do they encourage and protect either of these actions.

THE STRIKE HAS NOT BEEN EFFECTIVE

Another major inhibiting factor is the nature of hospital business, i.e., the voluntary, nonprofit status of the typical hospital. This unique position has molded the opinions of legislators, the courts, and the public to the extent that attempts at

---

[27] Figures computed from Tables 1 and 2c, Guide Issue, *Hospitals,* Part II, Aug. 1, 1965, pp. 431-452.

[28] Daykin, *op cit.,* p. 8.

[29] From an address by Ordway Tead to the ACHA, Aug. 17, 1958, Chicago.

unionization of hospital employes are met with hostile attitudes in many areas. The emotions connected with the service of the business of the hospital—caring for the sick—has been a factor. Any actions which might temporarily interfere with the operation of a hospital are thought of as being directed toward those persons lying ill in the hospital. An important deterring force is public sentiment which was illustrated in an organizational drive that was thwarted through an information campaign, including appeals in local newspapers.[30] In a leaflet prepared by the AHA for hospital administrators, one of the actions suggested to combat unionism was "Tell your story to the press."[31]

Finally, the strike—labor's ultimate weapon—has not been very effective in hospitals. In several instances, workers striking for union recognition have been victims of unfavorable public reactions, and they have failed to receive support from other labor unions or from the clergy. The available supply of volunteer workers to fill the vacated jobs, the refusal on the part of most other laborers to honor the picket line, and the hesitancy of strikers to insist that their picket line be honored have often made the hospital strike ineffective. These factors were instrumental in the defeat of the union in Chicago.[32]

SUMMARY

Many feel that hospitals are unique and, therefore, should be treated differently from other service and manufacturing industries when considering labor-management relations and other subjects. No unanimity of opinion exists, but in general the hospital administrators and hospital trustees are rather conservative and try to avoid any radical change from the past. Administrators and trustees receive support from professional groups (except for the nurses) which seem to be anti-union or anti-collective-bargaining-minded. However, as these groups mature and gain status, they will probably seek economic security as well as professional and educational benefits for their members.

A more liberal view of labor-management relations has recently emerged in the hospital administration field. The success of this group is rather limited at the present, but the group is increasing in number as the new and younger administrators assume leadership in the hospital field.

[30] John T. Foster, "Good Story Well Told Defeats Two Union Efforts at Wisconsin Hospital," *The Modern Hospital,* July, 1964, p. 36.

[31] "What to Do! A Checklist for the Individual Hospital," AHA, Chicago, Aug. 15, 1959.

[32] Robert B. McKersie and Montague Brown, "Nonprofessional Hospital Workers and a Union Organizing Drive," *The Quarterly Journal of Economics,* August, 1963, pp. 372-404.

25.
The Nurse as a Professional and as a Unionist

RICHARD L. EPSTEIN AND K. BRUCE STICKLER

Richard L. Epstein, J.D., is a partner and K. Bruce Stickler, J.D., is an attorney - with the firm Sonnenschein, Carlin, Nath, and Rosenthal, Chicago.

It has not been easy for the U.S. health care system to settle in to the new responsibilities imposed by coverage under the National Labor Relations Act. The nature and number of significant developments have already been such to warrant statistical reporting and analysis.[1] Perhaps the most important phenomenon of this past year has been the often painful awareness that professional personnel associated with health care institutions are no longer what they used to be. As a result, it would not overstate the case to observe that hospitals' relationships with all their professional personnel are undergoing profound change and that that change is likely to have greater impact on the executive resources and administrative behavior of a hospital than any other aspect of its labor relations.[2] This paper deals with the nurse portion of that picture.

THE PROBLEM

The developments that generate the special problem associated with nurses are essentially three-fold. First is the relationship among nurses, their hospital employer, and the regional, state, and national nurses' associations. Prior to labor law coverage,[3] nurses' associations were regarded more as a membership group of managers than of employees, and nurses were regarded by themselves and by others as occupying an employment status quite different from that of other hospital employees. As long as the notion of "hospital worker" did not include the "professional" nurse, the hospital could, and did, comfortably extend to the nurses, policies and practices that were not available to nonprofessionals and that were not, by and large, sought by other professionals.

The second development was the imposition of a new set of rules to govern the employment relationship. The enactment of the Taft-Hartley amendments in 1974

From *Hospitals, J.A.H.A.:* Reprinted, with permission, from *Hospitals, Journal of the American Hospital Association,* (Vol. 50, No. 1, January 16, 1976, pp. 44-48, 108). Copyright 1976 by the American Hospital Association. All rights reserved.

made it clear that the hospital is the nurse's "employer" under Sections 2(2) and 2(14),[4] that the nurse is the hospital's "employee" under Section 2(3),[5] that any representative of them, in whatever guise, is a "labor organization" under Section 2(5),[6] that different treatment for nurses raises problems under Section 8(a),[7] and that it matters whether a nurse with supervisory responsibility is included or not under Section 2(11).[8] It should be understandable that when a long-standing working relationship with established expectations became suddenly enmeshed in a panoply of specific regulation, legal consequences, case precedent, and enforcement proceedings, that relationship will require careful new study and considerable adjustment.

The third development was considerably more gradual but no less significant. In the decade preceding the 1974 amendments, we witnessed the evolution of the "professional" from a special type of employee, aloof from the turbulent style of labor organizations, to a full-blown union member. Teachers were the first to provide the lesson that special training for employment and a clearly acknowledged status as a professional no longer will separate them from the notion of joining a union, negotiating a contract, dealing through a representative, and striking for more wages, fewer hours, and changes in working conditions—not unlike a steamfitter or a steelworker.[9] Nurses and nurses' associations were the next to abandon the posture of the traditional professional and, in some jurisdictions, to don the trappings of a true labor organization.[10] But this development for the most part was nowhere as decisive and plain as in the teachers' history. In fact, among the problems we shall discover is the inability or unwillingness of the American Nurses' Association (ANA) to assume all the responsibilities as well as the privileges that go with becoming a part of organized labor, with consequent confusion to nurses who are members, to nurses who are not, and to the institutions that employ them.

These developments pose for hospital administrators these questions:

1. In the labor relations context, what is the nurses' association, at the national, state, and regional level and within the hospital?
2. How should they be treated?
3. How should their members be treated?
4. Where does the nursing service administrator fit in?

ANALYSIS OF PROBLEM

In focusing more sharply on the nature of the nurse problem, it would be well to define the entity we are dealing with and to identify the sections of the law that impinge on the hospital's response to that entity.

First, "labor organization" means "any organization of any kind, or any agency or employee representation committee or plan, in which employees participate and which exists for the purpose, in whole or in part, of dealing with employers concerning grievances, labor disputes, wages, rates of pay, hours of employment, or conditions of work."[11]

A professional association as defined by the authors is a formal organization of persons who share a common interest as employees or practitioners in a calling or vocation, the pursuit of which requires specialized knowledge, academic preparation, and extensive training.

Three things are evident. First, the ANA at all levels is a professional association within the meaning of the foregoing definition. Second, it is not inconsistent with that definition for such an association to be, as indeed the ANA and several of its affiliates have declared, a labor organization within the meaning of Section 2(5). Third, it is not necessary, however, for an affiliate of ANA to be a § 2(5) labor organization in order to be a professional organization.

There have emerged in the modern day nurses' association two separate identities. It is a professional association engaged with the concerns of health care, including education and training of nurses and the collecting, organizing, and imparting of information relating to the improvement of, and developments in, the delivery of health care.[12] It is a labor organization with the goals and structure that characterize the traditional representative of employees with respect to hours, wages, and working conditions.[13]

It is also the latter identity that triggers the problems that emanate from Taft-Hartley coverage. Several requirements of the act are fundamentally inconsistent with a number of practices that have been in wide use among hospitals. These practices have included hospital payment of dues to the nurses' associations; hospital encouragement of association membership; provision of meeting rooms, without charge, on the employer premises; and other tangible support of the association by the hospital employer.[14-16]

THE DILEMMA

The dictionary definition of "dilemma" appropriately describes the problem: "a situation involving [a] choice between equally unsatisfactory alternatives." Here, the unsatisfactory alternatives would be to treat a nurses' association solely under one or the other of its two identities. Taking these one at a time, we do have an entity that, whatever else it may be, is clearly a labor organization. To cast the nurses' association solely under the "union" label, however, would ignore those groups of nurses who do not so regard themselves and who endeavor to cooperate with one another and to organize together only for the purpose of enhancing their skills and education in dealing with the problems of health care delivery.[17] The labor organization label, by itself, also would ignore the fact that the association does hold wholly nonunion meetings in the form of educational programs, and that, indeed, it has a genuine commitment to the methods and quality of health care delivery and their improvement.[18] It is not surprising, therefore, that members of management, including directors of nursing service, traditionally have been association members[19] and that there are many other members of the national and state nurses' associations who have no interest in labor organization aspirations or activities.[20]

But neither may the nurses organizations be viewed solely as professional associations devoid of any labor union characteristics.[21] To ignore their "union" identity would be to ignore that they have thus declared themselves[22] and registered as such;[23] that they act in that fashion as certified representatives in the collective bargaining relationship;[24] that they make unhesitating use of the weapons and strategy historically characteristic of unions;[25] that they unmistakably view themselves as such;[26] and that the National Labor Relations Board has declared several state nurses' associations to be labor organizations.[27]

The two alternatives are, as dilemma implies, unsatisfactory. The fact is that for the hospital-employer to continue to regard nurses' associations as only professional organizations and to continue the favors and support that it has felt free to render the "professional association" would invite other labor organizations to seek, and not surprisingly, the same benefits of meeting space, dues payment, and other subsidies and assistance.[28] However, for the hospital-employer to adopt exclusively the alternative identity of labor organization would cause nurses and nurse groups who otherwise have no such inclination to act as a union in response to being treated as a union.

AN ANSWER

If it is true that the hospital's response should not be in terms of only one or the other of two association identities, we must be prepared to recognize that any good answer will likely be new, untried, and certainly untraditional. By no means does that necessarily signal an undersirable state of affairs. Rather, it conveys that a solution may need to be found in seasoned imagination instead of in tested precedent. The point is that hospital-employers may find it beneficial to avoid the either-or approach characteristic of the labor relations field and to address instead the matter of nurses' associations and their members on a selective basis—that is, to reciprocate the particular identity the nurse group is assuming at any moment in their relationship. Put another way, the hospital's response to nurses' organizations should be formulated on the basis of the organization's momentary function or activity rather than on the basis of seeking to divine the nature of an association or group as a whole. In other words, the hospital-employer should back off the issue of what the nurse group is or is not and should direct itself to what the nurse group is doing at a particular occasion or with respect to a particular matter. The determination then may be made by the employer that a specific occasion evidences the nurses' union identity, thus calling for certain appropriate responses pursuant to Taft-Hartley and the institution's general union policy; or, that a specific occasion evidences its professional identity, thus calling for an entirely different set of responses. In that manner the employer's response would be fashioned by its reciprocating the nurse group identity that is then being put forward.

This may be illustrated by these occasions:

• *Meeting on employer premises*—Hospitals have traditionally permitted nurses to hold meetings on the premises. In the past, when the meetings primarily involved health matters and took place prior to the effective date of Taft-Hartley coverage, there was no special problem.

Use of the reciprocal theory would proceed this way. Examine the occasion and purpose of the particular meeting and respond to it, not to all national, state, and regional nurses' associations. Look at the agenda and observe which of the two "identities" is holding the meeting—the health professionals, or the labor organizers—and then respond only to that identity.[29]

- *Time off to attend meetings of the nurses' association*—Here, too, the appropriate employer conduct may be determined by the particular purpose of the meeting, as disclosed by the agenda.

- *Payment of dues*—The meaning of "payment of dues" is twofold. One meaning is the mere deduction and transmittal of employee-authorized dues monies, commonly known as "dues check-off." A second meaning is the payment by the employer of the employee's dues obligations, with the employer providing the money, which we will refer to here as "dues payment benefit."

The employer's method of handling this matter should be determined by the nature of the recipient of the dues money. If the association to which dues are paid conducts any union-nature activities, as clearly do most nurses' associations, and if the revenue it receives remains commingled, all dues payments should be treated as dues to a labor organization. Accordingly, it would be improper and unlawful to provide or continue a dues payment benefit.[30] Whether to provide or continue a dues checkoff will be determined by the employer's judgment as to whether it would wish or be willing to do so for other labor organizations. Rather obviously, it would not, and so the response would seem clear.[31]

- *Director of nursing service also serving as a member or officer of a nurses' association*—The analysis of dues handling applies here as well. The employer's approach should be determined by the fact that, unlike the meeting occasion, it is the nature of the subject matter as a whole that will be determinative. That is, as dues had to be treated as "dues to a labor organization" because the association's treasury supports its labor union activities (as well as other activities), so too should membership in the association be treated as participation in the union activities of the association. It follows that as a member of management should not be a member of a union, the director of nursing service should not be a member of the nurses' association at any level.[32] The essence of objection here, as in the dues picture, lies in the fact that unlike meetings and unlike time off, the nurses' associations have not divided their treasuries and functions into the two separate identities that could then each merit a separate response. In short, the presently indivisible nature of membership in any nurses' association, as now constituted, disqualifies an employer's managerial employee from membership in that association.

The considerations that should be deemed to disallow a nursing director's membership in a nurses' association would obviously preclude holding office in the association.

- *Other supervisory and nonsupervisory nurses or members or officers of the association*—The response applicable to the director of nursing service is equally applicable to all the supervisory nurses. But as the line is crossed over to staff nurses, the need for discerning identities and for reciprocating falls away. Staff nurses, as employees covered under the Taft-Hartley Act, have all the rights and responsibilities that attend that status, and their classification as "professionals" is of no consequence in the matter of their membership or nonmembership in a nurses' association.[33]

• *Encouragement of membership*—Hospital and supervisor encouragement of nurse membership in nurses' associations has been widely practiced. This should be discontinued or avoided with respect to all levels of nurses, but, as seen earlier, for a somewhat different reason at each level.

• *Other activities*—There are various other occasions calling for similar judgments, such as employer payment of registration fees and of travel expenses for attendance at association meetings. The method for determining the appropriate reciprocal response has been illustrated earlier. That, plus the following observations, should afford the necessary benchmarks for reciprocal decision making.

MORE GROUND RULES

• *Tainting*—When an association includes union-identified activities, the association should be treated in its entirety as a labor organization for some purposes. In this context, these purposes include dues payments, holding office, and all other internal matters. The reason for treating either an activity or group as "tainted" is that the mere presence of the "union" identity, albeit in a larger setting, is sufficient to be pointed to by other labor organizations for precedent to obtain the same treatment for themselves, or to establish the basis for a successful unfair labor practice charge.

• *Deception*—There may be instances where, notwithstanding assurance to the hospital that a meeting or occasion is wholly of the health professional identity without labor organization taint, it develops that some aspect of the labor organization will emerge, intentionally or not. It has been suggested that this risk warrants the monitoring of meetings. Such monitoring is unnecessary and ill-advised. First, the presence of monitors undercuts the aspects of fairness and objectivity to be otherwise derived from the employer position recommended here. Second, the only risk of a tainted session is its use as a precedent for other organizations. To be able to prove that an assurance was received of it being a nonunion meeting is sufficient to overcome the concern about precedent. Third, an effective remedy is simply to withhold permission for all meeting requests thereafter. Moreover, not a great deal of harm will have resulted from one meeting having gone partially awry.

• *The concerned supervisory nurse*—Some high-ranking nurse managers respond to the proposition of denying them participation in their association by pointing out that this frustrates their desire to help shape and direct the nurses' associations. They have expressed their concern that the labor organization identity is being increasingly pursued by their associations at all levels. To the hospital administrator, this explanation for supervisors requesting that they be allowed to continue their association participation, and presumably influence, has an undeniable allure. The hard fact is, though, that the more valid the basis for this appeal by supervisors, the more violative would be their participation. A nurse manager is a part of the management of the employer, and employers may not interfere with or dominate the officers of what is without question a labor organization, at least in part.[34]

CONCLUSION

The ANA, along with its affiliates, has an opportunity to respond to the demands made upon it by new legal developments and by its new goals. This can best be done by the nurses' associations' realigning their internal structure to make absolutely and formally separate their educational function and their union identity.[35] It is important to nurses to have a resource for their continuing education, unfettered by union organizational matters. It is obviously important to the nurses' associations to promote their union aspirations. It has proven burdensome for one entity to do both. But as long as the nurses' associations fail to make the necessary reorganization, the best answer of the hospitals that employ their members is the reciprocal approach we have described here.

REFERENCES

[1] Rosmann, J. One year under Taft-Hartley Law, *Hospitals, J.A.H.A.* 49:64, Dec. 16, 1975.

[2] Section 2(12) of the National Labor Relations Act defines a professional: "(a) any employee engaged in work: (i) predominantly intellectual and varied in character as opposed to routine mental, manual, mechanical, or physical work; (ii) involving the consistent exercise of discretion and judgment in its performance; (iii) of such a character that the output produced or the result accomplished cannot be standardized in relation to a given period of time; (iv) requiring knowledge of an advanced type in a field of science or learning customarily acquired by a prolonged course of specialized intellectual instruction and study in an institution of higher learning or a hospital, as distinguished from a general academic education or from an apprenticeship or from training in the performance of routine mental, manual, or physical processes; or (b) any employee who (i) has completed the courses of specialized intellectual instruction and study described in clause (iv) of paragraph (a), and (ii) is performing related work under the supervision of a professional person to qualify himself to become a professional employee as defined in paragraph (a)."

[3] Prior to P.L. 93-360 (August 25, 1974), not-for-profit voluntary health care institutions were exempt from federal labor regulation under the Taft-Hartley Act by virtue of a provision in the Act which had existed since 1947. This provision has been deleted by P.L. 93-360.

[4] "2(2) The term 'employer' includes any person acting as an agent of an employer, directly or indirectly, but shall not include the United States or any wholly owned Government corporation, or any Federal Reserve Bank, or any State or political subdivision thereof, or any person subject to the Railway Labor Act, as amended from time to time, or any labor organization (other than when acting as an employer), or anyone acting in the capacity of officer or agent of such labor organization. 2(14) The term 'health care institution' shall include any hospital, convalescent hospital, health maintenance organization, health clinic, nursing home, extended care facility, or other institution devoted to the care of sick, infirm, or aged persons."

[5] "The term 'employee' shall include any employee, and shall not be limited to the employees of a particular employer, unless the Act explicitly states otherwise, and shall include any individual whose work has ceased as a consequence of, or in connection with, any current labor dispute or

because of any unfair labor practice, and who has not obtained any other regular and substantially equivalent employment, but shall not include any individual employed as an agricultural laborer, or in the domestic service of any family or person at his home, or any individual employed by his parent or spouse, or any individual having the status of an independent contractor, or any individual employed as a supervisor, or any individual employed by an employer subject to the Railway Labor Act, as amended from time to time, or by any other person who is not an employer as herein defined."

[6] "The term 'labor organization' means any organization of any kind, or any agency or employee representation committee or plan, in which employees participate and which exists for the purpose, in whole or in part, of dealing with employers concerning grievances, labor disputes, wages, rates of pay, hours of employment, or conditions of work."

[7] "8(a) It shall be an unfair labor practice for an employer—(1) to interfere with, restrain, or coerce employees in the exercise of the rights guaranteed in section 7; (2) to dominate or interfere with the formation or administration of any labor organization or contribute financial or other support to it: *Provided,* That subject to rules and regulations made and published by the Board pursuant to section 6, an employer shall not be prohibited from permitting employees to confer with him during working hours without loss of time or pay."

[8] "The term 'supervisor' means any individual having authority, in the interest of the employer, to hire, transfer, suspend, lay off, recall, promote, discharge, assign, reward, or discipline other employees, or responsibly to direct them, or to adjust their grievances, or effectively to recommend such action, if in connection with the foregoing the exercise of such authority is not of a merely routine or clerical nature, but requires the use of independent judgment."

[9] Alutto, A., and Belasco, J. Determinants of attitudinal militancy among nurses and teachers. *Indus. Labor Relations Rev.* 27:216, Jan. 1974.

[10] Stumptf, G. L. Labor relations among professional groups. *J. Amer. Diet. Ass.* 65:138 Aug. 1974. In 1946 at its annual convention the ANA passed the following resolution: "ANA believes that the several state and district nurses' associations are qualified to act and should act as exclusive agents to their respective memberships in the important fields of economic security and collective bargaining." In the ensuing years the ANA took the following action: 1950–adoption of a "no strike" policy. 1952–the economic security aims of 29 state nurses' associations had negotiated 87 agreements covering 199 health care institutions. 1957–43 state associations had officially accepted the responsibility for the ANA "economic security program"; however, only 17 had active programs. 1966–the "no strike" policy was rescinded. 1968–ANA offered technical staff assistance in financial and labor relations to states and districts, however, role of "exclusive agent" remained with the states and the districts. See also, *The Code For Nurses,* adopted by the ANA in 1950, revised in 1960 and 1968; specifically, article 8, which provides, in pertinent part, for "nurses' collective negotiations with employers" about economic conditions and general welfare.

[11] S 2(5) of the Act.

[12] Galloway, B. The nurse as a professional manager. *Hospitals, J.A.H.A.* 48:89, Nov. 1, 1974; Hampton, L. Evaluating continuing education programs. *Adult Leadership.* Sept. 1973, p. 105.

[13] For instance, the Code for Nurses, first adopted by the ANA in 1950, provides for collective bargaining; ANA's economic and general welfare department provides its members with a bibliography that includes literature on such topics as labor relations (generally), collective bargaining for nurses, and ANA's economic and general welfare program; and on Sept. 30, 1974, ANA's Commission on Nursing Services drafted a resolution to study the restructuring of ANA "to protect the right of each and every registered nurse to full and active membership" in the organization. This would include participation in labor relations representation and collective bargaining activities. In the area of white collar employees, the ANA's constituents won bargaining rights for more employees than any other union in the first nine months of 1975, winning 32 of 42 elections to represent 2,227 nurses. BNA *White Collar Report,* Nov. 28, 1975, No. 973.

[14] "Employees shall have the right to self-organization, to form, join, or assist labor organizations, to bargain collectively through representatives of their own choosing, and to engage in other

concerted activities for the purpose of collective bargaining or other mutual aid or protection, and shall also have the right to refrain from any or all of such activities except to the extent that such right may be affected by an agreement requiring membership in a labor organization as a condition of employment as authorized in section 8 (a) (3)."

[15] "14(a) Nothing herein shall prohibit any individual employed as a supervisor from becoming or remaining a member of a labor organization, but no employer subject to this Act shall be compelled to deem individuals defined herein as supervisors as employees for the purpose of any law, either national or local; relating to collective bargaining."

[16] "302(a) (1) It shall be unlawful for any employer or association of employers or any person who acts as a labor relations expert, adviser, or consultant to an employer or who acts in the interest of an employer to pay, lend, or deliver, or agree to pay, lend, or deliver, any money or other thing of value—(1) To any representative of any of his employees who are employed in an industry affecting commerce; or (2) to any labor organization, or any officer or employee thereof, which represents, seeks to represent, or would admit to membership, any of the employees of such employer who are employed in an industry affecting commerce; or (3) to any employee or group or committee of employees of such employer employed in an industry affecting commerce in excess of their normal compensation for the purpose of causing such employee or group or committee directly or indirectly to influence any other employees in the exercise of the right to organize and bargain collectively through representatives of their own choosing; or (4) to any officer or employee of a labor organization engaged in an industry affecting commerce with intent to influence him in respect to any of his actions, decisions, or duties as a representative of employees or as such officer or employee of such labor organization."

[17] We have heard many administrative, supervisory, and staff nurses working at health care institutions around the country express their views that their association is a professional one, not a labor organization. Moreover, these nurses' desire to remain active members of their state and district associations is for the stated purpose of improving educational and professional standards, not to engage in collective bargaining. In short, they do not perceive either their association or themselves as a union.

[18] The Code for Nurses, Article 7, provides: "the nurse participates in the efforts of the profession to define and upgrade standards of nursing practice and education."

[19] ANA recently (May 12, 1975) prepared a position paper in order to give direction to nursing service administrators when attempting to define their participation in ANA.

[20] Amundson, M. Labor relations and the nursing leader. *J. Nursing Admin.* 4:16, March-April 1974.

[21] Schrader, E. S. Editorial, *AORN Journal.* 21:192, Feb. 1975; O.R. nurse-betwixt union and management. *Hospitals, J.A.H.A.* 48:77, May 1, 1974; The ANA: can a professional association be a trade union too? *Hospitals, J.A.H.A.* 48:103, Sept. 1, 1974.

[22] "WHEREAS, The American Nurses' Association is the professional organization seeking to represent all registered nurses in the areas specified under Article I of the bylaws, including the promotion and protection of the economic and general welfare of nurses (section 3-g)..."ANA Commission on Nursing Services, resolution of Sept. 30, 1974.

[23] "WHEREAS, The collective bargaining activities of the ANA require its registration as a labor union under the Landrum-Griffith Act..." ANA Commission on Nursing Services, resolution of Sept. 30, 1974.

[24] Phillips, D. New demands of nurses—part 1. *Hospitals, J.A.H.A.* 48:31, Aug. 16, 1974; Phillips, D. New demands of nurses—part 2. *Hospitals, J.A.H.A.* 48:41, Sept. 16, 1974. During fiscal year 1975 (July 1, 1974 - June 30, 1975) 17 state nurses' associations participated in representation elections. The state nurses' associations affiliated with ANA won 21 of 28 representation elections gaining 1,319 new "union" members.

[25] See Phillips, D. San Francisco nurses' strike patient care issues and physician involvement. *Hosp. Med. Staff.* 3:10, Oct. 1974. The Ohio Nurses' Association engaged in a 53 day strike at Youngstown Hospital from December 1974 to February 1975; California Nurses' Association en-

gaged in a 21 day strike of approximately 40 San Francisco Bay area hospitals, June 7 to June 21, 1974; Montana Nurses' Association and its member registered nurses at St. James Community Hospital honored a teamster picket line at the institution in a strike lasting 25 days in June 1975.

[26] Schorr, T. Editorial: They'd better believe. *Amer. J. Nursing.* 74:11 (Aug. 1974). See also, The Code for Nurses, Article 8; on November 21, 1974 ANA-Nebraska Nurses' Association put on a joint workshop concerning ANA's economic and general welfare program. Topics discussed included: "professional organization unions," "bargaining rights," and "collective-action" (which is a euphemism for strike activity). See further, Indiana State Nurses' Association Manual on Economic and General Welfare Program, p. 11.

[27] *Anne Arundel Hospital,* 217 NLRB No. 148 (1975) where the Board found Maryland state nurses' association to be a labor organization within the meaning of Section 2(5) of the Act; see also *Oak Ridge Hospital of the United Methodist Church,* 220 NLRB No. 9 (1975) (Tennessee Nurses' Association).

[28] Granting favors to and requests of one labor organization while at the same time denying similar favors to or requests of another would subject the institution to charges of unlawful discrimination, assistance, or domination under Section 8(a) (2).

[29] The ANA has tacitly recognized its dual-identity makeup. In its May 1975 position paper on nursing service administrators' participation in ANA, the ANA spells out which activities an administrator may participate in and which functions a nursing administrator cannot either attend, promote, or join. Simply put, ANA states that its nursing administrators cannot participate on behalf of ANA in collective bargaining or union-related causes or events.

[30] This would be so under Section 8(a) (2) as well as Section 302 of the Act.

[31] Northeastern Vermont Regional Hospital responded in similar fashion when the Vermont State Nurses' Association (VSNA) filed a petition to organize the hospital's registered nurses. The hospital discontinued its practice of withholding from nurses' paychecks their dues and of sending the dues directly to the association. The VSNA filed an unfair labor practice charge against the hospital. The Regional Director refused to issue a complaint stating: "... the investigation has disclosed that the Employer did not violate the Act by discontinuing check-off and other concessions to the Charging Party when the latter became a labor organization by filing a petition for certification as representative which is currently being processed. By acting otherwise the Employer could have been charged with having violated Section 8(a) (2)." The regional director's refusal to issue a complaint against the hospital was sustained by the National Labor Relations Board's Office of Appeal. *Northeastern Vermont Regional Hospital,* 1-CA-10659 (June 30, 1975).

[32] This is recognized in part by the ANA. Thus the ANA's position paper on nursing service administrator's participation in ANA provides that "a nursing service administrator may not ... (b) be present, if holding office on the board of directors or other structural unit of the association, during discussion or decision making related to the collective bargaining activities of the association." We would go further by precluding, in the first instance, nursing supervisors, managers, and administrators membership in the association if any part of the association itself was union-related.

[33] Most of the early NLRB litigation involving representation of professionals has centered around whether certain classifications of nurses at health care institutions are supervisors or employees. In *Presbyterian Medical Center,* 218 NLRB No. 12 (1975), and *Northwestern Memorial Hospital,* 13-RC-13476 (1975), head nurses were excluded from the bargaining unit of RNs because in those institutions head nurses possessed substantial indicia of authority and control over staff RNs. However, in *Newton-Wellesley,* 219 NLRB No. 80 (1975); *St. Mary's Hospital,* 220 NLRB No. 92 (1975); *Doctors Hospital,* 217 NLRB No. 87 (1975); *Driftwood Convalescent Hospital,* 217 NLRB No. 183 (1975); and in several other institutions, head nurses, charge nurses, team leaders, coordinators, assistant coordinators, and the like were included in the bargaining unit. In each case the evidence demonstrated a lack of authority and supervisory criteria as re-

quired under Section 2(11) of the Act. These latter individuals, therefore, would be accorded their Section 7 rights to engage in activity on behalf of a labor organization and to participate in collective bargaining.

[34] This is prohibited by Section 8(a) (2) of the Act.

[35] Indeed, ANA may have attempted in part to do this. Its position paper which is supposed to serve as a guide to nursing administrators may be broadened both in terms of affected individuals (to include all nurse supervisors and managers) as well as in scope (to consider other permitted/prohibited activities).

26.
Solicitation Rules Will Need Revision

WILLIAM J. EMANUEL AND ALFRED KLEIN

William J. Emanuel, LL.B, is a labor relations attorney and partner in the Los Angeles office of Morgan, Lewis, and Bockius.

Alfred Klein, J.D., is an attorney with the Atlantic Richfield Company and was formerly with the NLRB - Los Angeles and San Francisco.

Most hospitals have rules regulating solicitation and related activities on hospital property. For the most part, these rules were adopted long ago because of recurring problems unrelated to union organizing activities.* However, because of the organizing tactics of many unions, these rules will have application to union organizing efforts and therefore must comply with legal requirements established by the National Labor Relations Board *(NLRB).*†

Accordingly, it is important that hospitals now reevaluate such rules, and the manner in which they are enforced, in order to ensure compliance with such requirements. Virtually all such rules that have not already been revised to comply with such requirements should now be revised.

Union organizing efforts are usually carried on by two types of organizers: the outside organizer and the employee organizer. The outside organizer is a person on the

---

*As used in this article, the term "union" includes all labor organizations, including associations that seek to represent registered nurses, laboratory technologists, or other hospital employees for purposes of collective bargaining.

†This article does not apply to government hospitals, as such institutions remain exempt from the National Labor Relations Act (NLRA).

From *Hospitals, J.A.H.A.:* Reprinted, with permission, from *Hospitals, Journal of the American Hospital Association,* (Vol. 49, No. 16, August 16, 1975, pp. 47-51). Copyright 1975 by the American Hospital Association. All rights reserved.

Since the original publication of this article, the National Labor Relations Board has issued a number of decisions which should be read in conjunction with this article. The most important of these decisions are *St. John's Hospital and School of Nursing, Inc.,* 222 NLRB No. 182 (1976); and *Tri-County Medical Center, Inc.,* 222 NLRB No. 174 (1976).

union's payroll whose job is to organize the hospital's employees. The employee organizer is an employee of the hospital who favors unionization and attempts to organize the hospital's employees for the union.‡

OUTSIDE ORGANIZERS

Outside organizers are not ordinarily entitled to access to the hospital's premises.[1] This includes the hospital's parking lot and cafeteria, even though such facilities may be open to members of the public who have business in the hospital.[2] Accordingly, if the hospital maintains a rule prohibiting solicitation or distribution by all outsiders, outside organizers may lawfully be excluded from the hospital's premises and may be treated as trespassers if they persist in entering the premises, including police arrest if necessary.[3]

This assumes that the union has other reasonable means of access to the employees; if the union does not have such access, it must be permitted to enter the premises.[4] However, this exception would apply rarely if at all in hospitals, as the union presumably can communicate with the employees by handbilling on public property adjacent to the hospital premises.[5]

The hospital's right to exclude outside organizers also assumes that the exclusionary rule is enforced in a nondiscriminatory manner. If outsiders are allowed, for example, to come on the premises to sell cosmetics or life insurance, the NLRB may require the hospital to grant the same privilege to outside organizers.[6] However, this does not apply to outsiders who visit the hospital on hospital business—for example, an insurance representative who visits the hospital to explain a hospital-sponsored insurance program to the employees.

An outside organizer would also be entitled to enter the premises for a legitimate purpose unrelated to union organizing, such as visiting a patient.[7] However, this exception is open to abuse, and, in the authors' opinion, the hospital could lawfully preclude solicitation or distribution by the outside organizer during such a visit.

Moreover, if hospital facilities, such as the parking lot or cafeteria, are open to the general public, as distinguished from members of the public who have business in the hospital, the hospital may incur a legal risk if it does not allow outside organizers to use such facilities. However, in the authors' opinion, the hospital could prohibit use of such facilities for purposes beyond those for which they are open to the general public. Of course, if the hospital permits the general public to use such facilities for solicitation or distribution of literature, it could not prohibit outside organizers from using them for the same purpose.

Outside organizers are entitled to use public sidewalks and streets for purposes of

‡Some unions also enlist the support of statutory supervisors to organize employees. Such supervisors are not considered "employees" under the NLRA and do not have the rights of "employee organizers" explained in this article. Organizing activity by supervisors may, and should, be strictly prohibited.

solicitation and distribution, as long as they do not physically block ingress or egress. Moreover, in rare cases a privately owned sidewalk, street, or parking lot may take on the character of public property and thus be considered "quasi-public."[8] In such instances the hospital may not be able to enforce its technical property right by excluding trespassers.

EMPLOYEE ORGANIZERS

Unlike outside organizers, employee organizers have a basic legal right to engage in union solicitation and distribution of union literature on hospital property, and broad rules prohibiting such activities are unlawful.[9] However, the hospital may adopt and enforce carefully drafted rules that restrict the times and, in part, the locations, at which employees may engage in such activities.

UNION SOLICITATION

Union solicitation is an *oral* appeal to an employee urging prounion activity—for example, to support the union, sign a union authorization card, attend a union meeting, or vote for the union. Solicitation is to be distinguished from distribution of union literature, which involves giving an employee *written* material conveying a prounion message. However, the distribution of union authorization cards, without other written material, is considered to be solicitation, not distribution of literature.[10]

A hospital rule that prohibits solicitation by employees on working time is presumed to be valid, absent evidence that the rule was promulgated for a discriminatory (anti-union) purpose or is enforced on a discriminatory basis.[11] However, a rule that prohibits solicitation by employees on nonworking time is presumed to be invalid, absent special circumstances that make the rule necessary in order to maintain production or discipline.[12]

Working time means the working time of both the solicitor and the employee being solicited, and the rule should be specific in this regard.[13] This term does not mean "working hours" in the broad sense, meaning all times when the hospital is in operation. In this regard, it is important that the rule be phrased in terms of "working time" rather than "working hours."[14] Other terms to be avoided are "hospital time" or "company time."[15]

Nonworking time includes all time when the employees in question are relieved of duty, including paid time such as rest periods. Thus the rule cannot be enforced when the employees are relieved of duty, even though they are on "paid time."[16] However, as explained later in this article, off-duty employees may normally be excluded from the premises.

In addition to the time during which solicitation may lawfully be prohibited, location is another important factor, especially in a hospital. Assuming that the employees involved are on nonworking time, a rule against solicitation in either working areas or nonworking areas is presumptively invalid.[17] Although the NLRB allows employers to prohibit solicitation during working time, it does not generally permit employers to prohibit solicitation in working areas. However, a prohibition applicable to working areas will be permitted if necessitated by "special circumstances."

An example of "special circumstances" is found in retail department stores, which may prohibit solicitation in selling areas and aisles, corridors, elevators, escalators, and stairways open to the public. However, solicitation in such stores must be allowed in other nonselling areas, such as public restrooms, waiting rooms adjoining private streets, and public restaurants, to the extent that solicitation is incidental to normal use and does not involve moving from one table to another.[18]

The NLRB has not issued a definitive decision as to how far the "special circumstances" exception will be applied in hospitals. However, it has adopted a general statement that "a hospital's right to ban union solicitation in working areas where patients and visitors are likely to be present is somewhat akin to that of retail department stores."[19] Thus, it appears that hospitals will be allowed to prohibit solicitation in working areas where patients and visitors are likely to be present, although exact guidelines in this regard are not yet available. However, there is a possibility that adoption of such a rule, coupled with "captive audience" speeches by the hospital during an organizing campaign, might result in a requirement that the hospital give the union "equal time" to respond on hospital property to the hospital's speeches.[20]

DISTRIBUTION OF LITERATURE

Rules that restrict the distribution of union literature may generally be more stringent than rules restricting union solicitation. A hospital rule that prohibits distribution of literature on working time or in working areas is presumed to be valid, absent evidence of discriminatory promulgation or enforcement. However, a rule that prohibits distribution when the employee is both on nonworking time and in a nonworking area is presumed to be invalid.[21]

In applying these principles, it should not be difficult to conclude that some areas of the hospital, such as the parking lot and employee lounges, locker rooms, or rest rooms, are nonworking areas and that some, such as patient care areas, are working areas. However, these principles are difficult to apply when the area involved has a mixed character, such as the cafeteria. In such cases, the NLRB will disregard the normal presumptions and balance the employees' right to organize against the hospital's right to prevent disruption.[22] Accordingly, unless the hospital can show disruption of the operation of the hospital or interference with patient care, the NLRB can be expected to find a violation if distribution is prohibited in such an area.

DISCRIMINATORY PRACTICES

An otherwise valid rule against solicitation or distribution will be invalidated if promulgated for a discriminatory (anti-union) reason.[23] Thus, if a no solicitation or no distribution rule is promulgated solely in response to a union organizing effort, the validity of the rule will be jeopardized.

This promulgation requirement does not mean that adoption of a validly drafted rule, or modification of an invalidly drafted rule, at the outset of an organizing drive would necessarily be precluded.[24] However, it may be more difficult to establish the validity of the hospital's action under such circumstances than if the rule had been adopted or modified prior to the organizing drive.

Furthermore, an otherwise valid rule will be invalidated if enforced on a discriminatory basis.[25] Therefore, if such a rule is not also applied to solicitation or distribution for causes unrelated to unions, the validity of the rule will be jeopardized.

The NLRB currently recognizes a limited exception to this "equal enforcement" requirement in the case of "isolated" instances of solicitation or distribution for causes unrelated to unions, especially if such isolated instances are of the beneficent (charitable) variety.[26] However, as the scope of this exception is not clear, it is recommended that solicitation or distribution for causes unrelated to unions be kept to a minimum.

ADMINISTRATIVE APPROVAL REQUIREMENTS

A hospital may not condition union solicitation or distribution on "approval of the administrator," as employees are legally entitled to engage in such activities on hospital property at the appropriate times and places.[27]

Although a no solicitation or no distribution rule requiring administrative approval might not be considered invalid if employees understand that such approval does not apply to union solicitation or distribution, such terminology should be avoided, as the hospital will have the burden of proving that such understanding was shared by the employees.[28]

RELATED PROBLEMS

A hospital rule excluding off-duty employees from the premises is presumptively valid, as long as all off-duty employees are prohibited from entering or remaining on the premises for any reason.[29] However, such a rule cannot be enforced against off-duty employees who wish to engage in union solicitation or distribution if other off-duty employees are permitted to enter or remain on the premises. Moreover, such a rule cannot be enforced if the union lacks other adequate means of access to the employees,[29] although this is unlikely in a hospital, as the union can presumably communicate with the employees by handbilling on public property adjacent to the premises.

A hospital may prohibit posting of union material on official bulletin boards, as long as posting by employees or outsiders for other causes unrelated to the union is not permitted.[30] However, posting of union material may not be prohibited on a bulletin board that is open to employees for general posting purposes.[31]

During some organizing campaigns, employees advertise their support of the union by wearing union buttons or other union insignia while at work. The NLRB has concluded that employees have a legal right to wear such insignia unless the employer can show "special circumstances" that would justify prohibiting such conduct.[32] The type of special circumstances needed to justify a ban against union buttons depends on whether the employees wearing them have regular contact with patients and the public.[33]

If the employees do not have regular contact with patients and the public, union buttons may be prohibited only if the hospital can demonstrate that the prohibition is justified by special circumstances relating to employee efficiency, safety, or discipline.[34]

If the employees have regular contact with patients and the public, a different standard may be applied. In this situation, if the hospital's image to its patients and the public is important and if a neat and professional appearance is an important part of the hospital's image, protection of its image will be treated as an additional special circumstance justifying a ban on some types of union buttons. Such a hospital may prohibit the wearing of union buttons if they are "conspicuous" or if their size or color detracts from the dignity of an employee's uniform.[35]

However, the wearing of union buttons may not be prohibited under any circumstances if employees are permitted to wear other types of nonwork-related insignia, such as "smile" buttons or religious or political buttons, although this does not apply to insignia such as name tags or school pins.[36] Thus if a hospital waits until a union organizing drive to adopt a "no adornment" rule, it will not be able to enforce such a rule against employees who wear union buttons.

RECOMMENDATIONS

While it probably is not realistic to expect that all discussion about the union on working time will be prevented by the existence of a rule limiting solicitation and distribution, the authors recommend that a lawful rule be maintained by the hospital, as this will make it easier from the legal viewpoint to deal with aggravated violations.[37]

If the hospital has an existing rule restricting solicitation or distribution that does not meet the NLRB's requirements, it should be revised without delay. The model rule shown in Figure 1 is suggested for this purpose, but it should not be adopted without careful review of the considerations discussed in this article, as it may not be entirely appropriate under all circumstances.

If the hospital is currently undergoing an organizing attempt, counsel should be consulted as to the appropriate means and timing of promulgating a new or revised rule.

If an invalid rule is included in the employee handbook, a revised rule should be posted on hospital bulletin boards and distributed to each employee pending revision of the handbook.[38]

Prior to adoption of a new or revised rule, existing practices as to solicitation and distribution by both outsiders and employees should be reviewed. It is important in this regard that the hospital not adopt a rule that it cannot enforce without discrimina-

Rule regarding solicitation and distribution of literature on hospital property

In order to prevent disruptions in the operation of the hospital, interference with patient care, and inconvenience to our patients and their visitors, the following rules will apply to solicitation and distribution of literature on hospital property.

Outsiders

Persons not employed by the hospital may not solicit or distribute literature on hospital property for any purpose at any time.

Employees of the hospital

Employees may not solicit for any purpose during working time. Employees may not distribute literature for any purpose during working time or in working areas.

"Working time" includes the working time of both the employee doing the solicitation or distribution and the employee to whom it is directed. If you have any questions as to the meaning of "working time" or "working areas," please ask the personnel office for clarification.

Employees may not remain on the premises for more than 30 minutes after punching out and may not come on the premises prior to 30 minutes before the scheduled starting time.

FIGURE 1

tion. If the hospital considers it necessary to permit beneficent or charitable solicitations by employees on working time, it may want to rely on the unclear "isolated instance" exception explained above. However, counsel should be consulted and such exceptions should be kept to a minimum. The hospital should also consider the feasibility of conducting such solicitations in a manner that would not raise possible discrimination problems—that is, without solicitation by nonsupervisory employees on working time or by outsiders.

For distribution purposes, an advance determination should be made as to which areas of the hospital will be considered working areas and which areas will be considered nonworking areas. If an area has a mixed character, distribution should be permitted unless it can be shown that this would seriously interfere with patient care or would disrupt the operation of the hospital.

In formulating the hospital's rule, a decision must be made as to whether solicitation will be prohibited in working areas under the "department store" exception. This is not normally recommended, as (1) such a rule will probably not be necessary in most cases and is likely to lead to litigation in the event of an organizing attempt and (2) as explained above, adoption of such a rule, coupled with "captive audience" speeches by the hospital, might give the union a right to "equal time." Moreover, if a rule that does not prohibit solicitation in working areas is adopted and the hospital later finds that such solicitation disrupts patient care or creates other operational problems, a more restrictive rule could be adopted at that time.

After the rule is formulated, a set of written guidelines should be prepared with the assistance of counsel for the hospital's supervisors in order to ensure proper enforcement of the rule. Training sessions for supervisors should also be held to provide instruction on proper enforcement.

The rule should include a prohibition against being on the premises more than a specified reasonable time before and after the employee's shift. If this is not considered feasible under the circumstances, off-duty employees should be restricted to specified areas, such as the cafeteria.

Most hospitals maintain no solicitation signs at their entrances. These signs should be modified to make it clear that they do not apply to employees of the hsopital. For example, a notation could be added in small print stating, "Solicitation and distribution by employees are governed by posted hospital rules."

Existing rules and practices regarding (1) posting of written material in the hospital and (2) wearing of nonwork-related insignia should be reviewed, and rules should be adopted or revised in accordance with the guidelines explained above.

The exercise of employee rights under the law should not be conditioned on "administrative approval."

FOOTNOTES

[1] *NLRB v. Babcock & Wilcox Co.*, 351 U.S. 105 (1956).
[2] *Central Hardware Co. v. NLRB.* 407 U.S. 539 (1972).
[3] *S.E. Nichols of Ohio, Inc.*, 200 NLRB No. 161 (1972).
[4] *Joseph Bancroft & Sons, Inc.*, 140 NLRB 1288 (1963); *S. & H. Grossinger's Inc.*, 156 NLRB 233 (1965), *enforced in pertinent part*, 372 F. 2d 26 (2nd Cir. 1967).
[5] *Monogram Models, Inc.*, 192 NLRB 705 (1972).
[6] *Priced-Less Discount Foods, Inc.*, 162 NLRB 872 (1967).
[7] *Heck's Inc.*, 156 NLRB 760 (1966).
[8] *Amalgamated Food Employees Union v. Logan Valley Plaza*, 391 U.S. 308 (1968); *Lloyd Corp. v. Tanner*, 407 U.S. 551, 556 (1972).
[9] *Republic Aviation Corp. v. NLRB.* 324 U.S. 793 (1945).
[10] *The Rose Co.*, 154 NLRB 228, 229, footnote 1 (1965).
[11] *Peyton Packing Co.*, 49 NLRB 828, 843 (1943).
[12] *Walton Manufacturing Co.*, 126 NLRB 697, 698 (1960).
[13] *Avon Convalescent Center, Inc.*, 200 NLRB No. 99 (1972); *Summit Nursing & Convalescent Home*, 196 NLRB 769 (1972); *Forbes Pavilion Nursing Home, Inc.*, 198 NLRB No. 113 (1972).
[14] *Essex International, Inc.*, 211 NLRB No. 112 (1974).
[15] *WIPO, Inc.*, 199 NLRB 649 (1972).
[16] *I. F. Sales, Inc.*, 82 NLRB 137, 138 (1949), *enforced*, 188 F. 2d 931 (5th Cir. 1951).
[17] *Stoddard-Quirk Manufacturing Co.*, 138 NLRB 615, 621-622 (1962).
[18] *Marshall Field & Co.*, 98 NLRB 88, 92-95 (1952).

[19] *Guyan Valley Hospital, Inc.*, 198 NLRB No. 28, JD p. 12 (1972).

[20] *The May Co.*, 136 NLRB 797, 799-802 (1962), *enforcement denied*, 316 F. 2d 797 (6th Cir. 1963); *Montgomery Ward & Co.*, 145 NLRB, 846, 848-849 (1964), *enforced as modified*, 339 F. 2d 889 (6th Cir. 1965).

[21] *Stoddard-Quirk Manufacturing Co.*, 138 NLRB 615 (1962); *Young Spring & Wire Corp.*, 138 NLRB 643, 646 (1962).

[22] *Willow Maintenance Corp.*, 143 NLRB 64, 67-68 (1963), *enforced*, 332 F. 2d 367 (2nd Cir. 1964). Cf., *NLRB General Counsel's Third Monthly Report on Health Care Institution Cases* (Feb. 1975), where the General Counsel authorized issuance of a complaint against a hospital that extended its no distribution rule to a cafeteria and coffee shop that were open to visitors and patients.

[23] *State Chemical Co.*, 166 NLRB 455 (1967).

[24] See, for example, *Whitcraft Houseboat Division*, 195 NLRB 1046 (1972); *Cussins & Fearn Co., Inc.*, 170 NLRB 1 (1968).

[25] See, for example, *Imco Container Corp.*, 208 NLRB No. 133 (1974).

[26] *Serv-Air, Inc.*, 175 NLRB 801 (1969); *Sequoyah Spinning Mills, Inc.*, 194 NLRB 1175 (1972).

[27] *J. R. Simplot Co.*, 137 NLRB 1552 (1962).

[28] *Ferguson-Lander Box Co.*, 151 NLRB 1615 (1965).

[29] *GTE Lenkurt, Inc.*, 204 NLRB No. 75 (1973).

[30] *General Motors Corp.*, 212 NLRB No. 45 (1974).

[31] *Challenge Cook Brothers of Ohio, Inc.*, 153 NLRB 92, 99 (1965).

[32] *Floridan Hotel of Tampa, Inc.*, 137 NLRB 1484, 1486 (1962).

[33] *United Parcel Service, Inc.*, 195 NLRB 441 (1972).

[34] See, for example, *Clover Industries*, 188 NLRB 252, 253 (1971); *Standard Oil of California*, 168 NLRB 153, 154-155, 159-162 (1967); *Campbell Soup Company*, 159 NLRB 74, 76-79 (1966).

[35] *Evergreen Nursing Home and Rehabilitation Center, Inc.*, 198 NLRB No. 101, JD pp. 10-11 (1972).

[36] *The Ohio Masonic Home*, 205 NLRB No. 65 (1973); *Evergreen Nursing Home, supra*.

[37] See *Selwyn Shoe Mfg. Corp.*, 172 NLRB 674, 676 (1968).

[38] *Barnes Hospital*, 217 NLRB No. 126 (1975).

27.

Grievance Procedure: Outlet for Employees, Insight for Management

ROD CLELLAND *

Rod Clelland M.B.A., is Administrative Superintendent of Central State Hospital in Milledgeville, Georgia.

In April 1966, 3500 registered nurses in New York City hospitals delivered an ultimatum threatening resignation if better working conditions and improved pay were not provided. Shortly thereafter, similar events occurred in Los Angeles, San Francisco, and Phoenix, Ariz. These events brought into sharper focus several questions about grievance procedures in hospitals and underscored the urgency of finding answers. Among these questions were: Are nurses and ancillary hospital personnel ready for union organization? How are hospitals preparing to deal with the new forces and new relationships that unionization suggests?

Heretofore, hospitals have been exempt from labor legislation requiring overtime pay and minimum wages. However, bills recently passed by Congress have put an end to these exemptions and suggest a need for reappraisal of all hospital personnel practices.

It is important to learn what is currently known, what is being done, and what is being planned in all areas of employee relations, but this is especially true in the area of grievance procedures, because such procedures are not only essential to a good personnel program, but also the best defense against unionization.

The need for a grievance procedure resides in the emotional makeup of human beings, particularly in their need for relief from frustrations. Unfair treatment of an employee, imagined or actual, can create an emotional block to his future usefulness. To relieve such situations, the best mechanism is a rare one, a supervisor gifted in human relations. Since more than half of hospital personnel are generally in nursing service, nurse training programs in hospitals and in colleges have a responsibility to emphasize supervisory techniques, but have not generally done so to any great extent to date. A newly appointed nursing supervisor usually has no training to help her deal with the complexities involved in the management of human resources.

Even if management subjects were taught in advanced nursing courses and hospitals did train nursing supervisors and prospective supervisors in the requirements of supervision, some means would still be needed to guarantee free expression of employee unhappiness.

From *Hospitals, J.A.H.A.*: Reprinted, with permission, from *Hospitals, Journal of the American Hospital Association*, (Vol. 41, No. 15, Part 1, August 1, 1967, pp. 58-60). Copyright 1967 by the American Hospital Association. All rights reserved.

*Current address: Larned State Hospital, Larned Kansas.

THE PROCEDURE DEFINED

A grievance procedure usually consists of a series of steps through which succeedingly higher levels of authority are called upon to resolve an employee's expressions of discontent over his relationship with any element of his employment.[1] The following is an example of a simple grievance procedure now in use in several medium-sized western hospitals:

A personnel relations committee is created to give employees an opportunity to take their problems to an important committee.

When a problem arises, the employee first takes that problem to his supervisor. If it is not resolved satisfactorily, he next makes an out and presents it to the personnel director, who attempts to resolve it.

If the problem still remains unresolved, the employee writes it out and presents it to the personnel relations committee, which investigates it thoroughly and reports its findings and recommendations to the administrator. The decision of the administrator is final.

In company-union contracts the grievance clause is usually more complex, carefully defining the participants on each side and the level of authority at which the problem is to be settled. In addition, time limitations are specified for considering a problem at a given level. Finally, various means of impartial outside arbitration, binding on both union and management, are provided in the event of an impasse throughout all of the internal steps. Adopting these steps can be beneficial to hospitals also, for they assure ultimate and bilateral fairness and they will compete well with the grievance program of any union.

Too frequently supervisors fear that their abilities will be judged on the very existence of employee expressions of unhappiness. Such fearful attitudes, which may be founded on past criticisms by the administrator or board, lead to a suppression of personal communication of dissatisfaction. It should be made clear that a supervisor will not be judged merely on the existence of grievances but rather on the volume of grievances and more particularly on their nature and on a determination as to whether or not they have been handled consistently in a fair and judicious manner.

Wendell French, in his analysis of the personnel management process, recommends such procedures for their value in fulfilling certain basic human needs:

"(The) procedure may give expression to a variety of human wants and needs. The self-esteem needs (independence, dominance, and achievement in particular) and the need for the esteem of others (recognition and attention) find expression in filing a grievance against management and pushing the complaint to a satisfactory conclusion."[2]

The best known text on hospital personnel administration lists the functions of grievance procedures among those essential to an adequate personnel department.[3] In

---

[1] Evans, J. J. *A Program for Personnel Administration* (New York: McGraw-Hill Book Co., 1945), p. 57.

[2] French, W. *The Personnel Management Process* (Boston: Houghton-Mifflin Co., 1964), p. 388.

[3] Bailey, N. D. *Hospital Personnel Administration* (Berwyn, Ill.: Physician's Record Co., 1959), p. 8.

[4] Ibid, p. 200.

pointing out that employees need more than wages, it looks upon good grievance procedures as essential to upward communication.[4]

In rationalizing the need for hospitals to set up grievance procedures, the following description of the initial effects of union organization may serve as an added incentive to establish them:

"When a firm is first unionized, what are the effects? A basic social change occurs in the structure of employer-employee relationships. A wedge seems to have been driven between the company and its employees. Many of these employees now profess an allegiance to an outside organization that, if it is affiliated with a national union, has broader interests and problems than those confronting an individual employer. In the initial stages of union relations, therefore, conflict is more probable than cooperation, especially if recognition of the union has followed a bitter period of name calling, electioneering, or possibly, a strike."[5]

THE SAFETY VALVE FUNCTION

A grievance procedure is also valuable as a safety valve, being a continuous means of avoiding arbitrary decisions and of providing justice. It can be an instrument for interpreting policy and perhaps discovering needs for policy changes. It is actually a formal expression of that much praised and desired thing—upward communication to management.

Edward W. Weimer has pointed out that some hospitals believe what is most unlikely—that their employees have no dissatisfactions.[6] A grievance procedure can enable first-line supervision to recognize anomalies in employee morale with the same kind of awareness that physicians possess in detecting symptoms and syndromes in patients. It permits them to find means to minimize the ill effects of grievances once they are discovered, for hospitals and industry both know that unrest is an overwhelming factor in the loss of productive effort. With Medicare, increased bed demand, chronic nurse shortages, and public reaction to increased hospitalization cost, administration must travel every path that can lead to a higher ratio of production per employee.

Robert E. Finley says we *need* some grievances. Forecasting what the enlightened personnel men of the future may bring about, he says:

"Labor relations men will not nearly as often be faced with grievances and troubles caused by managers who have no policies or objectives, who are not organized properly, who are arbitrary and insensitive leaders, or who perceive so poorly what is going on in their departments that they unjustly evaluate the work of certain people. There will, of course, always be grievances and to have a few is healthy. Some kinds of grievances, however, that now occupy so much ... time, will dwindle as managers become more knowledgeable."[7]

Not only does Finley believe that some grievances are needed, if for no other reason than to allow all personnel a channel of individual communication, but he also believes

[5] Pigors, P. and Myers, C. A. *Personnel Administration* (New York: McGraw-Hill Co., 1965), p. 188.

[6] Weimer, E. W. Grievance procedure. *Hospitals, J.A.H.A.* 38:36 Aug. 16, 1964.

[7] Finley, R. E. *The Personnel Man and His Job* (New York: American Management Association, 1962), p. 404.

that trained, knowledgeable, nonarbitrary, sensitive, organized managers and supervisors whose objectives are supported by policies are essential to grievance handling. It is now important that hospitals hold similar beliefs.

A limited survey among medium-sized hospitals in the western part of the United States on grievance procedures in use produced a number of informal procedures. Some institutions had no procedure; some are planning to develop one. At least two who had abandoned grievance procedures are preparing to reinstitute them. Of the procedures studied, none showed an awareness of the time urgency involved. The importance of this can be seen in formalized grievance procedures that provide for outside arbitration, where due to a delayed decision the employer can be required to reinstate a previously discharged employee, even after having filled the position during the discharged employee's absence.

There is need to learn the techniques for handling grievances that are most helpful. Some dangers in the application of such procedures should be noted and avoided. The trick of avoidance may lie in the drafting of the procedure, but more likely it lies in enlightened, alert administration.

BEGIN WITH SUPERVISOR

The supervisor or department head must not be bypassed in handling grievances unless one wishes to cut the ground from under him, with a resultant increase in the number of grievances. Employees must know the channels available to them in presenting a grievance and it has to begin with the supervisor.

The open-door policy sounds good to some, but it can rip the bottom out of the grievance procedure. For one thing, it can waste a remarkable amount of the administrator's time and it can embarrass and weaken the position of the supervisor.

In preparing to deal with unions, particularly with regard to handling the grievance clause, there are a great many tactics to anticipate: Unions may make use of the procedure as a "slowdown" weapon by encouraging the filing of multiple grievances; an employee may fail to state the real grievance, causing a second or third handling; grievances related to an outdated event of the past may be brought up; and grievances may be put forward that are really only efforts to bargain for a more advantageous condition of work than the contract provides.

SUMMARY AND RECOMMENDATIONS

The current situation makes it urgent that attention be given to the following:

1. Adequate training in supervisory skills should be given to all supervisory personnel, both in academic curriculums and on the job.
2. Workable procedures should be devised to allow employee expression of dissatisfactions.
3. Administration should study many related labor-management areas in preparation for the potential need to deal with employees through a union representative.

It is recommended that hospital associations and the larger hospital councils learn and teach the formulation of objectives, policies, procedures, methods, and the training needed to develop these skills in hospitals.

Part IV

QUANTITATIVE APPROACHES TO DECISION-MAKING

This part discusses the decision-making process and describes some quantitative techniques which can be helpful to the hospital decision-maker (Fries). Both the process and the quantitative techniques are linked to the resulting effectiveness and efficiency of the hospital. In a systems context, this linkage occurs in three primary areas. The first two include decisions related to determination of output(s) (objectives) of the hospital and the identification of the necessary input resources. The third area where linkage occurs is in the actual hospital management. That is, in addition to output-input determinations, decision-making is an integral part of the planning, controlling, organizing, and directing processes. All administrators, department heads, and supervisors make decisions. The scope, importance, and magnitude of these decisions is a function of the decision-maker's position in the hierarchy. The quality or efficacy of decisions that are made is often a result of the process used—whether it is systematic—and the amount and appropriateness of the information upon which those decisions are based. Quantitative techniques are particularly useful in providing critical information. Many of them have only been developed since World War II.

RESOURCE ALLOCATION

Today, external forces influence health care resource allocations to a greater degree than ever. Their impact results from attempts to influence health care resource allocation to meet societal objectives. An example is the 1974 National Health Planning and Resources Development Act (Rosoff). State health planning and development agencies (SHPDA) and local health systems agencies (HSA) created by the act were developed to: promote rational expansion of facilities; prevent duplication of facilities in geographic areas through demonstration of certificate-of-need; and foster shared services when possible. In essence, government has a societal objective of requiring more rational allocation of health care resources (facility, equipment, manpower) through the identification and comparison of needs to existing capabilities.[1] Similarly, the Health Maintenance Organization Act of 1973 attempts to shape the health care delivery system and, thereby, its allocation of resources. The establishment of professional standards review organizations (PSROs) in PL 92-603[2], and interest in the prospective reimbursement mechanism for federally funded health care services (Ellis) are attempts to reduce costs by eliminating unnecessary service. Though slightly different in emphasis, both add an important dimension.

OBJECTIVE FUNCTIONS

In terms of resource allocation, it is possible to look at the health care delivery system and individual hospitals from one of two objective functions: (1) "given the resources available, maximize output" and (2) "given an appropriate level of output, minimize the resources used."[3] These objective functions are obverse. As health care absorbs greater societal resources, there is emphasis on output. In fact, recent legislation demonstrates that resources are limited. The health care delivery system and its hospitals are asked, at least theoretically, to do more with no more.[4] Further, John D. Porterfield, III, former Director of the Joint Commission on Accreditation of Hospitals, has stated that there is increasing emphasis on quality assurance. His message is clear: forces in the supra system (consumers/government) are demanding that all components of the health care delivery system demonstrate an ability to provide care at an acceptable level of quality. Those forces must be informed of success or failure in meeting these objectives.

DECISION-MAKING

Simply, decision-making is choosing from alternatives. The administrator will make decisions alone or in consultation. These become the means to attempt to reach hospital objectives (outputs). Once established, this framework will guide decision-making on inputs required to accomplish the objectives. Further, decisions must be made on the organizational design, directing and utilizing manpower, and establishing control mechanisms to monitor work performed (Ewell).

Strategic-Operational Decisions

At high hierarchical levels, decisions are made by defining the means or strategies to be pursued to accomplish established objectives. The addition of a family practice center, contracting for emergency department services, and physical expansion of the hospital are only a few examples. These typically involve large amounts of resources. Thus, "strategy" decisions are major, enduring institutional commitments, and have a large impact on costs and internal resource allocation. When making these decisions, attention must be given to whether they will lead to accomplishment of objectives, if there is a better (less costly) way, what externally imposed constraints must be considered, whether the organization has or will have the financial and administrative resources to implement the strategy, and what impact implementation will have on other hospital subsystems.

In addition to decisions which are strategic in nature, there are others that do not involve major resource commitments, but are necessary for smooth hospital functioning. These operational decisions are made by personnel throughout the organizational hierarchy and may include among others, transferring employees, determining task assignment, vendor selection, scheduling activities, and determining which piece of equipment to purchase. In any case, strategic or operational decisions can be improved through the utilization of a systematic process.

Decision-Making Process

The decision-making process incorporates a number of activities ranging from problem definition to selection from among alternatives. Implementation follows the choice of an alternative. The specific activities are:[5]

1. Defining the problem.
2. Gathering relevant information.
3. Developing alternatives.
4. Evaluating those alternatives.
5. Choosing the most acceptable alternative.

Each of the activities comprising the decision-making process is important. However, depending upon the nature of the decision that must be made (strategic-operational), the experience of the decision-maker, the organizational support given, and the urgency or nature of the problem, a decision-maker may spend little time and effort on some and more on others.

Defining the problem is not always an easy task. It can be time-consuming; nevertheless, it is vital. Very often the efficacy of the whole decision-making process is functionally dependent upon how well the problem is conceptualized. Information is an additional requirement; not only information which helps define the problem, but also that which sets the parameters of possible choice and purpose of the choice. Those parameters can be viewed as solution criteria and solution constraints (Shell and Stelzer).

Solution criteria specify the ultimate purpose(s) for which the problem is being solved, e.g., patient care, employee morale, and cost containment. Solution constraints are the internal and external parameters within which the solution (alternative selected) is placed, e.g., authority, resource, cost, humanitarian, ethical, and political constraints. Decisions cannot be made in a vacuum. They must be considered within the context of the objectives to be fulfilled and internal and external constraints.

Once the problem has been defined and information collected, the decision-maker develops alternative courses of action. For example, a hospital in a locale with a declining birth rate may have the alternative of continuing obstetrical service (low occupancy), or developing a shared service with other area facilities.

Effective evaluation of alternatives is a decision-making activity often neglected, but extremely important. The ramifications of each alternative should be fully explored, both qualitatively and quantitatively. Quantitative techniques can be used successfully to assist the decision-maker. The information gathered should address three considerations. First, will the alternative contribute to the attainment of objectives, i.e., will it satisfy the solution criteria? Second, is the alternative feasible (can it be implemented)? This includes solution constraints and implementation as well as adequacy of available resources and consideration of the effect on hospital sub-systems. Third, does the alternative represent an acceptable degree of cost effectiveness? That is, does the proposed solution make maximum use of available resources relative to other uses of those resources; or, is there another less costly alternative?

Of course, there may be times when "least" or "lowest" cost should not be used as a criterion for decision-making. Often this is true in health care where quality considerations are so important. However, the costs involved relative to the benefits obtained cannot be totally ignored in light of external concern about resource allocation.

Following evaluation, one alternative is chosen. Typically there is no one "best" alternative; all have advantages and disadvantages. The decision-maker must judge which alternative has the fewest disadvantages or most advantages from both quantitative and qualitative standpoints.

QUANTITATIVE TECHNIQUES

There is a wide range of quantitative techniques which provide information to assist decision-makers. They range from simple ratio analysis (Snook and Sudell) to sophisticated simulation models. To present an overview of the variety of techniques, this section focuses on those particularly well-suited for planning, control, and evaluation of alternatives.

Planning

Characteristic of the planning process is the formulation and reformulation of objectives (outputs) and determination of the means or strategies to accomplish those objectives. All are dependent on one's assumptions about the future. Planning, either long-run or short-term, entails projecting into the future.

Regression analysis is a technique which can be very useful to the hospital administrator. Specifically, it involves collection and analysis of historical data so that trends can be identified.[6] This information, whether it concerns anticipated occupancy rate, employee turnover, inventory needs, cash flow, changes in demand by service, or likely governmental action, is of major importance to the decision-maker (Adam, et al.; Donlon). Depending on one's expectations of the future, decisions will be made about objectives, strategies (and resulting resource allocation such as expanding or not expanding services), and operational matters (hiring more staff). Another forecasting technique is model building. Gross national product forecasting models are the most widely known example. They are designed to predict future levels of economic activity. The disadvantage of large models is that they are macro in nature, expensive to develop and maintain, and do not have the ability to assist the individual hospital administrator—they do not focus on a specific organization within that system.

Control

The controlling process monitors organizational performance by measuring it and comparing it against standards which are a derivative of organizational objectives. The controlling process consists of collecting information, determining whether organizational activity is consistent with the standards, and taking corrective action should there be deviation. There are two points where control is typically focused: first on input resources used, and second, on outputs. Relative to the former, budgets (numerical representations of planned activity) can be standards against which resource utilization is compared. Examples are payroll, supply, and equipment budgets. Another relatively simple technique for measuring organization activity against standards is ratio analysis. Occupancy rate, turnover rate, overtime payroll expenditures relative to regular employee payroll, and average collection period are examples. These measures can indicate major deviation from standards and can be helpful in identifying the problem so that corrective action can be taken. For example, a large increase in the rate of employee turnover would have cost and quality of care implications. Additional information might reveal that the hospital's level of employee compensation is below that of other area facilities. If high employee turnover is unacceptable, a decision must be reached by evaluating available alternatives, e.g., increasing compensation.

The second area upon which control is focused is output. Statistical techniques can be used to monitor organizational output and determine whether it is the quantity and quality desired. Statistical analysis is a powerful tool available to the decision-maker (Daniel and Longest). For example, it is possible to test statistically whether an increase in the death rate was due to some assignable cause or simply due to chance. Also, it is possible to extract samples by making a limited number of observations and statistically draw inferences about a whole population.

Another control technique which incorporates planning is network analysis. Two similar methods, the Program Evaluation Review Technique (PERT) and Critical Path Method (CPM) are particularly suited for controlling one-time large scale projects such as facility expansion (Archer; Griffith, 1972, Chapter 8). The planning component entails determining various activities that must be sequentially and simultaneously carried out to complete a project. The control component includes monitoring the flow of events and the time to complete each event. As the project progresses, it is possible to monitor activities so that a delay in one, upon which others are dependent, can be identified. Then a decision can be made either to accept a longer completion time for the whole project, or to assign more resources to the activity in question so that it can be completed on time.

Evaluation of Alternatives

There are a number of quantitative techniques which can be used by the decision-maker to provide information pertinent to the evaluation of alternatives. Cost-benefit analysis, a generic term to denote the arraying of cost and benefits of various alternatives in numerical terms, is one technique. It is typically applied to program alternatives (comprehensive versus catastrophic national health insurance coverage), major alternatives involving commitments of large resources (facility expansion or adding services), and acquiring specialized equipment. Capital budgeting is one variation of this analysis.

Various techniques labeled Operations Research (OR) can be used to evaluate resource allocation alternatives.[7] Emerging from World War II, Operations Research (often called Management Science) is a discipline which focuses on the application of quantitative techniques to decision-making. Often the techniques attempt to maximize some objective function. Mathematical (linear) programming is an example (Rothstein; Warner and Prawda). However, OR also includes general model building (Amato and Nadler), inventory control models (Jennings), location analysis (Swoveland, et al.), scheduling (or queuing) analysis (Fetter and Thompson; Keller and Laughhunn; and McClain) and simulation (Schmitz and Kwak). Several of these techniques are described in the following selections. However, simulation will be briefly described to demonstrate this technique's power in providing information.

Simulation involves construction of a model representing a set of known phenomena by translating them into mathematical relationships. In essence, a mathematical representation of variables characteristic of an actual situation enables the decision-maker to alter the variable(s) and ascertain the resulting effect of change without actually having to change the situation that exists. For example, through simulation, Schmitz and Kwak (1972) were able to predict the recovery-room needs that would be required if an additional 144 medical/surgical (M/S) beds were added to the hospital. From historical data it was determined that 42 percent of M/S patients had surgery. The average lengths of stay in the operating and recovery rooms by type of surgical patient (ophthalmology, urology, orthopedic, etc.) were determined as were the proportion of surgeries by type. These variables were translated into mathematical equations. Random numbers were used to represent events—a surgical patient—in proportion to actual type (for example, ophthalmology represents 4.5 percent of all surgeries). Knowing the respective average length of operating and recovery room stay, they predicted the number of recovery room beds needed if M/S beds were increased to 144. As was observed, "the simulation model can facilitate planning, decision-making, and managerial control by providing management information."[8] The information provided was obtained without changing the actual situation, i.e., without actually increasing the number of M/S beds.

BIBLIOGRAPHY

Abernathy, William J., and Hershey, John C. "A Spatial-Allocation Model for Regional Health-Services Planning." *Operations Research* 20 (May-June): 629-642, 1972.

Adam, Everett E., Jr., Berry, William L.; and Whybrark, Clay. "The Hospital Administrator and Management Science." *Hospital Administration* 19(Winter): 30-41, 1974.

Amato, Frank C., and Nadler, Michael R. "Computer Simulation Models for Long-Range Financial Planning." *Hospital Progress* 56 (October): 52-56, 1975.

Ammer, Dean S. "Periodic Ordering for Inventory Control." *Hospitals* 48(June 16): 101-106, 1974.

Anderson, Ronald; Foster, Richard; and Weil, Peter. "Rates and Correlates of Expenditure Increases for Personal Health Services: Pre- and Post-Medicare and Medicaid." *Inquiry* 13(March): 136-144, 1976.

Archer, Sarah E. "PERT: A Tool for Nurse Administrators." *Journal of Nursing Administration* 4(September-October): 26-32, 1974.

Baligh, Helmy H., and Laughhunn, Danny J. "An Economic and Linear Model of the Hospital." *Health Services Research* 4(Winter): 293-303, 1969.

Bash, Paul L. "Can Capital Budgeting Work in Hospitals?" *Hospital Administration* 16(Spring): 59-64, 1971.

Bau, Martin A.; Bergwall, David F.; and Reeves, Philip N. "Planning Health Care Delivery Systems." *American Journal of Public Health* 65(March): 272-279, 1975.

Bauerschmidt, Alan D. "The Calculus of Hospital Administration." *Hospital Administration* 16(Fall): 50-68, 1971.

Bennett, Addison C. "New Thinking Required For Development of Management Effectiveness." *Hospitals* 50(February): 67-70, 1976.

Berki, Sylvester E. *Hospital Economics.* Lexington, Massachusetts: Lexington Books, 1972.

Berry, Ralph E., Jr. "Costs and Efficiency in the Production of Hospital Services." *Health and Society* 52(Summer): 291-313, 1974.

Brown, Max, Jr. "An Economic Analysis of Hospital Operations." *Hospital Administration* 15 (Spring): 60-74, 1970.

Curran, William J.; Steele, Richard J.; and Ober, Ellen W. "Government Intervention on Increase." *Hospitals* 49(May 16): 57-61, 1975.

Daniel, Wayne W., and Longest, Beaufort B., Jr. "Some Practical Statistical Procedures." *Journal of Nursing Administration* 5(January): 23-27, 1975.

Donlon, Vincent W. "Statistical Methods to Forecast Volume." *Hospital Financial Management* 29(April): 38-47, 1975.

Donnelly, Paul R. "Corporate Decision-Making and Information Flow Models." *Hospital Progress* 55(March): 33-39, 1974.

Dorsey, Joseph L. "The Health Maintenance Organization Act of 1973 (P.L. 93-222) and Prepaid Group Practice Plans." *Medical Care* 13(January): 1-9, 1975.

Ellis, Ce. "Prospective Reimbursement: Pain or Panacea?" *Modern Healthcare* 5(May): 31-36, 1976.

Etzioni, Amitai. "Alternative Conceptions of Accountability." *Hospital Progress* 55(June): 34-39, 1974.

Ewell, Charles M., Jr. "Setting Objectives: First Step in Planning." *Hospital Progress* 53(September): 68-71, 74, 1972.

Fetter, Robert B., and Thompson, John D. "Patients' Waiting Time and Doctors' Idle Time in the Outpatient Setting." *Health Services Research* 1(Summer): 66-90, 1966.

Fries, Brant E. "Bibliography of Operations Research in Health Care Systems." *Operations Research* 24(September-October): 801-814, 1976.

Gilbert, Neal. "Hospital Capital Budgeting Principles and Techniques." *Hospital Progress* 56(June): 56-59, 1975.

Glasser, Melvin R. "What Price Health Care?" *Hospital Administration* 20(Fall): 7-19, 1975.

Goodwin, Phil. "Bring Planning Into the Management Function." *Hospital Financial Management* 30(June): 24-32, 1976.

Griffith, John R. *Quantitative Techniques for Hospital Planning and Control.* Lexington, Massachusetts: Lexington Books, 1972.

──────. "Budgeting Process Integral to Effective Cost Control System." *Hospital Financial Management* 28(July): 12-28, 1974.

Grimes, Richard M.; Allen, Catherine L.; Sparling, Ted R.; and Weiss, Gerald. "Use of Decision Theory in Regional Planning." *Health Services Research* 9(Spring): 73-78, 1974.

Hax, Arnoldo C., and Wiig, Karl M. "The Use of Decision Analysis in Capital Investment Problems." *Sloan Management Review* 17(Winter): 19-48, 1976.

Heenan, David A., and Addleman, Robert B. "Quantitative Techniques for Today's Decision Makers." *Harvard Business Review* 54(May-June): 32-62, 1976.

Hershey, John C.; Abernathy, William J.; and Baloff, Nicholas. "Comparison of Nurse Allocation Policies—A Monte Carlo Model." *Decision Sciences* 5(January): 58-72, 1974.

Hodgetts, Richard M. *Management Theory Process and Practice.* Philadelphia: W.B. Saunders, Co., 1975.

Holder, William W. "Administrators Favor Prospective Reimbursement." *Hospital Progress* 57 (June): 71-73, 1976.

Jacobs, Philip. "A Survey of Economic Models of Hospitals." *Inquiry* 11(June): 83-87, 1974.

Jennings, John B. "Blood Bank Inventory Control." *Management Science* 19(February): 637-645, 1973.

Joseph, Hyman. "On Economic Theories of Hospital Behavior." *Journal of Economics and Business* 27(Fall): 69-74, 1974.

Kane, J.; Thompson, W.; and Vertinsky, I. "Health Care Delivery: A Policy Simulator." *Socio-Economic Planning Sciences* 6(June): 283-293, 1972.

Keller, T.F., and Laughhunn, D.J. "An Application of Queuing Theory To A Congestion Problem In An Outpatient Clinic." *Decision Science* 4(July): 379-392, 1973.

Knobel, Roland J., and Longest, Beaufort B., Jr. "Problems Associated With The Cost-Benefit Analysis Technique in Voluntary Hospitals." *Hospital Administration* 19(Winter): 42-52, 1974.

Kuzdrall, Paul J.; Kwak, N.K.; and Schmitz, Homer H. "Note on The Monte Carlo Simulation of Operating-Room and Recovery Room Usage." *Operations Research* 22(March-April): 434-440, 1974.

Lee, Maw Lin. "Theoretical Foundation of Hospital Planning." *Inquiry* 11(December): 276-281, 1974.

MacStravic, Robin E. "Provisions of the National Health Planning and Resources Development Act." *Hospital Progress* 56(April): 48-50, 80, 1975.

McClain, John O. "Bed Planning Using Queuing Theory Models of Hospital Occupancy: A Sensitive Analysis." *Inquiry* 13(June): 167-176, 1976.

McDonnell, John F. "The Human Element of Decision-Making." *Personnel Journal* 53(March): 188-189, 1974.

Milsum, John H.; Turban, Efraim; and Vertinsky, Ilan. "Hospital Admission Systems: Their

Evaluation and Management." *Management Science* 19(February): 646-666, 1973.
Morse, Edward V.; Gordon, Gerald; and Moch, Michael. "Hospitals Costs and Quality of Care: An Organizational Perspective." *Health and Society* 52(Summer): 315-346, 1974.
Moustafa, A. Taher, and Sears, David W. "Feasibility of Simulation of Health Maintenance Organizations." *Inquiry* 11(June): 143-151, 1974.
Phillips, Donald F. "Health Planning: New Hope for a Fresh Start." *Hospitals* 49(May 16): 35-38, 1975.
──────."American Hospitals: A Look Ahead." *Hospitals* 50(January 1): 73-81, 1976.
Pliskin, Joseph S., and Beck, Clyde H., Jr. "A Health Index for Patient Selection: A Value Function Approach with Application to Chronic Renal Failure Patients." *Management Science* 22(May): 1009-1021, 1976.
Porterfield, John D., III. "To The Defense of the System." *Hospitals* 48(March 1): 46-49, 1974.
Reeves, Philip N. "A Systems Approach to Development of a Health Services Plan." *Inquiry* 11(December): 247-255, 1974.
Robinson, Gordon H.; Wing, Paul; and Davis, Louis E. "Computer Simulation of Hospital Patient Scheduling Systems." *Health Services Research* 3(Summer): 130-141, 1968.
Rosoff, Arnold J. "Health Planning and Certification of Need Under the New Federal Health Planning Act." *Hospital Administration* 20(Summer): 60-72, 1975.
Rothstein, Marvin. "Hospital Manpower Shift Scheduling by Mathematical Programming." *Health Services Research* 8(Spring): 60-66, 1973.
Schmitz, Homer H., and Kwak, N.K. "Monte Carlo Simulation of Operating-Room and Recovery-Room Usage." *Operations Research* 20(November-December): 1171-1180, 1972.
Schulz, Rockwell I., and Rose, Jerry. "Can Hospitals be Expected to Control Costs?" *Inquiry* 10(June): 3-8, 1973.
Shell, Richard L.; and Stelzer, David F. "Systems Analysis: Aid to Decision Making: A Method of Investigation." *Business Horizons* 14(December): 67-72, 1971.
Shonick, William; and Jackson, James R. "An Improved Stochastic Model for Occupancy-Related Random Variables in General-Acute Hospitals." *Operations Research* 21(July-August): 952-965, 1973.
Shuler, Cyril O. "Some Unique Characteristics in Health Administration." *Hospital Administration* 17(Winter): 9-25, 1972.
Shuman, Larry J.; Hardwick, C. Patrick; and Huber, George A. "Location of Ambulatory Care Centers in a Metropolitan Area." *Health Services Research* 8(Summer): 121-138, 1973.
Snook, I. Donald; and Sudell, William B. "Financial Ratio Analysis, A Quick Simple Test." *Hospital Financial Management* 29(June): 16-19, 1975.
Starkweather, David B., Gelwicks, Louis; and Newcomer, Robert. "Delphi Forecasting of Health Care Organization." *Inquiry* 12(March): 37-46, 1975.
Stimson, David H., and Stimson, Ruth H. *Operations Research in The Hospital: Diagnosis and Prognosis.* Chicago: Health Research and Educational Trust, 1972a.
Stimson, Ruth H., and Stimson, David H. "Operations Research and the Nurse Staffing Problem." *Hospital Administration* 17(Winter): 61-69, 1972b.
Swoveland, C., Uyeno, D., Vertinsky, I.; and Vickson, R. "Ambulance Location: A Probabilistic Enumeration Approach." *Management Science* 20(December): 686-698, 1973.
Tersine, Richard J., and Riggs, Walter E. "The Delphi Technique: A Long-Range Planning Tool." *Business Horizons* 19(April): 51-56, 1976.
Toregas, Constantine, Swain, Ralph; ReVelle, Charles; and Bergman, Lawrence. "The Location of Emergency Service Facilities." *Operations Research* 19(October): 1363-1373, 1971.
Torrance, George W. "Health Status Index Models: A Unified Mathematical View." *Management Science* 22(May): 990-1001, 1976.
Vora, Jay A. "Heuristics and Optimizing Techniques Applied to Long Range Facility Planning for Hospital Ancillary Departments." *Management Science.* 21(December): 409-417, 1974.

Warner, D. Michael, and Prawda, Juan. "A Mathematical Programming Model for Scheduling Nursing Personnel in a Hospital." *Management Science* 19(December): 411-422, 1972.

Young, Stanley. "Organizational Decision-Making." *Hospital Administration* 10(Fall): 38-65, 1965.

Zilm, Frank; Calderaro, Luci; and Del Grande, Madlyn. "Computer Simulation Model Provides Design Framework." *Hospitals* 50(August 16): 79-85, 1976.

FOOTNOTES

(See Bibliography for full citation as necessary)

[1] For an interesting presentation predicting the future of health services in the United States and the role of the hospital see Phillips (1976).

[2] For a full treatment of PSROs see Selection 37.

[3] For presentation of these two concepts and related presentations from an "economics" perspective see Berki chapters 4 and 5; Berry; Brown; Jacobs; and Joseph.

[4] For an interesting evaluation of the objectives/limited resources point of view see Schulz and Rose.

[5] There are some variations to these activities. See Donnelly; Hodgetts; McDonnell; and Young.

[6] For a non-quantitative method of forecasting, the Delphi technique, see Starkweather, et al.; Tersine and Riggs.

[7] For an excellent presentation of OR in the hospital setting see Stimson and Stimson (1972a). For one of the most up-to-date bibliographies on OR applications to health care see Fries. It is strongly recommended to the reader who wishes to explore this subject further.

[8] Schmitz and Kwak (1972), p. 1171.

Decision-Making

In Selection 28, "THE ANATOMY OF A DECISION" by Edward J. Spillane, the author characterizes the primary role of the hospital administrator as that of a decision-maker who must achieve results (output) by allocating the hospital's limited resources for maximum payoff, at minimum cost. Further, he states that constructing a decision model (process systematization) is critical to making appropriate decisions.

Five elements basic to the decision-making process (DMP) are mentioned. Some described in the preceding text are not included, e.g., defining the problem, but the writer includes the essential points. Determining what is to be maximized or minimized is the first DMP element mentioned. This element is identified as the focal point of the DMP and constitutes determining and linking the objective function and solution criteria. After these are determined, the second element involves identification of resources available for allocation. The third element is identification of non-resource constraints. These are the internally and externally imposed solution constraints (political, ethical, legal) which provide the framework for the decision. The fourth element, identification of the risk factor, is one not mentioned previously. There are few situations where there is complete certainty; therefore, the writer advocates incorporating risk and probability within the DMP. The fifth element is determining and comparing the "payoff value with input costs" among the alternatives, i.e., evaluating them.

28.

Anatomy of a Decision

EDWARD J. SPILLANE

Edward J. Spillane is Assistant Director of The Catholic Hospital Association.

In the complex situation of today's hospital, there is a great need to identify the administrator's primary function in terms of his objectives or output. Too often, in practice, if not in theory, hospital management specialists consider the administrator's *work* more important than his *objectives*. His identity seems to "melt" into and become synonymous with certain activities—loosely labeled management functions—such as planning, coordinating, delegating authority and reviewing financial statements.

But the administrator is primarily a decision-maker. He is not adequately described in terms of specific tasks. Rather, he is concerned with achieving results, with accomplishing objectives. His principal goal is to allocate the hospital's limited resources in such a way as to achieve maximum payoff at minimal cost in terms of realizable hospital objectives. To accomplish this task he must continually make decisions. Decisions, then, comprise the major part of an administrator's output. Through them he either achieves or fails to achieve his and the institution's objectives.

Because decisions *per se* are so important, they must be carefully analyzed. An analysis of a past decision can furnish guidelines for the future; an analysis of a "constructed" or "in-the-making" decision can often mean the difference between success or failure of a yet-to-be-launched project.

ANALYSIS VITAL TO UNDERSTANDING DECISION-MAKING

This article attempts to identify and briefly describe the vital factors which comprise a managerial decision. Unless these parts are understood the administrator and his subordinates will be unable to:

1. Analyze a decision or learn from such an analysis.
2. Be certain that the decisions they "construct" meet the requirements of a complete decision.
3. Fully understand, let alone use, the new concepts, techniques and procedures of the management sciences as recommended by management specialists.[1]

·Reprinted by permission from *Hospital Progress: Journal of The Catholic Hospital Association,* St. Louis, Vol. 50 (April, 1969), 47-50, 68. Copyright 1969 by The Catholic Hospital Association. All rights reserved.

Conversely, an understanding and appreciation of the essential elements of a decision will enable the administrator to more correctly identify and concentrate on his role (decision-maker), and thus better fulfill his responsibility (achieving results). Moreover, it will help him to better coordinate and evaluate his efforts of allocating available resources and thus achieve more efficiently his and the organization's goals.

Included with a brief description of the essential elements of a decision model will be a question outline that the administrator can use to judge the adequacy of each part of a decision. Elementary, but hopefully adequate, examples of each vital element will also be given.

THE ANATOMY OF A DECISION

The following paragraphs may appear to deal only with the decision itself to the exclusion of the administrator's real challenge of implementing the decision. However implementing the decision as well as abstracting relevant facts from the empirical situation are correlative activities and dependent upon effective decisions. Since the success of these activities depends directly on a decision(s), the decision is the key or initiative factor. Admittedly, it is often difficult to distinguish *the* decision from the many supporting decisions that precede and follow the major, output-oriented "go" or "no go" decision. Once again, it is not the activities *per se* that need analysis and emphasis. It is the decision(s), or more correctly the construction of the decision model, that in most instances really spells success or failure in the administrator's efforts to achieve his and his organization's many and varied objectives.

The anatomy of each management decision model is comprised of five vital elements. They are:

1. A clear idea of what is to be maximized or minimized based upon a problem or question.
2. An identification and appreciation of the resources to be allocated.
3. An identification and appreciation of non-resource constraints.
4. An identification of risk factor(s)—imperfect knowledge situation.
5. A comparison of payoff "value" with input "costs."

Although these elements are essential to every decision, they are not all-inclusive. In concentrating on the vital elements, one must not lose sight of the whole. No part is meaningful by itself and each is fully understood only in its relation to the other parts. Likewise, no decision should be made and/or acted upon apart from its relationship to other decisions made or contemplated.[2] A decision lacking one or more vital elements may result in an inefficient allocation of hospital resources in terms of potential payoffs.

---

[1]For a more detailed application of some of these tools and techniques to hospital administration, see the excellent article "Modern Management Concepts, Tools," by George R. Wren, Ph.D., *Hospital Topics,* January, 1968, p. 37.

[2]"Rational decision-making depends on having a full range of rational options from which to choose. Successful management organizes the enterprise so that this process can best take place." Robert S. McNamara.

MAXIMIZATION-MINIMIZATION

The focal point of every decision is the determination of that factor which is to be minimized or maximized. Describing and understanding this factor is the most difficult aspect of "constructing" a decision. This factor must be subject to some degree of quantitative or qualitative measurement and translated into terms of output or objectives. In making this determination, community analysis (market research), exit interviews, attitude surveys, sampling techniques and many other data-gathering tools are helpful. An understanding and utilization of such managerial concepts and techniques as value analysis, management by objectives, payoff tables, simulation and systems management is not possible unless the administrator can clearly define that which he is attempting to maximize or minimize in each decision situation. Vague platitudes (e.g. maximize the quality of patient care, minimize the costs of patient care, good personnel policies), stated in purely descriptive terms, are too general; only precise definition will meet the requirements of determining the maximization-minimization factor.

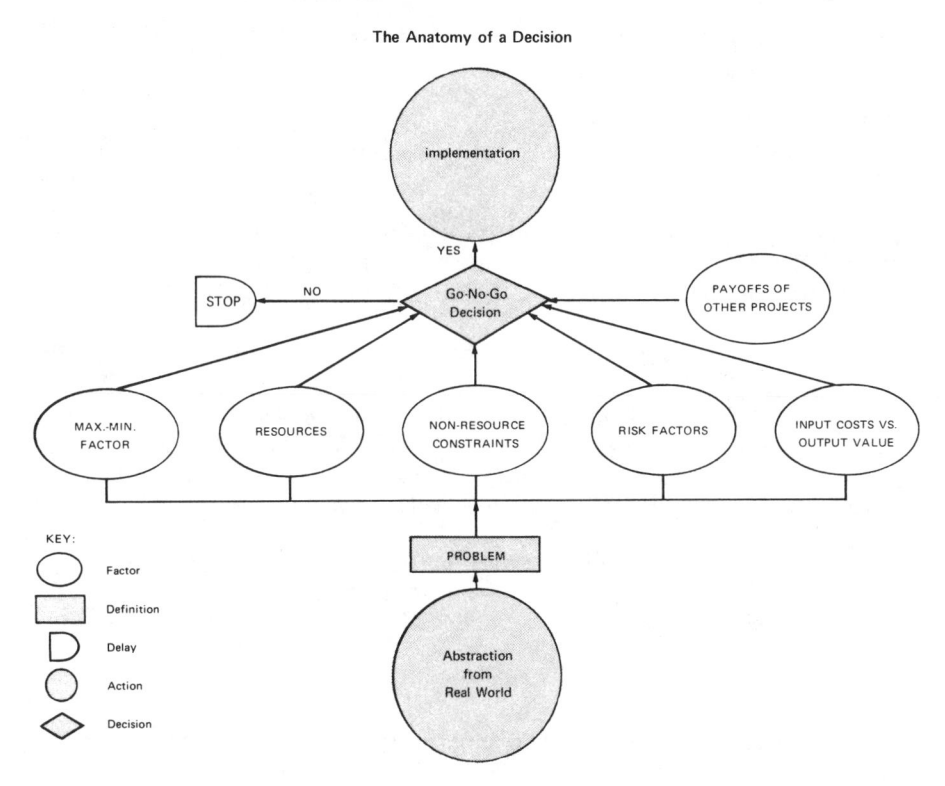

The Anatomy of a Decision

In identifying this factor, the administrator should attempt to answer the following questions: What is to be maximized or minimized, and to what degree? For example: 1. Labor turnover *(what)* is to be minimized to a target level of two per cent *(degree)* a month; 2. Medication errors *(what)* are to be minimized to a target level of 12 *(degree)* per month; 3. The productive time of all physicians while in the hospital *(what)* will be maximized so that no physician will ever have to wait *(degree)* for an open line in order to dictate medical records information.

Although strict definition is necessary, the dynamics of the situation also require flexibility. The maximization-minimization factor can and will be changed as other parts of the decision take shape. Its significance lies in two areas: 1. Its relation to the other parts of the decision model and its ability to furnish the administrator with a clear objective or base upon which to proceed in the decision-making process, and 2. its use as a standard for future evaluation and control.

LIMITED RESOURCE ALLOCATION

This decision factor is used to identify the quantitative and qualitative characteristics of the resources available and required. In each decision, limited (scarce) resources will be programmed for allocation via some type of organizational structure to some project or activity. These limited resources must be calculated in terms of cost, quantity, quality, possibility for and degrees of substitutability. In addition, the relation of payoffs in terms of output resulting from various mixes of resources (together with associated input costs) to that which is to be maximized or minimized should be identified and analyzed. Understanding what is needed to accomplish this part of the decision will make industrial engineering science and such managerial concepts as linear programming, break-even, labor-capital substitution and discounted cash flow analysis more meaningful and useful to the administrator.

In analyzing this part of a decision, the administrator must answer the following question: What least expensive mix of scarce resources will achieve a payoff that is consistent with the maximization-minimization requirement?

LEAST EXPENSIVE MIX OF SCARCE RESOURCES

An example of a limited resource allocation could be algebraically expressed as follows: To achieve a given target of 1000P level of clean linen inventory (output) during an eight-hour period, two possible combinations of resources (inputs) and production functions can be proposed, which will achieve the same output.

A. $1000P = f(1800L + 300X + 8Y + Z)$
B. $1000P = f(1200L + 800X + 4Y + Z)$

Where

L = Linen at a unit cost of $1.
X = Labor at a unit cost of $2.
Y = Capital equipment (allocated expense) at a unit cost of $50.
Z = Other indirect costs of $5 per eight-hour period.

Assigning costs to the variables (inputs) in the above equations (production functions) and solving the equations will give the lowest cost needed to achieve the target output of 1000P per eight-hour period.

One can readily see from the payoff analysis that combination A is the preferred mix of resources. Substituting capital (L and Y) for labor resources (reduction in units of labor) makes the difference in costs possible. Without such a substitution analysis the administrator may overlook various options and a less than efficient allocation of the hospital's scarce resources could result. This assumes, of course, a "payoff at minimal cost" rationale.

NON-RESOURCE CONSTRAINTS

Each decision usually includes certain identifiable constraints on the allocation, organization and use of resources that are non-resource in nature. These non-resource constraints can be classified as legal, social, psychological, religious or political in nature, and, often, they do not lend themselves to quantification or certain prediction. The administrator must recognize these constraints, estimate their impact on other parts of the decision and the final output and then incorporate this knowledge into the decision model.

Various federal, state and local laws regulating the use of labor resources are tangible examples of non-resource constraints. The psychological impact of change on labor units is less known and more difficult to estimate. Another possible constraint would be the significance that findings and recommendations of local planning agencies, in terms of the need or lack of need for additional hospital beds, might have on the administrator's decision to expand or not expand the inventory of hospital beds. In terms of labor resource allocation and use, union contracts present a definite constraint on the administrator's decision-making.

RISK FACTOR

Every decision-maker attempts to achieve certainty in the decision-making process, but seldom in major decisions is this goal realized. Neither the constraints nor the chances of achieving the objective as reflected by the element to be maximized or minimized are known with certainty. The administrator must make estimates and base subsequent actions upon them. An understanding of the aspect of risk will make such things as the Bayesian probability theory, decision trees and joint probability tables more meaningful and useful to the administrator.

Being aware of the degree of risk is the first step toward reducing the risk factor. The administrator must determine the degree of risk by attempting to decide whether the activity or project will actually meet or surpass the desired payoff. One example of the element of risk or uncertainty facing the administrator can be seen in the following situation: A proposal to purchase a pulmonary function test machine costing $1,500 has been made. The risks involved in this project might include, but are not limited to, some of the following: Will the physicians use the machine enough to recover the cost before the machine becomes obsolete? Can necessary personnel be obtained to help the physician in the operation of the machine? Will other hospitals purchase these machines and reduce the volume of use? In deciding whether or not to purchase the PFT machine, the risks or uncertainties must be analyzed, evaluated, considered and incorporated into the total decision.

COMPARISON OF THE PAYOFF VALUE WITH THE INPUT COSTS

In constructing this part of the decision the administrator is actually asking: "Given the costs of inputs (resources) and the value of the output factor to be maximized or minimized is the allocation of resources to this project justified?" In other words, the payoff must be equal to or greater than the costs of the resources allocated to achieve this payoff. The probability of success factor will, of course, alter this balance. For instance, in the laundry production example given previously it was found economical to substitute capital for labor. However, the probability of success factor could change the picture drastically. If the probability of achieving 1000P by substituting capital for labor was only 50 per cent (A) because of machine downtime and lack of an adequate maintenance department, while the probability of achieving 1000P in the labor intensive situation (B) was 90 per cent, one would naturally reconsider the choice of resource mixes.

An administrator would not readily incur X costs for a payoff value of X-1, especially when the same combination of resources could be allocated to other projects and achieve an X + 1 value payoff.

An example of the cost input vs. value output analysis is as follows: labor turnover in a given situation is calculated to cost a hospital $500 per terminating employe. Thus the total value to the hospital for a reduction in turnover could be expressed $500X (X being the reduction in turnover units). An estimate is made that labor turnover can be reduced by 10 units or roughly 12 per cent for a 200-bed hospital during a 12-month period. If the cost to achieve this objective, in terms of a better employe selection program, increased salaries and fringe benefits and more inservice education, was equal to or greater than $5,000, one would question the wisdom of the allocation of resources. Although other factors might indicate that reduced turnover, inservice education, department head meetings, etc., would be desirable, they should not be initiated because such action cannot be justified, in this instance, by the cost of input-value or output-analysis.

"GO" OR "NO GO" OUTPUT

All of the decision factors coalesce in the action or no action judgment. In making this judgment, the decision-maker must compare the payoff resulting from the allocation of the resources to one project with the payoff that might result from allocating the resources to another project or activity. An example of this would be as follows: Assume that $3,000 worth of resources could result in a $5,000 payoff via reduced labor turnover. But assume also that the $3,000 worth of resources could be allocated to improve the doctor's parking lot with a payoff value of $8,000. Under a results-oriented management with limited resources, and assuming that computations of cost and payoff values are correct, the labor turnover project would in all probability be put aside in favor of the parking lot project.

SUMMARY

Better decisions through improved technology result in increased hospital efficiency. Improved technology can be explained as follows:

$$OP = f(A, B, C, D) \text{ when}$$
$$(A + B + C + D) = X \text{ costs (present situation)}$$
$$OP = f(A_1, B_1, C_1, D_1) \text{ when}$$
$$(A_1 + B_1 + C_1 + D_1) = X - Y \text{ costs}$$
$$\text{(improvement through technology)}$$

That is, the same payoff using less resource input costs or a required greater payoff using the same or less resource input costs is essential to improved technology.

This article has analyzed the decision-making process and has given the manager a brief conceptual framework within which the various concepts and tools of modern management can be fitted and understood in relation to the decision-making process. Without such an outline the newer "scientific" methods of managerial problem-solving will not be understood, let alone utilized. Although analyzing decisions and using modern management techniques cannot solve all of the administrator's "real world" problems, such activities can give him a new way of looking at his job—the job of making decisions capable of achieving objectives. A better understanding of the nature of a decision can help him achieve his primary goal—allocating the hospital's limited resources in the most efficient way possible. This is what technology and increased efficiency in hospital operations is all about.

Hospital decision-making must be considered within the context of reimbursement formulas. Unlike the competitive environment, the hospital environment does not demand adherence to maximization and minimization requirements. Reimbursement formulas tend to allow a decision-making process not subject to unlimited resources. Changes in the reimbursement formulas requiring more efficient uses of hospital resources via technology in the future will make this decision-making process more relevant to hospital decision-makers.

Quantitative Techniques

Operations Research (OR) is presented in Selection 29, "OPERATIONS RESEARCH IN HEALTH AND HOSPITAL ADMINISTRATION" by Ronald L. Gue. OR is characterized as a discipline which incorporates the systems perspective and application of quantitative methods in solving complex problems. The writer identifies various applications—inventory control, waiting lines, and scheduling.

The next three selections describe three specific quantitative techniques in the hospital setting: linear programming, queuing, and a variation of capital budgeting. In Selection 30, "THE APPLICATION OF LINEAR PROGRAMMING TO DECISION-MAKING IN HOSPITALS" by William L. Dowling, the writer states that many decisions made by hospital administrators involve resource allocation. Such decisions have three elements. First, an objective (solution criteria) is to be maximized or minimized. Second, there are alternative ways to accomplish that objective. Third, resource constraints exist—facility, equipment, and personnel.

The writer presents linear programming as a quantitative technique useful in making resource allocation decisions. He contends that it is not important for the administrator to know the mathematics of the various equations used to solve a problem. A general awareness of the technique permits recognition of its use and an ability to understand and interpret results obtained by technical experts. The writer illustrates the application of linear programming with a hypothetical surgical problem. He mathematically sets up the objective function (maximize the number of surgical patients serviced), the production coefficients (the amount of each type of resource required to service each type of surgical patient), and the resource constraints (available operating room hours, recovery room bed hours, and surgical service bed days). Given resource availability (constraints) and resource consumption by type of surgical patient, the problem is translated into mathematical equations to solve the objective function (maximize the number of surgical patients serviced). This selection also presents a literature review of various other applications of linear programming.

Another quantitative technique helpful to the decision-maker is presented in Selection 31, "ESTIMATING BED NEEDS BY MEANS OF QUEUING THEORY" by James K. Cooper and Timothy M. Corcoran. The problem addressed is the determination of the number of acute and intermediate coronary care beds needed to service expected demand without misallocating resources by having too many beds. The technique used is queuing. It has the elements of arrivals for service, service time, and a determination of the waiting line, i.e., queue and waiting time, should those requiring service arrive faster than they can be serviced. Many situations, given certain assumptions involving these elements, can be analyzed by using this technique. Examples are the admissions desk, cashier unit for discharges, cafeteria, operating room, and emergency department. By establishing the acceptable length of the line or waiting time, the decision-maker can add more service resources, such as a second cashier.

In the application presented, the acceptable standard was that there be a sufficient number of beds so that the probability of a coronary patient having to wait for a bed did not exceed .05. Analysis of historical data determined that 60 percent of patients admitted have a false myocardial infraction and require an average service time of three acute-care days. The remaining 40 percent require an average of six acute-care days as well as an average of five days of intermediate care. With assumptions on the rate of death and estimated arrivals (400 to 800) per year at random intervals, it was determined that 11 acute-care and 6 intermediate care beds would be required.

The last Selection, "CAPITAL BUDGETING DECISION-MAKING FOR HOSPITALS" by Richard F. Wacht, presents a technique for making hospital resource allocation decisions. It is a hybrid between cost-benefit analysis and industrial capital budgeting. The writer calls it hospital capital budgeting. Basically this technique involves evaluation of alternatives requiring investment expenditures by determining the present value of all benefits (monetary and non-monetary) less costs. The presentation is interesting because it seeks to measure as part of the analysis, the non-monetary benefits accruing to society (saving lives/correcting some malformation or malfunction of the patients). These benefits are represented by the future productive earnings of patients to be served and are considered an integral part of the analysis.

29.
Operations Research in Health and Hospital Administration

RONALD L. GUE

Ronald L. Gue, Ph.D., is a Professor of Hospital Administration at the University of Florida in Gainesville.

What can operations research (O.R.) mean to hospitals? Some hospital administrators may be well familiar with the field; others may view it as some foggy area of endeavor that is cited once in a while in the literature and mentioned in a convention every now and then; a few may have been involved, in one way or another, with an operations research study. In any case, because O.R. can have an indelible impact on hospitals, it is important for the hospital administrator of the present—and of the future—to become as familiar with it as possible. To this end, we present a brief sketch of operations research as a discipline, illustrate its use in several problem areas in the health field and discuss its potential in the future growth of health and hospital administration.

Hospitals have felt the impact of scientific and technical developments in industry, the military and related areas throughout hospital history. The industrial revolution, based on the development of power-generating equipment and machine tools, has benefited hospitals in many ways. Large scale production and the development of national transportation have allowed new economies. The concept of division of manual labor felt so strongly in industry has prompted redefinition of the duties of nursing and ancillary activities.

The division of manual labor in industry was followed by a division of managerial labor. A parallel development has been seen in hospital administration. In industry the continued development of technology and managerial segmentation caused new problems concerning control and decision-making, the complexity of which continues to grow. This complexity has caused a keen awareness that the changes in management and developments in technology in the past have not been followed by parallel advancements in administration and in the executive function.

Throughout these developments, parallel progress in the health field has lagged behind similar progress in industry and the military. In this paper we will attempt no rationalization of this, but will only point out that in the late forties and early fifties operations research was born in response to the need to handle some of these new and complex problems in industry and the military, and that the health field is just beginning its parallel development of O.R. and its application to complex problems of coordination and control. As an example of the time lag involved, one needs only note that papers similar to this one were appearing in various industrial and trade journals about ten years ago (12, 13).[1] It's interesting to note that one of the earliest references to the use of "scientific management" in hospitals comes from the military (21).

During and since World War II hospitals have suffered from severe public pressures from without, as well as troubles from within. Flagle (10) has cited rising costs, shortage of key professional personnel, internecine strife between physicians and administration, inadequacy and decay of physical plant as being among the more acute problems facing hospitals since World War II. The development of operations research in the health services has been in response to the growing complexity of the administrative function in the face of these problems.

OPERATIONS RESEARCH AND DECISION PROCESSES

Operations research has several characteristics that serve to differentiate it from other disciplines. Its most distinguishing feature is its concern with whole problems or its system orientation. The idea here is that activity by any part of an organization has some effect on other activities within the organization. We all are aware of the occasional conflict of opinion among the medical staff, nursing service and administration in a hospital system. For example, some hospitals in the country have recently been examining the feasibility of using disposable bedpans. From the standpoint of nursing, their use seems to be highly desirable since it replaces the undesirable task of emptying and handling soiled bedpans. Administration, on the other hand, while aware of the implications to improved nursing satisfaction and improved nursing care must consider the cost of the disposables. If the unit cost of the disposable bedpan proves to be more than that of the reuseable bedpan there may be some question in the administrator's mind about the value of adopting the disposables. There could be a basic conflict between nursing and administration in deciding whether or not to use disposable bedpans. In making a decision that is oriented toward the hospital as a system, rather than nursing satisfaction or dollar cost, both factors must be considered.

The basic concept of the systems orientation, while accepted in theory, is seldom used in practice. This is generally due to practical limitations on time and resources, or due to the fact that the theoretical techniques available for use are not sufficiently developed to be applied under a systems orientation.

MIXED RESEARCH TEAMS

A second characteristic of operations research frequently cited is that the research is conducted by a mixed team of scientists from many disciplines. This mixed character of the research teams was necessitated during the early years of O.R. because there was no one formally trained to do operations research. The value of this mixed approach

---

[1] Numbers in parentheses refer to references in the Bibliography at the end of the paper.

to problem-solving that was born of necessity has come to be recognized as the heart of any operations research effort. In O.R. studies in the health field we may find physicians, administrators, engineers, statisticians, economists and many other disciplines. For example, a recent article on the evaluation of recurrent medical examinations (28) was authored by a mathematician and a physician. There are many such examples in the literature of the wedding of health service personnel and other diverse disciplines.

A third distinguishing characteristic of O.R. is its method and approach to problem solving. Operations research is generally concerned with complex decision problems—problems related to determining how people should act in order to reach a satisfactory or best decision. Decisions are usually made because the decision-maker wants to attain some goal or objective. Generally he will choose an action that will help him attain his objective. The word "decision" implies a choice, and there must be more than one course of action available to the decision-maker; otherwise, there is no choice.

Consider, for example, the hospital administrator who must decide what quantities of linen inventory he should keep on the hospital floor. His objective might be to minimize the total cost to the hospital. How should the administrator choose one course of action (a single supply level) from all the courses of action (all possible supply levels) available to him? How does operations research help him make his decision?

In order to make his decision the administrator must have some measure of the effect of choosing each course of action—a measure of effectiveness. In our example, this would probably be an expression of the dollar cost to the hospital for each course of action. However there are certain uncontrollable factors which may affect the total cost to the institution. For example, the demand for linen is uncontrollable since it is governed by such things as census on the floor and the nature of the patients' ailments. Thus, the measure of effectiveness will depend on the administrator's choice of a course of action and the state of various uncontrollable factors in the system.

The operations researcher usually resorts to the use of a model of the system that expresses the measure of effectiveness as a function of the alternative courses of action and the uncontrollable variables in the problem. This might be a mathematical model of the form:

$$E = f(C_i, U_j)$$

This equation says symbolically that the measure of effectiveness (E) depends upon the controllable variables, or courses of action (C_i), and the uncontrollable variables (U_j). Operations research, as a discipline, helps the decision-maker to decide which course of action (C_i) will yield the "best" measure of effectiveness. In our example, it would help the administrator to determine which linen supply level would minimize the total linen supply cost to the hospital.

The decision-making framework and the example discussed above are admittedly oversimplified, but they do serve to illustrate the framework used in O.R. Operations research is not only concerned with how to make best decisions, but is concerned with every facet of the decision-making process from actually defining the problem to determining what the best decision really is. The reader who would like to do more study of the framework for decision-making is referred to Miller and Starr (8) or Ackoff and Rivett (2).

Although operations research is a distinct discipline in its own right, its presence in a research activity is usually in combination with certain associated areas of science and engineering. For example, the quantitative measurement techniques of industrial engineering are frequently used in the data collection phase of the O.R. study. The theory of mathematical statistics is frequently used in designing the data collection system and in the analysis of the data. Digital computers are often used in facilitating computations in the data analysis, as well as playing a significant role in storing, retrieving and processing information in the management system that evolves as a consequence of the operations research study. Because of its close association with these and other disciplines, any discussion of the applications of O.R. will necessarily include studies in some of these related areas. In the problem areas discussed below, these related studies as well as research that is clearly O.R. will all be classified as operations research. Certainly each piece of work cited has played, or will play, an integral part in an O.R. study.

DECISION PROBLEMS

There is no single classification of problems that falls in the realm of operations research, but there are certain problems that have repeated themselves in the past few years. Ackoff and Rivett (2) have suggested that many of these problems seem to fall in a classification similar to the eight areas listed below:

1. Inventory
2. Allocation
3. Waiting Lines
4. Scheduling
5. Competition
6. Replacement
7. Search
8. Sequencing

We will use these areas to discuss the types of problems of concern to O.R. and then discuss selected applications in the health field. The applications mentioned do not constitute an exhaustive list of health research, but only serve to indicate the character of past and current activity.

INVENTORY PROBLEMS

Inventory has been defined as idle resources, and resources "are anything that can be used to obtain something else of value" (2). Men, drugs, supplies and equipment are resources that hospital administrators are involved with. Decisions in inventory problems are made in terms of time and quantity, and in response to the following questions:

1. When should the inventory be replenished?
2. How much should be added to inventory?

Time and quantity are usually controllable variables, while such factors as demand and time between order and delivery are uncontrollable.

The administrator will see certain obvious inventory problems in a hospital system related to drug inventory, supplies, stores and linen. In the most thorough study of these problems to date, Smalley et al. (25, 34 and 35) have been studying the inventory problems that exist in hospital supply decisions. They have studied cost factors, design of cost prediction instruments, hospital inventory policies and the various costs associated with these policies. Differential costs associated with a shift in usage from one supply item form to another (e.g., reusable to disposable) have been identified and measured. Methods of establishing reorder points, economic lot sizes and other inventory policies in a multi-item hospital inventory system have been studied and compared. Various methods for measuring order costs and carrying costs have also been examined.

In a less traditional application, Rockwell *et al.* (33) have formulated the demand and supply of whole blood in a hospital as an inventory problem. They have analyzed the effect of various ordering policies on the blood inventory level. Attempts have been made to minimize the risk of storage and to maximize the effective utilization of available blood within a community.

ALLOCATION PROBLEMS

An important class of decision problems is concerned with the allocation of limited resources so that some measure of effectiveness is maximized or minimized. If there are enough resources to go around, the problem is greatly simplified. Usually the resources are limited in such a way that they cannot be used in the most effective manner.

Studies at The Johns Hopkins Hospital (23) have been concerned with the allocation of nursing resources to meet the variable demands of patient care. Their initial concern was with the amount of bedside care a patient actually received from nursing personnel of all types. After concluding that the demands of an individual patient vary with his degree of illness, a classification scheme was developed that categorized patients into three homogeneous classes. The average amount of bedside care required by patients in these classes was found to vary widely from one category to another. Using this classification scheme, a bedside care index was developed to indicate the total amount of time required for bedside care in an eight-hour day. Once nursing requirements are thus established, nursing personnel are allocated among the hospital floors.

A group at Tulane University (18) has studied the allocation of basic food ingredients in hospital menu planning. Their efforts have been toward the planning of menus that satisfy basic dietary and taste requirements, while minimizing the total cost of the meal to the hospital. It is hoped that research in this area will lead to a system for planning menus through the use of digital computers, that will be practical for use by many hospitals in the country.

WAITING LINE PROBLEMS

Queuing, or waiting line problems, are concerned with the design and planning of facilities to meet a randomly fluctuating demand for services. If service facilities are not adequate to meet demand, this causes congestion to occur at the service facility and incurs certain associated costs. However, increased service capacity to reduce congestion usually causes increased idleness in the service system, thus incurring a cost of idle service facilities. Waiting line problems usually strive to design systems that balance the aggregate costs of idleness and congestion and minimize the total cost of the service system.

Analysis in this problem area of health research has been more extensive and probably more sophisticated than any other. Outpatient departments, as service facilities, have been analyzed in this country (43) and abroad (14). Several appointment systems have been considered in an attempt to reduce the time patients spend waiting for service while maintaining a low level of physician idle time.

The hospital system itself may be viewed as a large and complex service facility. Congestion occurs in the form of waiting lists or patients who go to another hospital when they cannot be immediately admitted. Increasing the capacity of the hospital may cause an excess of idle service facilities in the form of idle beds, excess staff and other services. Balintfy (17) and Young (44) have developed explicit descriptions of the hospital as a service facility and have examined the effect of various admission and service policies on reduction of waiting lists as well as a reduction in idle facilities.

SCHEDULING PROBLEMS

Scheduling problems are concerned with the timing of arrivals (or departures) of units at a service facility in such a way that costs associated with total time taken to complete a project, idle service facilities and waiting time for service are minimized. There is a good deal of similarity between waiting line and scheduling problems. In fact some authors (1, 2) have classified both as waiting line problems. We personally feel that separating the two will make our arguments a little easier.

Studies at the University of Florida Hospital (24) have been concerned with the scheduling of operating room staff and facilities in the face of highly variable demand. Statistical methods have been devised so that the variation between predicted and actual operating room utilization is reduced along with subsequent costs.

Two relatively new techniques are currently being considered for scheduling and isolating key activities in planning construction and in research and development. The techniques are called PERT (Program Evaluation and Review Technique) and the Critical Path Method. They may be used by architects, engineers and administrators to plan construction and finance large scale hospital projects in such a way that costs are minimized, time schedules are maintained and potential bottlenecks are located. A recent article by Nalon and Ballinger (30) discusses the use of these techniques by hospitals.

COMPETITION PROBLEMS

Competition problems involve two or more individuals or organizations with conflicting objectives trying to optimize (maximize or minimize) some measure of effectiveness. These are problems where a decision made by one decision-maker can affect a decision made by one or more of the remaining decision-makers. Examples of competitive problems range from two players struggling to win at chess to two large companies striving for a greater share of their market.

An important extension of the competition problem is the consideration of Nature and its effect on decision-making. These are viewed as competition problems with one or more decision-makers in competition with Nature. This formulation has evolved to handle the random and uncontrollable character of certain variables in decision problems. Ledley and Lusted (28) have suggested the formulation of the diagnostic process as a competition problem against Nature. Warner (39) has reported the application of these concepts in the diagnosis of congenital heart disease. Flagle and Lechat (27) have reported on the use of the concept of competition against Nature in the selection of diagnostic and therapeutic strategies in public health. All of these studies have taken a step forward in increasing the accuracy and developing a better understanding of diagnoses.

OTHER DECISION PROBLEMS

The remaining decision problems in our classification of problem areas in operations research have seen limited application in the health services. In order to complete our discussion of the nature of O.R., we will just briefly summarize the character of the remaining areas.

Replacement problems are of two general classes, depending on whether the equipment involved deteriorates gradually or does not deteriorate but is subject to failure. In the case of deteriorating items, the problem is concerned with balancing the cost of new equipment against the cost of maintaining the efficiency of the old equipment. For items that fail, the problem is one of determining which items to replace and how often to replace them.

Search problems are concerned with looking for "things" where the search is subject to two kinds of errors: (a) failure to find the "things" and (b) failure to find the "things" although one has looked in the right place. These "things" can be symptoms of a disease, information in a medical record and others.

Sequencing refers to the order in which units requiring service at some service facility are serviced. In terms of queuing problems, the order in which members of the waiting line are served is called the queue discipline. The sequence of units to be served is chosen in such a way that the sum of the pertinent costs is minimized.

Very few problems found in operations research fall uniquely into one of the categories above. O.R. problems may include many of the decision models discussed. For example, the work of Connor et al. (23) at The Johns Hopkins Hospital on the allocation of nursing resources included problems in scheduling, replacement and waiting lines, among others. In their work on the reasoning foundations of medical diagnosis, Ledley and Lusted first define a diagnostic problem as a competitive problem and then formulate certain search problems in order to efficiently apply the analysis through the use of data processing.

The sketch of decision problems in O.R. that has been presented above can offer, at best, only a gross indication of the nature of the field. A recent book by Ackoff and Rivett (2) is recommended to the administrator who wishes to learn more about operations research.

CONTENT OF FUTURE RESEARCH

The decision problem framework in the discussion above was used primarily as a method of presenting the nature of operations research. In summarizing the accomplishments of operations research and associated areas, and in projecting the content of future research, we will use a classification that is probably a little more familiar to the hospital administrator.

NURSING

Previous work in this area has firmly established the character of nursing activity or time allocation (e.g., 23, 39). Measures sensitive to variations in the amount of self sufficiency of the patient population have been developed and subsequently used to allocate nursing time to various patient areas (23). Current research at The Johns Hopkins Hospital is concerned with developing a method of distributing nursing tasks among nurses, students and aides in such a way that the effectiveness of nursing care is maximized. The random and variable nature of nursing care has been studied and the effect of this variation on patient waiting time and the allocation of nursing resources has been predicted (42). Studies related to the measurement of patient care are underway at Ohio State University (27).

A research project at the University of Florida Hospital is concerned with a quantitative analysis of a unit manager system: a system that assigns many administrative and non-professional tasks formerly performed by nurses to a non-nurse. Exploratory studies are underway to examine the effect of the unit manager system on the allocation of nursing time, supply consumption and personnel costs associated with patient care. The long-run goal of the project is to establish a quantitative basis for the evaluation of the unit manager and similar systems throughout the country.

Most O.R. studies in nursing eventually point out the need for a measure of the effectiveness of nursing care. This measure has been called a measure of the quality of nursing care with increasing frequency. In order that more advanced decision problems related to nursing can be solved, this measurement problem must be tackled. Studies of the quality of nursing care and related areas are underway at a few hospitals in the country (e.g., 31, 32). The future should see an expansion of research in this area. Once adequate measures of effectiveness of nursing care have been formed, research activity in nurse scheduling and allocation, assignment of tasks and other related activities can proceed at full speed.

HOSPITAL PLANNING AND DESIGN

With increased federal support of hospital expansion and growing community health needs, the need for advanced concepts in the planning and design of health facilities becomes more apparent. The utilization of existing hospital facilities has received extensive study (14, 38, 45). These studies have concerned themselves with more efficient use of the hospital system. For example, Young (45) has predicted the effect of various admissions policies on the hospital census. In a related piece of work, Balintfy (17) has predicted daily discharges and admissions and has examined the effect of seasonal and chance fluctuations in occupancy levels.

LACK OF COMMUNICATION

Although there have been several articles in the literature concerning the use of operations research in planning new facilities (e.g., 20, 38), there is little evidence that O.R. has had a profound effect on hospital planning and design. There is a distinct need for improved communication between the researchers in this area and those doing the hospital planning. On the other hand, operations research in this area is still in a virgin stage. Still to be answered are questions such as: What criteria should be used in deciding where to locate a hospital? When is a hospital too large? Where should ancillary services be located within the hospital?

LOGISTICS

Problems in this area are concerned with the demand for and supply of quantities of people, equipment and auxiliary supplies. The relationships between highly variable demand, limited supply and its movement, and consumption have not been fully explored. Problems related to optimum inventory levels of supply, distribution systems and purchase quantities have been studied and in a few cases implemented (33).

Unlike most of the problem areas discussed in this paper, there is not an overwhelming need for new theoretical developments in the study of logistics; there is simply a need to apply the existing knowledge of operations research in the area. Smalley, *et al.* (34, 35) have led the way with their work on supply decisions mentioned earlier. The future should bring an increased concern for supply and logistics and the implementation of research results to analysis of optimum inventory levels and purchase quantities.

COMMUNICATIONS

Flagle (10) cites three major areas of concern for communication in hospital systems: management information, electronic monitoring of patient conditions and computer-aided diagnosis.

Hospitals, like other organizations, require adequate and rapid communication to facilitate the management function. Although some claim that hospital systems are unnecessarily bogged down with paperwork (the physical form of communication), they are probably no more bogged down than similar organizations found in industry or the military. Regardless, there is currently deep concern in the health field for management information systems. Automation of these systems has been a frequent subject of discussion. The so-called "total system" concept has evolved through a concern to automate the entire hospital communication system. One of the more noteworthy studies in this area is taking place at Bolt, Beranek and Newman, Inc. (19). Their effort is to "design, construct, apply and evaluate" a computer system specifically for use in a general hospital. They are in the process of developing computer programs that will allow efficient communication between the various parts of the hospital system and the computer.

ELECTRONIC MONITORING OPERATION

The advent of space medicine technology has fostered a growing interest in the electronic monitoring of patient conditions. The monitoring operation has been limited to certain vital signs, including temperature, pulse rate, and respiration rate. The efforts in this area are aimed at precision in patient care, more precise ways to diagnose illness and more precise ways to anticipate treatment needs (36).

Medical data processing presents a problem of increasing magnitude to hospitals throughout the country. New data is formed continuously by the physicians' daily examinations and interviews. These visits to the physician generate other data including doctors' orders, medication records, X-rays and laboratory reports. This flood of information filtering into the medical records system causes enormous problems in both storage and retrieval of medical information. Current research is concerned with utilization (in terms of quantity of records and what information in the record is used), prediction of space requirements, and the design of automatic data processing systems (33).

The computer obviously plays an important role in future plans for research in hospital system communication. A recent article by Spencer, *et al.* (36) summarizes past work in the automation of hospital functions and projects the need for future research. They point out that operations research is needed to study the decision processes in hospital operation and the implications of these decision processes on the requirements for communication systems.

SCREENING AND DIAGNOSIS

A recent and most intriguing application of operations research has been in the logic of screening and diagnosis. Mathematical models of diagnosis have been formulated by Ledley and Lusted (30). Their original concern was caused by an increasing interest in the use of computers in medical diagnosis. Before computers could be used there was a need to know more about how a physician makes a diagnosis. As an example of the use of these mathematical models, together with the digital computer, Warner (39) has reported their application to the diagnosis of congenital heart disease.

The screening of patients in hospitals with large out-patient facilities presents a major problem. Walton (33) has developed models of the decision processes involved in ascertaining the need for medical attention and has used these models to direct patients to proper specialty clinics.

Of all the problem areas discussed, modeling the diagnostic process stimulates the imagination more than any other. A concentrated effort is certain in this area in order to increase the accuracy of diagnosis, to develop an understanding of diagnosis and to facilitate the use of computers in the diagnostic process.

RESEARCH LEADERSHIP

Without question, national leadership in the application of operations research in the health field has come primarily from the federal government. Specifically, the Hill-Burton Act of 1954 provides that:

... the Surgeon General shall encourage, cooperate with, and render assistance to appropriate authorities, scientific institutions, and scientists, in the conduct and coordination of research, investigations, experiments, demonstrations, and studies relating to cause, diagnosis, treatment, control, and prevention of the physical and mental diseases and in impairments of man.

A good part of the operations research activity, partly in response to this government support, has developed in various academic institutions in the country. Operations research projects in universities such as The Johns Hopkins University, Case

Institute of Technology and Yale University are supported, in part, by grant funds from the Public Health Service. Other universities, such as the University of Florida, have fostered a spontaneous interest in the use of O.R. in health problems without grant support.

UNIVERSITY LEADERSHIP

We must look to the universities of the country for future leadership for at least two reasons: first, the existence of the required physical facilities such as hospitals and clinics, libraries, computing facilities and competent researchers, together with the atmosphere and traditions of research excellence, all in one geographical location, make the university the ideal setting for health research activity. Secondly, the dearth of competent health researchers is concomitant with each day's growing needs; the university, while participating in a health research program, will take a step in the direction of fulfilling the research needs of the country and in the direction of training researchers in the proper laboratory setting.

On the other hand, the wedding of the federal government and the university in a health research partnership breeds problems. For example, at least one experienced consultant in the field has said that he could count on one hand the number of hospital research studies conducted at various universities in the country that have actually been implemented. This is a danger signal. The root of the problem is found in the basic properties of this government-university partnership. First, the fact that the research activity in the university hospital is usually not dependent on the hospital for financial support may cause a lack of incentive to achieve practical results through implementation. Secondly, hospital administration, while realizing that there is a lack of implementation of the research activity in the hospital, may feel that the prestige that accompanies having an O.R. group outweighs this lack of implementation. Thus, the O.R. group may be tolerated without solid accomplishments.

Another point to be considered is that operations research groups in the university setting are staffed primarily by academic personnel. These researchers tend to seek problems of intellectual interest as well as problems that merit publishable research. However, many problems of practical significance to the hospital will satisfy neither of these requirements. A related problem is that many of the university O.R. groups employ graduate students. As a consequence of the limited resident time of these students, many research activities lack continuity and follow-through, thus compounding the problem of lack of implementation. We don't claim to know the answer to these problems, but we do feel that the implementation of certain O.R. studies may be sufficiently rewarding to hospitals in the country to justify the expenditure of hospital funds for operation research and related research activity. A second method of stimulating implementation may be for the operations research group to have certain non-academic staff members—who are primarily concerned with implementation of research projects and with certain pragmatic problems that are of little interest to faculty and graduate student—participating in the project.

These problems of implementation and continuity are indicative of the rapid expansion of operations research in the health field, and of the awareness of hospital administration to the need for new techniques to aid decision-making in the increasingly complex executive function. This is reason enough for optimism; these problems will ultimately be resolved.

CONCLUSION

Although operations research is intimately associated with decisions and decision problems, its major contribution to the health services has not been the identification of optimal or best decisions. Flagle (5) points out that where operations research has made a contribution

> ... has often been in revealing to administrators the true nature of the system with which they are dealing. Most often than not, the "true nature" has been the (chance) aspects, which have been misunderstood or not formally recognized in the existing management systems. The criteria for decision and change have not been in mathematical optimization, but simply a motivation for compatibility between the management procedures and the organizational phenomena they seek to control.

Advances that have been made are advances in understanding rather than in the identification of best decisions. A benefit of improved understanding is an ability to better formulate and define the real decision problems facing the health administrator. Hopefully, the future will bring a more explicit definition of decision problems in health administration together with subsequent solutions.

BIBLIOGRAPHY

This bibliography is intended to suggest further reading in operations research to the health or hospital administrator. Most publications cited have been chosen for their clarity, brevity and lack of technical detail. In the case of certain articles concerning applications, technical detail is unavoidable. These cases will be noted.

Introductory Reading in Operations Research:

1. ACKOFF, RUSSELL L. "The Development of Operations Research as a Science,"*Journal of Operations Research Society of America,* Vol. 4, No. 3, June 1956.
2. ——— and PATRICK RIVETT. *A Manager's Guide to Operations Research.* New York: John Wiley and Sons, Inc., 1963.
3. BOEHM, GEORGE. "Helping the Executive Make Up His Mind," *Fortune,* April 1962.
4. CAYWOOD, THOMAS E. "Operations Research as a Management Resource," *Hospital Administration,* Vol. 3, No. 2, Spring 1958.
5. FLAGLE, CHARLES D. "Operations Research in Community Services," Chapter 13 in Hertz, David B. and Roger T. Eddison. *Progress in Operations Research.* Vol. II, New York: John Wiley and Sons, Inc., 1964.
6. ———, WILLIAM H. HUGGINS and ROBERT H. ROY. *Operations Research and Systems Engineering.* Baltimore: Johns Hopkins Press, 1956 (See Chapters 1, 2 and 6).
7. MCCLOSKEY, JOSEPH F. and FLORENCE TREFETHEN. *Operations Research for Management.* Vol. 1, Baltimore: Johns Hopkins Press, 1954 (See Part I).
8. MILLER, DAVID W. and MARTIN K. STARR. *Executive Decisions and Operations Research.* Englewood Cliffs, N.J.: 1960 (See Chapters 1-4).
9. WAGNER, HARVEY M. "Practical Slants on Operations Research," *Harvard Business Review,* Vol. 41, No. 3, May-June 1963.

General Reading with a Little Mathematic Sophistication:

10. FLAGLE, CHARLES D. "Operations Research in the Health Services," *Journal of Operations Research Society of America,* Vol. 10, No. 5, 1962.
11. ———."Operations Research in a Hospital," Chapter 25 in reference 6.

Applications of O.R. in Industry:

12. ACKOFF, RUSSELL L. "Operations Research—New Tool of Industrial Science," *Industrail Laboratories,* November 1953.
13. HICKS, DONALD. "Operational Research in the Coal Industry," *Operational Research Quarterly,* December 1951.

Case Studies in Health and Hospital Administration: (Starred numbers indicate those articles with technical detail.)

14. BAILEY, N. T. J. and J. D. WELCH. "Appointment Systems in Hospital Outpatient Departments," *Lancet,* May 31, 1952.
15. ———. "Operational Research in Hospital Planning and Design," *Operational Research Quarterly,* Vol. 8, No. 3, September 1957.
16.* ———. "Queueing for Medical Care," *Applied Statistics,* Vol. 3, No. 3, November 1954.
17.* BALINTFY, JOSEPH L. "A Stochastic Model for the Analysis and Prediction of Discharges and Admissions in Hospitals," *Management Sciences,* Vol. 2, New York: Pergamon Press, 1960.
18. ——— and C. RALPH BLACKBURN. "A Significant Advance in Hospital Menu Planning by Computer," *Institutions,* July 1964.
19. BARUCH, J. J. "Hospital Research and Administration with a Digital Computer," *Circulation Research,* Vol. 11, No. 3, September 1962.
20. BLUMBERG, MARK S. "D P F Concept' Helps Predict Bed Needs," *The Modern Hospital,* Vol. 97, No. 6, December 1961.
21. BLUMBERG, MARK S. "Hospital Automation: The Needs and the Prospects," *Hospitals,* Vol. 35, No. 15. August 1961.
22. BECKMAN, MAJOR FRANKLIN P. and CAPTAIN ROLAND C. KENNEDY, "Pioneering 'Scientific Management' in U.S. Army Hospitals," *Hospital Management,* Vol. 70, No. 5, 1950.
23. CONNOR, ROBERT J., *et al.* "Effective Use of Nursing Resources: A Research Report," *Hospitals,* Vol. 35, May 1, 1961.
24. DAVIS, GORDON J. and RUDDELL REED, JR. "Variability Control is the Key to Maximum Operating Room Utilization," *The Modern Hospital,* Vol. 102, No. 4, April 1964.
25. FREEMAN, JOHN R., *et al.* "Carrying Costs," *Hospital Management,* Vol. 97, No. 5, May 1964.
26. FLAGLE, CHARLES D. "Criteria of Effectiveness for Selection, Training, Motivation of Hospital Personnel," *Journal of Operations Research Society of America,* Vol. 5, No. 4, August 1957 (Abstract).
27. ——— and M. F. LECHAT. "Statistical Decision Theory and the Selection of Diagnostic and Therapeutic Strategies in Public Health," presented at the meeting of the International Federation of Operations Research Societies, Oslo, July 1963.
28. HOWLAND, DANIEL. *The Development of a Methodology for the Evaluation of Patient Care,* Progress Report, Systems Research Group, Ohio State University, 1961.
29.* LINCOLN, THOMAS L. and GEORGE H. WEISS. "A Statistical Evaluation of Recurrent Medical Examinations," *Journal of Operations Research Society of America,* Vol. 12, No. 2, March-April 1964.
30.* LEDLEY, ROBERT S. and LEE B. LUSTED. "Reasoning Foundations of Medical Diagnosis," *Science,* Vol. 130, No. 3366, July 3, 1959.
31. NALON, PAUL F. and ROBERT I. BALLINGER, JR. "Critical Path Method of Scheduling and Financing for Hospitals," *Hospital Management,* Vol. 97, No. 5, May 1964.
32. Nurse Utilization Project Staff, State University of Iowa, *An Investigation of the Relation Between Nursing Activity and Patient Welfare,* 1960.
33.* Operations Research Division, The Johns Hopkins Hospital, *Progress Report,* 1962.

34.* ROCKWELL, THOMAS H., et al. "Inventory Analysis as Applied to Hospital Whole Blood Supply and Demand," *Journal of Industrial Engineering,* March-April 1962.
35. SMALLEY, HAROLD E., et al. "Cost Factors in Purchasing," *Hospital Management,* Vol. 97, No. 2, February 1964.
36. ———, et al. "Inventory Policies," *Hospital Management,* Vol. 97, No. 3, March 1964.
37. SPENCER, W. A., et al. "Requirements and Applications of Automation in Hospital Functions," *Journal of Chronic Disease,* Vol. 17, 1964.
38. THOMPSON, JOHN D., et al. "How Queueing Theory Works for the Hospital," *The Modern Hospital,* Vol. 94, No. 3, March 1960.
39.* TORGERSEN, PAUL E. "An Example of Work Sampling in the Hospital," *Journal of Industrial Engineering,* May-June 1959.
40.* WARNER, HOMER R., et al. "A Mathematical Approach to Medical Diagnosis," *Journal of the American Medical Association,* Vol. 177, No. 3, July 1961.

Dissertations and Theses:

41. DAVIS, J. GORDON. "A Model for Improvement of Operating Room Utilization," Master's Thesis, University of Florida, 1961.
42. GUE, RONALD L. "A Stochastic Description of Direct Patient Care and Its Relation to Communication in a Hospital," Doctoral Dissertation, Johns Hopkins University, 1964.
43. SONNENDECKER, J. R. "A Model for Forecasting Whole Blood Requirements of a Hospital Blood Laboratory," Master's Thesis, Ohio State University.
44. SORIANO, A. "A Comparative Study of Block and Individual Appointment Systems in the Outpatient Department, Wilmer Opthalmological Clinic," Master's Thesis, Johns Hopkins University, 1960.
45. YOUNG, JOHN P. "A Queueing Theory Approach to the Control of Hospital Inpatient Census," Doctoral Dissertation, Johns Hopkins University, 1962.

30.
The Application of Linear Programming to Decision-Making in Hospitals

WILLIAM L. DOWLING

William L. Dowling, Ph.D., is Associate Professor and Director - Graduate Program in Health Services Administration and Planning - School of Public Health and Community Medicine - The University of Washington

Many of the decisions an administrator must make in managing his hospital involve the allocation or assignment of personnel and other resources to alternative ends or uses to accomplish certain objectives. The allocation of available operating room personnel and facilities to meet the demand for different surgical procedures, and the assignment of available RN's, LPN's, Aides, and Unit Managers to the different tasks which must be performed in caring for patients are examples of this type of decision.

Decisions of this type, called *resource allocation decisions,* deal with the problem of determining the most efficient way to use resources to accomplish objectives. All such decisions have three common elements. First, the decision-maker has an *objective* in mind. In the nursing example, the objective may be to determine the nurse staffing pattern that minimizes the cost of meeting the needs of patients on a given nursing unit. Second, there are *alternative ways to accomplish the objective.* RN's can be assigned to tasks requiring their level of skill or less levels of skill. LPN's and Aides can also be assigned in different ways. Unit Managers can be assigned some of the tasks usually performed by nurses. Third, there are *constraints* on the decision. All essential tasks must be performed. All personnel must be fully utilized. Certain tasks must be performed by RN's. Only so many nurses are available for each shift. When confronted with a problem of this type, the decision-maker seeks the *optimal solution.* That is, he seeks the solution which maximizes the results that can be produced with a given set of resources, or minimizes the resources that must be used to produce a given result.

Resource allocation decisions are made frequently in hospitals, often by department heads and supervisors guided by established criteria and policies. In many cases, good judgment is all that is required to find a solution that is optimal or near optimal.

Reprinted by permission from *Hospital Administration* (currently *Hospital and Health Services Administration): Quarterly Journal of the American College of Hospital Administrators,* Vol. 16 (Summer, 1971), pp. 66-75. Copyright 1971 by the American College of Hospital Administrators. All rights reserved.

However, in more complex situations, where there are many resources, many tasks, many alternative ways of assigning resources to tasks, and many constraints on the acceptable assignments, it is difficult to make optimal decisions. In such situations, especially where non-optimal decisions result in a substantial waste of resources, more structured decision-making techniques should be considered.

One such decision-making technique is *mathematical programming*. Mathematical programming involves the formulation of a mathematical model to represent the resource allocation problem. The problem is then solved by a process (usually performed by a computer) of systematically searching for the optimal solution from among the alternative feasible solutions. *Linear programming* (1-6)* is the simplest form of mathematical programming, but because many problems can be approximated by linear equations or functions, it is applicable in a great variety of situations. Linear programming has been used successfully in industry since the late 1940s, and in recent years it has been applied with increasing frequency to hospital problems.

THE ADMINISTRATOR'S ROLE

The administrator need not know the mathematics required to transform a problem into a set of equations or the computer technology required to obtain a solution. Industrial engineers and operations researchers have the required training. However, it is important that the administrator be able to recognize problems, such as those discussed above, which are amenable to solution by linear programming. Otherwise opportunities to improve hospital efficiency may be missed. The administrator is also the person to specify the objectives of problems and to point out the institutional demands and policies that constrain their solution.

Specifying the *objective function* of a linear programming problem is often the most difficult aspect of applying this technique, and it is here that the expertise and judgment of the administrator are critical. If the specification of the objective of a problem does not reflect the real objectives of the hospital, the solution may impede or be irrelevant to the attainment of these objectives. The objective function must be expressed in terms of a set of *decision variables* (i.e., variables over which the hospital has control and to which the resources to be allocated can be related). For example, if a firm seeks to maximize profit, the objective function might express total profit (to be maximized) as a function of the unit profits of each of its products. The decision to be made is the amount of each product the firm should produce to maximize profit, given its fixed resources. Alternatively, the objective function might express total cost (to be minimized) as a function of the unit costs of producing a product by alternative processes. The decision to be made is the amount of each process the firm should use to minimize cost, given that it must produce so many units of the product.

---

*Numbers in parenthesis refer to bibliographic citations at end of article.

A HYPOTHETICAL HOSPITAL PROBLEM

The concepts of linear programming can be illustrated by a hypothetical hospital problem. Note that in applying this technique it is necessary to

1. Specify an objective function in terms of a set of decision variables.
2. Specify the relationships between resources and decision variables.
3. Specify the constraints that limit the acceptable values of the decision variables.

Suppose an administrator wishes to determine the maximum number of surgical patients that can be admitted and treated in his hospital during a given period of time, given the fixed (in the short-run) capacities of hospital resources to produce the services required by these patients. Assume, for the sake of simplicity, that there are only three types of surgical patients, appendectomies, cholecystectomies, and tonsillectomies, and let x_1, x_2 and x_3 represent the number of each type of patient. Assume, again for simplicity, that there are only three resources that might constrain the number of surgical patients treated, operating rooms, recovery room beds, and surgical service beds, and let c_1, c_2 and c_3 represent the capacity of each resource expressed in terms of units of service (i.e., operating room hours, recovery room bed hours, and surgical service bed days). The decision that must be made is to determine the optimal number of each type of patient to be treated. Therefore, the x's are the decision variables. The relationships between resources and decision variables are the quantities of the different services required to treat the different types of patients. The constraints are the capacities of the different resources.

Since the hospital seeks to maximize the number of surgical patients treated, the objective function may be expressed as follows:

$$\text{Maximize Surgical Patients} = x_1 + x_2 + x_3$$

This equation simply states that total surgical patients is the sum of the number of each of the three types of surgical patients. The objective is to determine the combination of patients that maximizes total patients while at the same time taking into account the constraints imposed by the service requirements of the patients and the service capacities of the resources. More complex objective functions could be specified if different values are associated with different types of patients. For example, more value might be placed on patients who have the most serious illnesses, or who represent the best teaching cases, or who are admitted by certain physicians. In such cases, the objective would be to

$$\text{maximize } V = v_1 x_1 + v_2 x_2 + v_3 x_3$$

with the v's reflecting the benefit or value to the community or hospital associated with each type of patient.

PRODUCTION COEFFICIENTS

Let us assume that the quantities of the different services required to treat each type of patient are as follows:

	x_1	x_2	x_3
Operating room hours	1	2	1
Recovery room bed hours	3	5	1
Surgical service bed days	6	9	2

These values, called *input-output* or *production coefficients*, represent the average quantity of each service required by each type of patient.* They can be obtained from hospital records, reports (e.g., the last row of coefficients, which are simply average lengths of stay, can be obtained from PAS reports), or from special studies.

MATHEMATICAL EXPRESSION OF THE PROBLEM

Finally, the capacities of the resources for the period of time under consideration can be estimated from past output levels or special studies. Let us assume that

$$c_1 = 1000 \text{ operating room hours}$$
$$c_2 = 2000 \text{ recovery room bed hours}$$
$$c_3 = 3000 \text{ surgical service bed days}$$

All of the information required to formulate the linear programming problem is now available, and the problem may be expressed as follows:

$$\text{Maximize Surgical Patients} = x_1 + x_2 + x_3 \tag{1}$$
$$1x_1 + 2x_2 + 1x_3 \leq 1000 \tag{2}$$
$$3x_1 + 5x_2 + 1x_3 \leq 2000 \tag{3}$$
$$6x_1 + 9x_2 + 2x_3 \leq 3000 \tag{4}$$
$$x_1, x_2, x_3 \geq 0 \tag{5}$$

Equation 1 is the objective function. Equations 2 - 4 are constraints which state that the total quantity of each service consumed by the three types of patients cannot exceed (must be equal to or less than) the service capacity of the corresponding resource. Equations 5 are non-negativity constraints. Obviously, the hospital cannot treat negative numbers of patients, but since the computer does not know this without being

---

*The assumption of linearity, which is central to linear programming, simply means that these coefficients are fixed and independent. That is, (1) there are no economies in treating additional patients (e.g., if six patient days of care are consumed in treating one patient, twelve will be consumed in treating two) and (2) treating more or less of one type of patient does not affect the service requirements of the other types.

instructed, non-negativity constraints must be included in any linear programming problem. The solution to this problem would indicate the combination of patients the hospital should admit and treat to maximize total surgical patients.

To make this problem realistic, many more types of patients and many more resources would be included in the model. In addition, constraints would be added to reflect institutional demands and policies. For example, the model could include constraints to prevent the hospital from exceeding its budget, or to prevent it from exceeding its desired occupancy level, or to require it to treat no less than some minimum number and no more than some maximum number of each type of patient.

The solution of linear programming problems yields two additional types of information which, for some problems, may be more important than the solution values of the decision variables. First, the *imputed value or shadow price* associated with each resource indicates the increase in the optimum value of the objective function (i.e., in the total number of patients treated) that could be obtained by increasing the capacity of the resource. For example, the shadow prices for this problem would indicate the number of additional surgical patients that could be treated with a one unit increase in the capacity of each of the resources. Positive shadow prices are given only for resources which are binding or constraining at the optimal solution. If for example, the optimal number of patients fully used the capacity of the operating rooms but not that of the surgical service beds, the shadow price attached to the former would be positive, and that attached to the latter would be zero, since increasing the supply of beds would not enable the hospital to treat any more patients. This information could be useful in facility and personnel planning.

ANOTHER PRACTICAL APPLICATION

Second, the *opportunity cost* or *tradeoff* associated with each decision variable indicates the decrease in the optimal value of the objective function (i.e., in the total number of patients treated) that would be required by an increase in the decision variable. That is, starting from the optimal combination of surgical patients, how many patients would have to be discharged to make room for an additional patient of each type? This information could serve as the basis for scheduling admissions.

Finally, *sensitivity analysis* can be used to evaluate the effects of hypothetical or planned changes in hospital policies. This technique is applied after the optimal solution has been found to determine the impact on the optimum values of the objective function and decision variables of changes in individual input-output coefficients and constraints. Sensitivity analysis would allow the administrator to ask, "How many more surgical patients could be treated if another operating room was added, or if the average length of stay of appendectomy patients was reduced by one day, or if tonsillectomy patients were taken directly back to the nursing units after surgery?" Sensitivity analysis is also useful in determining the degree of accuracy required in specifying the input-output coefficients and constraints. If the optimal solution is sensitive to small changes in these values, sufficient data must be collected to determine them quite accurately; if not, estimates will give satisfactory results.

A VARIETY OF USES FOR LINEAR PROGRAMMING

Linear programming has been applied to a variety of hospital problems. Balintfy (7-9) has used linear programming in hospital menu planning. The problem is to minimize the cost of meals subject to constraints on the nutritional adequacy, balance, frequency, and portion size of the foods combined to make up meals. Gue (10) has conducted further work in this area. Wolfe (11) has applied linear programming to the assignment of nursing personnel to the activities that must be performed on a nursing unit. The problem is to determine the assignment pattern that minimizes personnel cost subject to a number of constraints reflecting the value of assigning different categories of personnel to different tasks and the requirement that every task be performed. Kant (12) has suggested the use of linear programming in planning the allocation and location of hospitals in one of the territories in Russia so as to provide optimal preventive medicine service for the population. Earickson (13) has demonstrated the potential usefulness of linear programming in selecting a location for a branch of Cook County Hospital in Chicago so as to minimize the aggregate cost of travel by users of the branch. He suggests that the same approach could be used to determine the optimal number and location of neighborhood health clinics. Holland (14) has worked on developing methods to evaluate the location of hospitals in rural areas. Park and Freeman (15) have used linear programming to determine the most effective allocation of community health resources.

Feldstein (16) has applied linear programming to the problem of determining the combination of cases that should be treated by hospitals in the British National Health Service. Hospital output is measured by the number of cases treated in each of nine medical specialties. Four inputs—bed days, doctors, nurses, and purchasables—are included in the model. The objective is to maximize the weighted sum of the number of cases treated, subject to the quantities of inputs available during the planning year. The solution indicates the number of cases of each type that should be treated, the excess quantity of each non-constraining input, and the shadow price of each constraining input.

Hobbs and his associates (17) have applied linear programming to analyze the admission scheduling policy at Presbyterian-University Hospital. The objective is to determine the number of patients in each of 24 elective surgery categories that should be admitted per month to maximize the total number of surgery patients treated. Bed capacity and operating room capacity constraints, as well as constraints reflecting hospital policies concerning occupancy levels, costs, specialization requirements, and teaching requirements are included in the model. The problem is also solved for the objective of minimizing the cost of treating surgery patients. Dantzig (18) and Resh (19) have also applied linear programming to the admission scheduling problem.

THE BALIGH AND LAUGHHUNN STUDY

Baligh and Laughhunn (20) have developed a linear economic model for planning hospital admissions, although they make no attempt to operationalize the model. The model is based on the concept of "equivalence classes" of patients, each of which is defined by a set of requirements for hospital services and by a value or weight assigned by the hospital to treating the class of patients. The problem is to maximize the weighted sum of the number of patients treated, subject to available resources, budget, and hospital policy regarding the minimum number of patients in each class that are required for teaching purposes.

Dowling (21) has applied linear programming to model the production of patient care by a 275 bed community hospital. Hospital output is measured by the number of patients treated in each of 55 PAS diagnostic categories. The treatment of each category is viewed as a separate production process requiring a specific combination of diagnostic and therapeutic services. The constraints on output are the capacities of the hospital departments to produce these services. The problem is to determine the mix and volume of patients that maximizes the total number of patients treated per year, subject to the capacities of the departments and to certain maximum and minimum patient requirements. Actual hospital output is compared to optimal output as a measure of hospital efficiency. Gurfield and Clayton (22) have demonstrated the value of linear programming in planning the expansion or reorganization of hospital facilities to meet changes in patient load or innovations in patient care by modeling the care of adult and pediatric cardiac patients at U.C.L.A. Hospital.

BIBLIOGRAPHY

(Citations with identifying numbers have appeared in Abstracts of Hospital Management Studies.*)*

1. Dorfman, Robert. "Mathematical or 'Linear' Programming," *American Economic Review,* Vol. 43, December 1953.
2. Henderson, A., and Schlaifer, R. "Mathematical Programming," *Harvard Business Review,* Vol. 32, May-June 1954.
3. Baumol, William. *Economic Theory and Operations Analysis* (2nd ed.), Englewood Cliffs, New Jersey: Prentice-Hall, Inc., 1965, pp. 70-128 and 270-294.
4. Dantzig, George. *Linear Programming and Extensions,* Princeton, New Jersey: Princeton University Press, 1963.
5. Dorfman, R.; Samuelson, P.; and Soslow, R. *Linear Programming and Economic Analysis,* New York: McGraw-Hill Book Company, Inc., 1964.
6. Gass, Saul. *Linear Programming: Methods and Applications,* New York: McGraw-Hill Book Company, Inc., 1964.
7. Balintfy, Joseph. "Linear Programming Models for Menu Planning," in Smalley, H.E., and Freeman, J.R. (eds.), *Hospital Industrial Engineering,* New York: Reinhold, 1966, pp. 402-408.
8. Balintfy, J. and Vetter, E. "Computer Writes Menus," *Hospital Topics,* Vol. 42, June 1964.

9. Balintfy, J. and Nebell, E. "Experiments with Computer-Assisted Menu Planning," *Hospitals,* Vol. 40, June 16, 1966.
10. Gue, Ronald. *Mathematical Programming in Institutional Menu Planning,* Southern Methodist University, Dallas, Texas, 1968. (DI2-5327).
11. Wolfe, Harvey. *A Multiple Assignment Model for Staffing Nursing Units,* Operations Research Division, The Johns Hopkins Hospital, Baltimore, Maryland, 1964. (NU1-3694).
12. Kant, V. I. "The Use of Linear Programming in Perspective Planning of Preventive Medicine," *Zdravookhranenie* (Kishinev, USSR), No. 2, 1964.
13. Earickson, Robert. "The Case for Decentralizing Cook County Hospital," Working Paper #111.4, Chicago Regional Hospital Study, January 1968. (AR-2102).
14. Holland, Max. "An Efficient Allocation of General Hospital Facilities in Rural Areas: A Computer Algorithm Methodology," Ph.D. dissertation, Clemson University, Clemson, South Carolina, 1970. (AR0-5617).
15. Park, K. and Freeman, J. *Community Health Resource Allocation with Linear Programming Methods,* Health Systems Research Division, University of Florida, Gainesville, Florida, 1969. (MN-2040).
16. Feldstein, Martin. *Economic Analysis for Health Services Efficiency,* Chicago, Illinois: Markham Publishing Company, 1962, pp. 168-182.
17. Hobbs, Terrance, *et al.* "Linear Programming as Applied to the Admissions of Elective Surgery Patients at Presbyterian-University Hospital," Department of Industrial Engineering, University of Pittsburgh, Pittsburgh, Pennsylvania, 1963. and "Some Mathematical Techniques Applicable to Presbyterian-University Hospital," Department of Industrial Engineering, University of Pittsburgh, Pittsburgh, Pennsylvania, 1963, (MN-1004).
18. Dantzig, George. *A Hospital Admission Problem,* Operations Research House, Stanford University, Palo Alto, California, 1970. (AM1-5533).
19. Resh, Michael. "Mathematical Programming of Admissions Scheduling in Hospitals," Ph.D. dissertation, The Johns Hopkins University, Baltimore, Maryland, 1967. (AM-2011).
20. Baligh, H. and Laughhunn, H. "An Economic and Linear Model of the Hospital," *Health Services Research,* Vol. 4, Winter 1969.
21. Dowling, William. "A Linear Programming Approach to the Analysis of Hospital Production," Ph.D. dissertation, The University of Michigan, Ann Arbor, Michigan, 1970. (MN2-6294).
22. Gurfield, R. and Clayton, J. *Analytic Hospital Planning: A Pilot Study of Resource Allocation Using Mathematical Programming in a Cardiac Unit,* The Rand Corporation, Memorandum RM-5893-RC, April 1969 (SC1-6837).

Bibliographic citations for this commentary were compiled through the resources of the Cooperation Information Center for Hospital Management Studies at The University of Michigan. Subscriptions to *Abstracts of Hospital Management Studies,* the quarterly publication of the Information Center, are available at $25 per year from The Center at Room 420, City Center Building, 220 East Huron Street, Ann Arbor, Michigan 48108.

31.
Estimating Bed Needs By Means of Queuing Theory

JAMES K. COOPER AND TIMOTHY M. CORCORAN

James K. Cooper, M.D., is a Policy Analyst in the Office of the Assistant Secretary for Health - Department of Health, Education, and Welfare and Assistant Clinical Professor - Department of Health Care Sciences - George Washington University School of Medicine.

Timothy M. Corcoran is Deputy Director - The Housing Allowance Office of St. Joseph County, South Bend, Indiana and was formerly an Operations Research Specialist with the Rand Corporation.

Recently, a major urban hospital planned to increase and improve its cardiac-care services. The hospital desired an increase in the number of acute coronary-care-unit beds; it also planned to establish an intermediate-care facility so that patients with infarction could be discharged into a unit that provided less care than the acute unit, but more care than the general-hospital beds. Planning required an estimate of the number of beds necessary for both acute and intermediate coronary care.

Since the admission of a patient with a suspected acute myocardial infarction is an event that cannot be expected to occur at regularly spaced intervals, it became apparent that the problem of estimating the number of required beds could not be solved by simple arithmetic, Hospital planners requested an estimate based on operations-research techniques. The solution to this problem should be of general interest.

The problem resembles the standard multiple-server queuing model of operations-research theory. However, it is complicated by the restriction that the patients in the first unit (coronary-care unit) are of two kinds (true and false myocardial infarction), each kind staying a different length of time, and that a second service area (intermediate-care facility) receive a certain portion of the patients discharged from the first unit. For the first complication, differing lengths of stay, an exact mathematical solution was found; for the second complication, sequential service units, an approximate solution was used.

It was recognized that it was not possible to have a bed available every time it was required. The problem was solved for the requirement that a bed would be ready when needed in each unit at least 95 percent of the time. The hospital requested that plans

---

Reprinted by permission from *The New England Journal of Medicine,* Vol. 291 (August 22, 1974), pp. 404-405. Copyright 1974. All rights reserved.

assume 600 suspected cases of myocardial infarction per year. To broaden applicability, the problem was also solved for expected admissions from 400 to 800.

In the general queuing model, patients are assumed to arrive at a service facility, in this case a specialized-care unit, at varying and random intervals. The patients arriving in the first unit are of two kinds depending on clinical diagnosis—i.e., the overall population of patients suspected of having myocardial infarction can be regarded as consisting of two subpopulations, those with a true and those with a false infarction. It was assumed that 60 percent of the patients admitted would turn out not to have a myocardial infarction—a figure based on the history of the existing coronary-care unit. It was further assumed that the patterns of care for the unit would not change, and that the patients with true infarction would remain in the unit for an average of six days and those with false infarction would be discharged at the end of an average of three days. The time within the unit represents the service time for each group. The average service time for the intermediate-care facility was expected to be five days.

Of the patients with true myocardial infarction, it was assumed that 20 percent die in these two facilities, half in the first facility, and half in the second. Time from admission to death is assumed to have the same type of distribution as time from admission to discharge for those who do not die. This assumption predicts the fatality rate to follow an exponential pattern, which is consistent with actual data. All patients with true myocardial infarction on discharge alive from the coronary-care unit would be sent to the intermediate-care facility.

The above figures established the dimensions of a triangular queuing system with two types of customers, true and false myocardial infarction. Further assumptions of the model are that the interarrival time between patients and the service distribution times are exponential. Details of the proof of the solution of this model are beyond the scope of this paper.* Briefly, the various possible states of the system and the transition rates from one state to another were described. With use of the differential-difference equation method, seven linear equations were derived to describe the probability of the system in each state.

The probability that a newly arriving patient will have to be turned away from the acute-care unit is shown in Figure 1. As the number of beds increase, there is less chance that a patient will be turned away. To achieve the desired probability of 0.05, more than 10 beds are required. Since a partial hospital bed does not exist, this produces a requirement for 11 beds. Also shown in Figure 1 is the probability that a patient with true myocardial infarction will be turned away from the intermediate-care facility, assuming that 11 beds are available in the acute coronary-care unit. To achieve the requirement that less than 5 percent of such patients will be turned away requires six intermediate-care beds. The results for different admission rates are shown in Table 1.

This analysis has value on three levels. First of all, it should be useful to anyone planning a new or expanded progressive coronary-care-unit system. Secondly, because

---

*The detailed solution is available from the authors.

Figure 1

PROBABILITY OF TURNAWAY vs **NUMBER OF BEDS**

(Curves shown for ACUTE CARE and INTERMEDIATE CARE)

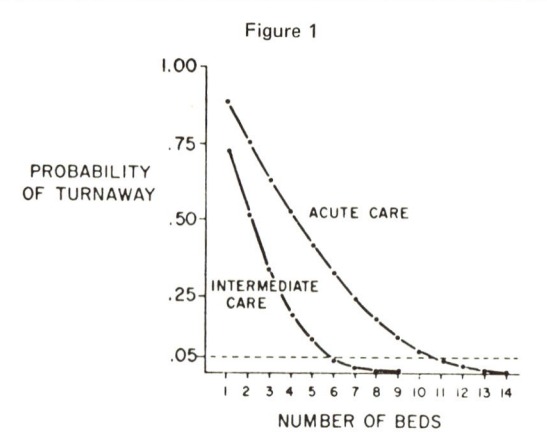

TABLE 1.

Bed Requirements for a Coronary-Care-Unit System According to Number of Annual Arrivals and Loss-Rate Requirements.*

No. of Beds Needed

Hospital Arrivals/Yr	Acute Coronary Care	Intermediate Coronary Care
400	9	5
500	10	6
600	11	6
700	13	7
800	14	8

*It is assumed that 40% of arrivals have myocardial infarction; 4% die in each service facility. The average stay for patients with infarction is 6 days in service area 1 & 5 days in service area 2. That for patients without infarction is 3 days in service area 1. Bed requirements are given to provide a bed when needed 95% of the time.

the formulas are general, they can be applied in any medical situation in which there is one service unit (two-customer queuing theory) or two units serving patients in sequence (sequential queuing). The inclusion of patients, those who die or who leave the system for any reason, further generalizes the applicability. Finally, the analysis represents a concrete example of the potential value of operations-research theory to health-care planning.

We are indebted to Dr. Joseph Lindsay, Jr., who provided encouragement and data for this analysis.

32.

Capital Budgeting Decision Making for Hospitals

RICHARD F. WACHT, PH.D.

Richard F. Wacht, Ph.D., is an Associate Professor of Finance at Georgia State University in Atlanta.

There has been a considerable amount of work accomplished in the area of cost-benefit analysis applied to health programs. Some of the more notable efforts have been by Weisbrod[1] and Mushkin,[2] and other authors who have made contributions in supporting areas, such as Reynolds in his study of the cost of road accidents in Great Britain.[3] Most of this work, however, has been directed toward the aggregate costs and the aggregate benefits to society of eradicating disease and saving lives, and the main interest has been concentrated on the problem of valuing the benefits per life saved or per illness avoided.[4]

EXPENDITURE BY SOCIETY AS A WHOLE

Implicit in these efforts to develop a theory of human capital formation and the attempts at statistical measurement of the benefits to be derived by allocating economic resources to health programs is the assumption that their primary concern should be with the analysis of an expenditure *by society as a whole* earmarked for the elimination or cure of a specific disease. This assumption, however, suggests that the application of cost-benefit analysis is performed by what may well prove to be the wrong unit; instead of analyzing an expenditure by *society*, the unit that should perform the analysis is the individual *hospital*—the ultimate investor of society's health program funds and the ultimate dispensor of health services to society. This follows from the fact that hospitals are financed at the margin by public-type funds (e.g.,

[1] B. A. Weisbrod, *Economics of Public Health: Measuring the Economic Impact of Diseases* (Philadelphia: University of Pennsylvania Press, 1960).

[2] Selma J. Mushkin, "Health as an Investment," *Journal of Political Economy,* Vol. LXX (Supplement), October 1962.

[3] D. J. Reynolds, "The Cost of Road Accidents," *Journal of the Royal Statistical Society,* Vol. 119, Part 4, 1956.

[4] A. R. Prest and R. Turvey, "Cost-Benefit Analysis: A Survey," *The Economic Journal,* Vol. LXXV, December 1965, p. 721.

Reprinted by permission from *Hospital Aministration* (currently *Hospital and Health Services Administration): Quarterly Journal of the American College of Hospital Administrators,* Chicago, Vol. 15 (Fall, 1970), pp. 14-27. Copyright 1970 by the American College of Hospital Administrators. All rights reserved.

public grants, gifts, donations, etc.) and they attempt to serve the health needs as demanded by the communities in which they are located. In addition, the hospitals generate income by billing patients for services rendered and, consequently, are sometimes in a position to supplement public funds with their own internally generated funds which may be made available for additional investment in health programs. Therefore, it would appear that the individual hospital, rather than society, ought to be charged with allocating those resources placed at its disposal among health programs not presently provided by it or else provided on only a minimal basis.

A SET OF DECISION RULES

Since a change in focus may in fact be required, and since the current state of the art of hospital capital budgeting can be described as primitive at best, the purpose of this paper is to develop a set of decision rules for applying existing cost-benefit theory and technique to the problem of maximizing the return on health program investment (made by hospitals). The applications in the field are legion, but the scope of the following discussion will be limited to investment in plant and equipment.[5]

THEORETICAL FRAMEWORK

Cost-benefit analysis, which is also known as investment planning and project appraisal, is a practical way of assessing the desirability of public projects in terms of short- and long-run benefits accruing from all affected economic entities.[6] It has as its counterpart in the private sector what is termed capital budgeting theory. With the aid of this similar approach, the profit-seeking corporation assesses its proposed capital investment expenditures in order to eliminate from consideration those projects which fail to meet some predetermined *profit* criterion.[7] The aim of both approaches is identical; i.e., to maximize the present value of all benefits less that of all costs, subject to specified constraints.

NEITHER APPROACH ADEQUATE IN ITSELF

In spite of the very great similarities between cost-benefit analysis and capital budgeting, neither approach is adequate in itself to provide the basic framework for capital budgeting decision-making in hospitals. This is because of the unique position hospitals occupy in our economy—halfway between the public sector and the private sector. Hospitals operate on the margin with public funds and mainly for the public good; therefore, cost-benefit analysis is especially applicable in the area of measuring non-monetary benefits derived from saving lives and from correcting mental and

---

[5] Included here under the term *plant* and *equipment* will be project planning, which encompasses necessary outlays for and benefits from capital and non-capital (e.g., personnel, medical and non-medical inventories, etc.) items for installing a new health service.

[6] Prest, *op. cit.,* p. 683.

[7] See Ezra Solomon, ed., *The Management of Corporate Capital* (Chicago: The Free Press of Glencoe, 1959), and Harold Bierman and Seymour Smidt, *The Capital Budgeting Decision,* 2nd ed. (New York: The Macmillan Co., 1966).

physical disabilities of people so that they may become more productive members of society.

It must also be recognized that, to a great extent, hospitals act like profit-seeking corporations. Hospitals must attempt to cover operating costs in order to survive and in order to continue to improve the health services that the public demands of them. Society may be willing to pay for the health care of people who are unable to pay for it themselves, but it should not be asked to bear the burden of waste or inefficiences in the management of hospitals. Thus, maximum benefit (in both the financial sense and social sense) should be sought for each dollar of expenditure by each hospital. Consequently, capital budgeting, designed as a microeconomic tool where money costs and money returns are involved, is just as applicable for hospital financial management as cost-benefit analysis.

Given that a combination of both approaches is needed, it is now necessary to spell out as precisely as possible the general principles of this hybrid approach, which shall be called *hospital capital budgeting.*

Very briefly, the object of analyzing an expenditure within the framework of hospital capital budgeting is to determine the numerical value of the ratio of the present value of benefits expressed in dollars to the present value of money costs. In order that society realize a net gain from the investment, this ratio should be greater than unity; that is, the present value of the benefits should exceed the costs.

As a practical matter, the major difficulties in applying this tool will be in defining and measuring the benefit; and costs associated with a hospital project. In most cases the scope and nature of the projects which are to be submitted for analysis are clear, but *for the sake of definition,* it might be well to enumerate the various elements that would go to make up these costs and benefits:

CAPITAL BUDGETING COSTS

(a) *Costs.* There are two types of costs with which hospital capital budgeting will be concerned: (1) the cost of acquiring, assembling, and making ready for operation all the necessary material required by the project, which cost shall be referred to as the *investment;* and (2) the costs associated with the normal functioning of the project once it has commenced operation. The latter costs will be called *operating costs.*

Investment is defined here to include the delivered cost of the plant and equipment, installation costs, any increase in inventories and accounts receivable attributed directly to the functioning of the project under consideration, and any other expense that would normally be capitalized and subsequently written off over the expected life of the equipment.[8]

Operating costs are those expenses which are directly associated with the project's operation, such as wages and salaries, electricity, and any increase in overhead expenses brought about by the adoption of the projects. Non-cash expenses, such as depreciation, are ignored however, since most hospitals are either state-supported institutions or non-profit corporations. Consequently, the effect of depreciation on tax liability need not be considered.

[8]The total of these items is the amount which is analogous to the principal or market value of a bond or certificate of indebtedness which should be returned to the investor (with interest) at maturity.

(b) *Benefits*. The benefits from new projects can be separated into two parts: (1) monetary benefits; and (2) non-monetary benefits. The *monetary benefits*, obviously, accrue from offering a service to the public at a price and collecting a sum of money once the service has been rendered. It is hoped that the money thus collected would be sufficient to cover the operating costs. If so, the *net cash benefits* arising from the investment in the project will be positive and can be expressed in terms of dollars received monthly, quarterly, or annually. If, however, operating costs exceed the collections, net cash benefits will be negative, but they will still be expressed in the same terms, but will be deducted from total benefits.

The *non-monetary benefits* arising from hospital investments are those with which cost-benefit analysis is mainly concerned; that is, the benefits to society arising out of saving lives or correcting some sort of malformation or malfunctioning of human bodies either totally or in part. One very definite result of this type of activity is that society retains (or gains) a productive member or realizes a gain from a productive member being made even more productive. Such benefits should be included in hospital capital budgeting, even though they are not directly expressed in money terms.

VALUATION OF COSTS AND BENEFITS

Hospital capital budgeting is concerned with costs and benefits which are either directly expressible in terms of money or, are capable of being expressed in terms of money. In applications such as these, all items should be valued at their *current* market value without adjustment for expected changes in the general price level. The reasoning here is that the valuation of all costs and benefits must be determined on the same basis, and for convenience the current price-level is generally employed.[9]

The more difficult problem, however, is to measure the value of those non--monetary benefits accruing to society from the investment in plant and equipment by hospitals. The basis for this type of measurement for health care benefits in general has been the subject of much of the literature of cost-benefit analysis, and the concensus is that economic resources devoted to health care represent in some part an investment in health; the resource gained as a result of dollars spent in order to prevent or cure sickness (including injury) is human labor. Thus, the attempt to value this resource gain in dollars must necessarily be directed toward estimating the output added by health care.[10]

Unlike much of the previous work in this area, the effort here must be directed toward labor product measurement not in the aggregate but as it applies to a given capital expenditure by an individual hospital.

RELATIVE WORTH ANALYZED

The effects of sickness or injury on human labor available for productive purposes can be classified under three headings: (1) death (permanent loss of labor); (2)

[9] Prest, *op. cit.*, p. 691.

[10] Mushkin, *op. cit.*, p. 138. For a more complete discussion of labor product measurement in the aggregate, see S. J. Mushkin and Francis d'A. Collins, "Economic Costs of Disease and Injury," *Public Health Reports*, LXXIV (September 1, 1959), pp. 795-809.

disability (temporary or permanent loss of labor); and (3) debility (temporary or permanent decrease in the productivity of labor).[11] In order to measure the value that hospital capital spending provides, an estimate of gain in productive work time brought about by the capital expenditure must be made, and a money value must be assigned to the output that this added work time represents. The resultant dollar figure will be an estimate of the non-monetary benefits arising out of the capital expenditure which, when added to the net cash benefits, will provide a figure that can be used to analyze the relative worth of the proposed capital acquisition.

MAN-YEARS AS A MEASUREMENT

The gain in resources derived from human labor made available for productive purposes through hospital capital expenditures must first be stated in terms of some basic unit which can then be assigned a value. Perhaps the most convenient unit of measurement would be man-years added to production since any smaller unit would tend to compound the arithmetic without making a corresponding contribution to the accuracy of the estimates. Reduction in deaths and long-term disabilities can be expressed directly in terms of additions of man-years on the job, and, in the case of debility, an improvement of efficiency on the job can readily be converted to full-time equivalents.[12]

EARNINGS AS A GUIDE

The estimate of the dollar value of the economic benefits from saving lives begins by determining earnings of the average person whose life is saved (productive capacity is enhanced) as a result of the capital expenditure being made by the hospital. The use of earnings, defined here to exclude any income resulting from a return on property or capital, can be justified on the grounds that the product of human labor benefits society and that this benefit should be measured by the market value placed on the units of labor.[13] The use of the earnings of the average person is also justified since the facilities acquired by hospitals will continue to yield benefits over a number of years by serving a cross-section of those people who are likely to succumb to the particular disease being treated.

The value of the total benefits, expressed as an annual figure, will therefore be

$$(1) \qquad B_t = B_m - C_o + \sum_n (e_t Y) (1 + r)^{-n}$$

where B_t represents total benefits at time t; B_m, monetary benefits received per year; C_o, annual operating costs; e_t, annual earnings at time of the average person benefiting from the capital expenditure; Y, estimated number of man-years added to production per year; and r, the rate of discount used to determine the present value of future

---

[11] *Ibid.*

[12] *Ibid.*, p. 140. Full employment can be assumed since there can be no loss of production in an unemployment situation and since unemployment should be considered as having its own costs.

[13] The value of the *product* is not used since this value is the result of the joint efforts of land, capital *and* labor. The benefits to society from saving lives is only that part of the product created by labor and should be valued by what labor receives in compensation.

earnings over the next n years, n being the number of years remaining of the life expectancy of the average person mentioned above.

PRESENT VALUE OF TOTAL BENEFITS

Equation (1) requires that the *present value* of future earnings of the average man be used as the non-monetary benefits. In addition, the estimated future benefits from the capital expenditure must be discounted at some rate of interest in order that all costs and benefits be reduced to comparable terms. In other words, what is required is the present value of total benefits, B_t. In equation form, this would be

(2) $$\text{Present value of total benefits} = \sum_t B_t (1 + r)^{-t}$$

where t would equal the expected economic life of the capital investment. Thus, there are two requirements for which an interest rate is needed to discount future benefits.

The literature on selecting the proper rate of interest for *public* investment projects is voluminous, and what is infinitely clear from a survey of this literature is that the proper method of determining this interest rate is at present unclear.[14] If such a method could indeed be developed, it would no doubt be of great value. But lacking such a ready-made tool, the best anyone can do is depend on a value judgment in selecting an interest rate.[15] It would appear satisfactory, however, to use the cost of acquiring borrowed funds for hospital capital budgeting purposes since this rate of interest is (1) meaningful to the individual hospital in terms of real costs, (2) easily determined or determinable, and (3) convenient. No defense of this rate on theoretical grounds will be offered here since, as Prest and Turvey so aptly put it, "whatever one does, one is trying to unscramble an omelette, and no one has yet invented a uniquely superior way of doing this."[16]

HOSPITAL CAPITAL BUDGETING TECHNIQUE

The technique of hospital capital budgeting can best be described with the aid of a hypothetical situation. The case problem that will be examined is one involving the establishment of a new hospital wing designed to cure hemophilia by means of organ transplant.[17]

---

[14] Otto Eckstein, "A Survey of the Theory of Public Expenditure Criteria," in James M. Buchanan (ed.) *Public Finances: Needs, Sources, and Utilization* (Princeton: Princeton University Press, 1961), pp. 458-460.

[15] For purposes of hospital capital budgeting, the problem of finding r becomes at once simpler and more complex than that for strictly public expenditures. On one hand, the monetary returns to the hospital take the form of corporate earnings which, in this sense, should be discounted at the hospital's cost of acquiring capital funds. This is simply the cost of borrowing for private institutions or, for state-supported institutions, the cost of funds borrowed by the state at the margin. On the other hand, the non-monetary benefits are actually returns to society expressed in money terms and should be discounted at a social rate of interest, which figure cannot be agreed upon. Thus, the choice of r must be a value judgment.

[16] Prest and Turvey, *op. cit.*, p. 700.

[17] No claim is made for the accuracy of any dollar figures presented here, nor should these figures be considered as even rough estimate of actual cost and income. The figures are for illustrative purposes only.

NET INVESTMENT REQUIRED

TABLE 1
CASH OUTFLOW FOR INVESTMENT IN PLANT AND EQUIPMENT FOR ORGAN TRANSPLANT PROJECT

($000)

ITEM	YEAR 1	YEAR 2
Construction Costs	$1,052	$ 80
Equipment Costs	48	168
Installation Costs	0	42
Working Capital	0	10
TOTALS	$1,100	$300

The first step is to determine the net investment required in order to build, equip, and otherwise ready the new wing for the acceptance of its first patient. It is important to determine both the total cash outlay for the project and the timing of such outlays. For example, it can be assumed that the new wing will take one year to build and another year to accumulate and install the necessary equipment once the decision has been made to undertake the project. The expenditures on the building and equipment contracts are to be paid continuously over the two-year period, except for the supplies inventories (which will be called working capital), so that the initial cash outflow can be shown in Table 1.

OPERATING COSTS

The next step is to estimate the operating costs which would likely be incurred at the projected level of activity for the new wing. These would consist of all utilities for the wing, personnel (both staff and administrative), housekeeping, supplies, etc. In other words, any actual increase in current operating costs associated with the new wing and its functioning should be considered. Allocated costs, however, such as administrative overhead, should be ignored unless these costs actually increase as a result of the project. For present purposes, let it be assumed that annual operating costs total $120,000 (and are incurred and paid continuously throughout each year, beginning in year three).

Another important consideration is to estimate the useful life of the combined investment. The building may last forever, but since it was designed for a special purpose (organ transplant) its maximum utility is realized only so long as it is used for the purpose for which it was designed. The equipment, on the other hand, will last for only a relatively short time before it will have to be replaced. But replacement of existing equipment is an investment decision in itself, so the useful life of a project extends from the time the first patient is accepted until the facility can no longer serve its primary purpose because of deterioration or obsolescence. In the present example, this period will be from year three through year ten or an expected useful life of eight years.

ESTIMATING THE RESULTING BENEFITS

The final bit of information needed is an estimate of the benefits—both monetary and non-monetary—that will result from the investment in the project. Measurement of the monetary benefits is relatively simple. It is merely the estimated annual number of non-indigent patients times the expected per patient charges. An estimate of the average length of postoperative care must naturally be made, along with the ancillary services that will be provided during the patient's stay. To these billings should be added any receipts from other sources on behalf of indigent patients. For the present case, it can be assumed that total monetary benefits are estimated to be $3,500 per average patient (including indigent for determining the average) and that it is expected that twenty patients per year will be treated successfully in the new wing.

MEASURING NON-MONETARY BENEFITS

Several steps are involved in measuring non-monetary benefits. The first is to determine the characteristics of the patients who will directly benefit from the investment expenditure made by the hospital. Hemophilia, for example, is almost exclusively a male disease. The disease can cripple as well as kill, and although its crippling effects can be treated on a temporary basis, no method has yet been devised to prevent their recurrence. As a consequence, a person with hemophilia, if he avoids the crippling effects of the disease and survives long enough to enter the labor market, is limited as to the type of employment he may engage in and probably will not reach the maximum productive capacity he would have achieved without the disease.

MAKING AN ESTIMATE

If it can therefore be assumed that the organ transplant will cure the hemophiliac, the investment in the project will result in preventing death, disability, and debility (in some ratio) in twenty people per year. It can also be assumed here that the time to perform the organ transplant for the patient would be at as early an age as practical, since the slightest bump may be fatal or permanently damaging to the hemophiliac. Finally, let us assume that a search of existing data shows that 5 per cent of all those suffering from the disease enter the labor market, 65 per cent die partially as a result of the disease prior to entering the labor market, and the remaining 30 per cent become permanently disabled.

Based on these assumptions, an estimate of the non-monetary benefits can now be made. The first step is to determine the average annual earnings at each age (for males only in this case) beginning from the age of the average patient, and discount these earnings to the present at the proper rate of interest.[18] The *present value* of the lifetime earnings of an average American male, age one year, discounted at 7 per cent

---

[18]The rate used here is 7 per cent.

is $19,266.[19] Without the organ transplant, 19 of 20 males would never enter the labor market, and the one who will, will earn, say, only two-thirds of his potential. Thus, the annual non-monetary benefits of investing in the new hospital wing will total about $378,000. Table 2 summarizes the timing and size of all the costs and benefits over the relevant period.

BENEFITS OVER COSTS

The final step in the process is to discount the net benefits (and costs) at the proper interest rate and compare the present value of the net investment with the present value of the net cash benefits plus the non-monetary benefits.[20] In this case, the present value of the net investment, discounted at 7 per cent is $1,362,000, and the present value of the net benefits from years three through ten total $1,498,000. The excess of benefits over costs is therefore $136,000 and the project should be undertaken, since the rate of return on investment by the hospital exceeds the cost of acquiring the funds. If the present value of the net investment had exceeded that of the benefits, however, the project should be rejected on the grounds that this particular allocation of resources would tend to make society less well off in the long run.

TABLE 2

COSTS AND BENEFITS ASSOCIATED WITH ORGAN TRANSPLANT PROJECT

($000)

Year	Investment*	C_o Operating Costs	B_m Monetary Benefits	$e_t Y$ Non-monetary Benefits	B_t Net Benefits (Costs)
1	($1,100)†				($1,100)
2	(300)				(300)
3		($120)	$70	$378	$ 328
4		(120)	70	378	328
5		(120)	70	378	328
6		(120)	70	378	328
7		(120)	70	378	328
8		(120)	70	378	328
9		(120)	70	378	328
10	10‡	(120)	70	378	338

*From Table 1.
†Parenthesis denote costs or cash outflows.
‡Represents the retention of working capital after project life is ended (See Table 1).

[19] Based on 1960 census figures. U.S. Senate, 88th Congress, 1st Session, *Hearings Before the Committee on Labor and Public Welfare on Bills Relating to Equal Employment Opportunities,* July-August 1963, p. 334.

BEST APPLICATION

Again, it should be stated that perhaps the best application of this tool would be in deciding among alternative investments, given a budget constraint or otherwise mutually exclusive projects under consideration by a hospital. In this type of application, the hospital would select the project(s) which promised the greatest excess present value or the greatest ratio of the present value of net benefits to present value of investment.

SUMMARY

In summary, the steps that one should take in applying the technique of hospital capital budgeting developed in this paper are as follows:

1. Determine the size and timing of cash expenditures on the required investment in plant and equipment.
2. Estimate the operating costs involved in the project.
3. Estimate the life of the project.
4. Estimate the monetary and non-monetary benefits.
5. Discount the costs and benefits with the proper interest rate and compare.

This technique will provide the hospital with an objective criterion that can be used in capital budgeting decision-making processes. Existing criteria on which such decisions are now being based, such as need or urgency,[21] persuasiveness or bargaining skill of individuals, and other similar approaches, obviously are not totally responsive to the hospital's environment as expressed in terms of the economics of health and medical care of the community which it serves. This is not to suggest, however, that the technique of hospital capital budgeting presented here should be used as the sole criterion for such decisions. The hospital's policy statements and long-run objectives should provide the framework for all activities, regardless of their nature, but it must be recognized that objective criteria are also necessary for rational decision-making.

SUGGESTED FURTHER READING

Robert Dorfman, ed., *Measuring Benefits of Government Investments* (Washington, D.C.: The Brookings Institute, 1965). Outlines some of the current thinking about criteria useful in measuring returns in the Public Sector.

Samuel B. Chase, Jr., ed., *Problems in Public Expenditure Analysis* (Washington, D.C.: The Brookings Institute, 1968). A much broader approach to the problems discussed in the Dorfman book.

Burton A. Weisbord, *Economics of Public Health* (Philadelphia: University of Pennsylvania Press, 1961). The most often quoted book in the field—a real classic.

Herbert E. Klarman *Economics of Public Health* (New York: Columbia University Press, 1965). Another classic.

---

[20] The present value tables used here are found in Jerome Bracken and C. J. Christenson, *Tables for Use in Analyzing Business Decisions* (Homewood, Illinois; Richard D. Irwin, Inc., 1965).

[21] *American Hospital Association, Budgeting Procedures for Hospitals* (Chicago: AHA, 1961), p. 38.

Part V

HEALTH CARE POLICY ISSUES AND TRENDS

No informed observer can deny that relations between society and the health care system are strained. Some of this difficulty is attributable to changes in societal perceptions—health care is now considered by many to be a "right." Are all persons regardless of economic or social circumstances entitled to health care? Compounding this are expectations of positive, even miraculous, results from an encounter with the health care system.

But more than artifacts, there are real problems. The Committee on the Costs of Medical Care, in its 1932 report, identified a number of unmet needs and shortcomings in the delivery and financing of health care.[1] Reading that report gives one an uncanny feeling—changing dates would make it current. Shortcomings have clearly existed for several scores of years and contextual and perceptual changes have exacerbated them.

Critics have suggested that the free enterprise system is not capable of dealing with problems of the scope and magnitude found in the health care field. For many, the federal government should be the prime mover in any attempted solution. Such involvement is not necessarily undesirable; but there is substantial evidence available by analogy, e.g., education and welfare, or from experience in other countries where there is large scale government involvement. It dramatically shows that governmental action offers no panacea; that at best one set of problems is exchanged for another, and the second set may well be no more amenable to solution than the first.

GOVERNMENT INVOLVEMENT—ISSUES AND BASES

The Constitution

Significant government involvement in health care is a very recent phenomenon. No evidence of federal concern with health, public or individual, can be found in the Constitution, or the debates surrounding it. The United States Constitution drew heavily upon a view of nature supported both by Christian traditions and by seventeenth century science. John Locke's philosophy made a major contribution to the Constitution. He postulated: by nature men are born equal and have a right to life, freedom, and the fruits of their labor. But there is the difficulty that each man is a judge of his own rights and that some men refuse to accept their obligations. To defend his natural rights, therefore, man has to give up his natural condition and form a political society which will protect these same rights.[2]

It was through the Constitution that a group of autonomous states mutually agreed to relinquish part of their sovereignty to a central authority. Consequently, the Constitution is primarily concerned with organization of the federal government and the limits of its powers with respect to the states and citizens.[3] Another major reason for establishing the Constitution was to provide economic stability among the states. The first ten amendments (Bill of Rights), added when it was found that a specific statement of rights was needed, address the question of liberty or legal rights of the individual.

It should be emphasized that "natural rights" in eighteenth century thought meant liberty or legal rights. The Constitution of the United States does not mention those which later were to be distinguished as distributive (benefit) rights, i.e., rights associated with needs such as income, housing, food, and health care, and which are now widely deemed basic to minimal levels of human existence. Those who speak of a health care right, or these other distributive rights, implicitly base their arguments on a "natural rights" philosophy.* This is a substantial enlargement and possibly a distortion of the traditional view since Locke's philosophy was formulated on the premise that liberty or legal rights were man's only "natural rights."

Unfortunately, there is often an implied or even explicit assumption that distributive rights may be granted on the same basis as liberty rights. This is not the case. Providing the citizen with distributive rights requires that part of a society's productivity be used to guarantee them. The allocation will vary with the distributive right involved, but it usually amounts to significant proportions. Besides the obvious qualitative distinction, liberty rights require far less of society's output in order for them to be guaranteed by government. With few exceptions, guaranteeing liberty rights for one group does not make them less available for another.

Education would be considered a distributive right, but like health care, there is no reference to education in the Constitution. It is useful to draw an analogy between education, which was considered by the Constitutional Convention, and health care, which was not. One constitutional scholar noted that federal aid to educational institutions was proposed during the Convention, but the matter was not pursued further.[4] The Constitution, therefore, provides no guidance for federal involvement in education, and the power to legislate concerning education was seen as one inherently belonging to state government.[5] This was consistent with the distrust of strong central government generally exhibited by the Founding Fathers.

Similarly, no mention of the terms, health and medicine, is found in either the Constitution or the debate surrounding its adoption by the Constitutional Convention.[6,7] Furthermore, the Amendments ignore them. Constitutional justification for

---

*The phrase "right to health care" must be distinguished from what is inaccurately termed a "right to health." Society can make substantial efforts to guarantee access to "health care." But "health" has so many components beyond society's reach, e.g., genetic makeup and lifestyle, that it cannot guarantee "health."

federal activities in public health and medical care has usually come from the commerce and the general welfare clause. The commerce clause was initially used to legitimatize federal involvement in quarantine legislation. The general welfare clause has justified broad federal involvement in health, education, and welfare activities. It is found in Article 1, Section 8, Clause 1:

> The Congress shall have Power to lay and collect Taxes, Duties, Imposts and Excises, to pay the Debts and provide for the common Defence and general Welfare of the United States...

The general welfare clause has been interpreted as a limitation on the federal power to lay and collect taxes, rather than a distinct power.[8] This view was expressed by James Madison in Federalist Paper #41 and reiterated in a letter from Madison to Andrew Stevenson written in 1830.[9] There was, however, a school of thought which advanced the opposite view of the general welfare clause—that it was a distinct power. This concept was adopted by the Supreme Court when it upheld the constitutionality of the Social Security Act of 1935.

It seems appropriate to conclude that had health care been discussed when the United States was founded, it would have been left to the states, as was education. Responsibilities for public health were exercised by the states through their police power, and local governments had organized and financed some health care for the indigent.

Curative Medicine and Public Health

Eighteenth century medicine had relatively little to offer. Curative medicine, especially, was to have a dormant period of another 100 years before it began to approach efficaciousness. Public health had not advanced further theoretically or technologically. However, unlike curative medicine, it had developed some general principles vis-à-vis a king or other governmental authority. For example, the principle that the sovereign was responsible for the protection and promotion of public health had precedent in England, and was brought by the colonists to America. "As early as 1648, ... Massachusetts Bay Colony passed an Act for Maritime Quarantine, and various other health laws were promulgated by different colonies before the Revolution."[10] The sovereign power over sanitation goes back substantially further, and has been traced to Hammurabi, during whose reign (2123 to 2080 B.C.) a Code of Laws was promulgated.[11] This same tradition is carried on to the proclamation of sanitary laws in the Old Testament, Leviticus, Chapters 11-15. The ancient Greeks and Romans also recognized the value of sanitary measures and there is evidence they used health officials.[12]

Thus, with the discovery and colonization of the New World, there were several precedents for government involvement in public health measures. At the time the United States was established these measures were primarily devoted to development, promulgation, and enforcement of quarantine laws. Although little was known about communicable diseases, there was sufficient empirical evidence to conclude that separating the ill (or those who might become ill) from the community could prevent spread of disease.

The early period of the Federal Republic was also a time for delineating the limits of power which the Constitution had granted to the federal government and divided among its three branches. In terms of future federal government intervention in matters related to health, especially quarantine, the Supreme Court ruling in *Gibbons v. Ogden* (1824) was a landmark decision.[13]

The first 150 years of the United States show that government efforts regarding public and personal health care were diverse, but extremely limited in the latter. During this same period the vast majority of total personal health services was provided, organized, and financed through efforts of the private sector. Government influence, especially at the federal level, developed very slowly and had been so inactive and unchanging that its role had assumed predictable proportions and characteristics. That involvement was to remain substantially unchanged until at least the 1930s. However, that is not to say no evolutionary changes took place.

EVOLUTION OF FEDERAL INVOLVEMENT

Pre-Medicare and Medicaid (1965)

By 1900 government had developed extensive interests in two areas which may generally be characterized as being on opposite ends of a public and personal health care continuum. At one extreme were the public health efforts such as quarantine, immunization, and sanitation. Local and state governments carried the majority of this burden. At the other extreme were the special groups of beneficiaries such as military personnel, veterans, Indians, and merchant mariners, for whom federal government had come to accept responsibility. In the first decade of the twentieth century these traditional areas of interest and delineation continued.

During the early years of the twentieth century rapid strides in health care were not available to significant numbers of Americans. Rejection of large numbers of World War I draftees for medical reasons, many of which could have been remedied with adequate care, dramatized this discrepancy, and, in a real sense, this can be considered the first national health survey. Evidence of congressional interest in another specialized group, mothers and children, came with passage of the Sheppard-Towner Act in 1922. Documentation of unmet needs and problems in organization and financing of medical care was formally made in the report of the Committee on the Costs of Medical Care (1932). This evidence mounted with the formal national health survey during the 1930s. Mobilization and conduct of World War II further emphasized unmet health needs at military induction centers.

The Depression, followed by American involvement in World War II, provided unique circumstances which resulted in federal government intrusion into areas which previously had been state, local, or private enclaves. Primarily, it was a matter of money; federal government had access to seemingly unlimited funds through personal and corporate income tax structures, while state and local governments clung to the far less lucrative or flexible sales and property taxes. Inability of the states to cope with the severe problems brought about by the Depression was forcefully noted by Justice Cardozo in the *Steward Machine Co.* case, one of three which held the Social Security Act of 1935 constitutional. Thus, as areas of need became manifest, federal government seemed to be the appropriate governmental unit to assist. Traditional groups, veterans, Indians, and merchant mariners, continued to receive care. However, during a fifteen-year period beginning in the mid-1930s, federal government was to become committed to financial support in other diverse areas. The federal role in medical sciences research, after small starts with the National Institutes of Health during the 1930s, was to become preeminent in the 1940s and 1950s. Passage of the Hill-Burton Act in 1946 continued and increased federal activity in health facility construction which had begun in the 1930s.[14] During the 1950s federal programs concerned with education of manpower in health and medical care developed.

It is apparent that no planned, general policy with specific goals was developed in the areas where federal health care interest and intervention occurred. It was a matter of participation as required by need and circumstance. However, this does not mean that an informal policy failed to develop from the attempts, successful and unsuccessful, through which government became involved in health care activities. The policy varied under the influence of diverse economic and political factors. Each further acceptance of responsibility can be viewed as recognition that government has a duty to provide something to which the people consider themselves entitled (Alford; Cater and Lee).

Except for substantial losses of men and material, the United States emerged from World War II economically strong and politically sound. The postwar era was to mark emergence of big federal government. Its growth was experienced by most sectors of the economy; health care as delivered by hospitals was one. At the outset, in the immediate post-World War II era, this involvement was primarily one of providing assistance to hospitals. Federal government paid for hospital construction and remodeling, training physicians and paramedical personnel, building health centers and clinics; in 1965 it began to pay for large groups of beneficiaries through the Medicare and Medicaid programs.

Post-Medicare and Medicaid

In the mid and late 1960s, state and federal government began the first, sometimes faltering, efforts to regulate hospitals. This was attempted through various health planning legislation beginning with the Comprehensive Health Planning Act of 1966. These early efforts proved to be unsuccessful primarily because, as some observers have argued, these laws had few teeth, i.e., there were inadequate means of forcing or prohibiting certain actions by health care providers. Therefore, beginning in the early 1970s federal legislation increasingly had sanctions which could be applied against institutions.

Hospitals have been the uneasy recipients of this increased attention, primarily because of the large proportion of national health care expenditures which they absorb. While the experts might disagree over the efficiency of the services delivered, there is little doubt that in sum it is the best available anywhere in the world. Hospitals today are being probed and prodded and poked by cadres of various experts in operations research, systems analysis, data processing, and auditing; of course, the politician is becoming increasingly ubiquitous. More importantly, hospitals have been cast into a political arena where they are not only uncomfortable, but unprepared (National Council, 1976). They have in the past consistently prided themselves on being nonpolitical, i.e., they provided an almost sanctified service which transcended such boundaries. Before the politicization of health care, this approach was relatively risk free. Now, singly or in groups, they are being forced to choose sides. They are put in a position of having friends and enemies and it is unlikely that they can emerge from the current conflict over national health insurance unscathed. However, to do nothing leaves them without a voice in the decision-making process, and ultimately in the final outcome (Jones).

NEW ENVIRONMENT FOR HOSPITALS

Today's hospitals find themselves in a land of paradoxes and contradictions. Hospital regulation is often cited as one means of reducing costs; clearly, this also limits independence and freedom of action. Yet, at the same time there are demands for more initiatives to reduce costs and demands to make patient care more efficient. Another paradox is that hospitals are told to be humanistic and show compassion, at the same time they are urged to be more cost conscious and business-like in their activities. Implicit in the latter is that the product should be measured by the dollar value. These demands do not come from the same sources, but hospitals nonetheless are put in awkward, contradictory, and sometimes untenable positions.

Traditionally, hospitals have primarily focused their efforts on care of the sick and injured and education of medical personnel. To a lesser extent they have conducted research and engaged in preventive activities. Some experts have suggested that the hospital should become the center for an emerging comprehensive health care system. They argue that hospitals are organizational entities—bricks and mortar institutions already in place, and they provide substantial portions of all health care.

However, a major consideration, increasingly recognized, is that prevention and health education are essential elements in an effective health care system. Hospitals are not well-prepared to provide these types of services; and new emphases on social, environmental, psychological, and genetic aspects of health problems will exacerbate this deficit. Changed emphases will also require different organizational arrangements and personnel. The historical institutional and in-patient orientation, as opposed to programmatic and out-patient emphases, may cause inadequate response in an era where adaptability and flexibility are essential. It is possible that hospitals may not be as responsive or able to provide these services as would a new entity. On balance, however, it is probably desirable that hospitals become the center for community health care of all types. The extent to which this actually occurs will depend on how willing and/or able the hospital is to provide a leadership role and to respond to demands and expectations of the community it serves (Creditor; Epperson and Juedeman; Somers).

REGULATION AND NATIONAL HEALTH INSURANCE

Hospitals are being subjected to increasingly stringent limitations on their freedom of action (Phillips and Sprague). This control has primarily come from state and federal governments, and secondarily from private groups, e.g., Blue Cross and the Joint Commission on Accreditation of Hospitals. Writers have argued this is appropriate because of the ultra-important role hospitals play in society. In an attempt to put this control into a meaningful conceptual framework, it has been suggested that they fit one of two existing models; regulated industry, e.g., airlines; or a public utility, e.g., telephones. These regulatory analogies have some attractive features and are a tribute to hospitals' recognized and emerging importance (Kauffman; Kovener).

However, regulation also raises significant policy questions. The record of both the regulated and the regulators in various sectors of the American economy is not enviable. Critics have charged that in some agencies the regulated control the regulators, and that this is facilitated by common and frequent personnel exchanges between them. There is also evidence that regulation often causes increased costs for industry and consumer, both directly and indirectly. The truth or falsity of these charges, and their extent, if true, is outside the scope of this introduction. However, they should raise warning signals for society and hospitals alike.

There are difficulties in attempting to compare by analogy the hospital delivery of health care with services provided by public utilities. Health care services and therefore hospitals are unique. This uniqueness results from an increasingly common attitude that receiving health care is a matter of right. For no public utility is this the case. The contexts from which views of these industries spring are different, i.e., implicit in the assertion of a right to health care is that an absence of money is not a barrier to receiving the service. However, when dealing with a utility the quantity of service available, e.g., electricity, is limited by the amount of money the consumer has; it has not been suggested that all must be provided with unlimited telephone or electric service. The same limitations have not been identified for health care services. Thus far the commitment suggested for a governmentally guaranteed right to health care is open-ended. The potential cost alone makes this unrealistic. Even government ownership, the only logical concomitant to a "right to health care," would not provide unlimited services for all.

Except for minimal (by comparison) private efforts, welfare and educational systems are governmental monopolies. In the first instance they occurred at the state level, but both are becoming federal responsibilities. Most people consider education and welfare rights to be appropriately guaranteed by government. Conceptually, there is little to distinguish health care from education or welfare, either in terms of current public attitudes about them, or in terms of their historical trends. In the long run, this development should cause little optimism for the future of the voluntary hospital system in the United States. A reasonable case can be made that the incremental federal involvement now being experienced is a transition stage through which we are passing. It is necessary because the health care system is so large and complex that this is the only way it can be absorbed. It would be paranoid to suggest that this is a thought-through, officially sanctioned, but secret federal policy. Yet, total federal control is not an unlikely end result of increasing involvement in the health care field.

In much of this increase in federal government activity, the encouragement of hospitals is apparent. Hospitals have taken the position that they should be helped in solving a particular problem. The flow of money is welcomed, but the recipients argue there should be no attempts to regulate its use. An obviously unrealistic distinction.

If government seeks to implement the societal view that health care is a right, i.e., through national health insurance (NHI), substantial consideration must be given to how these services would be financed (Harris; Lindsay). Payroll and perhaps income taxes will have to be levied to pay the cost of such a program. If it is a payroll tax similar to the social security tax, it will be labelled regressive since all persons will pay similar amounts for the coverage. To the extent that NHI is linked to a progressive income tax structure it will have social impact through income redistribution. Generally, the level of income taxation will determine how much discretionary spending remains for consumers. The resulting limitation on choice is likely to have its most substantial impact on the middle income groups. The poor never had a real choice, and the wealthy will continue to purchase services from any remaining private sector.

In the health care field, a major split of responsibility exists between federal and state government. Currently, state government is responsible for specific regulation of providers, e.g., licensure of both institutional and personal providers, and certificate of need regulation of institutional providers. Federal government has taken responsibility for large scale investment in plant, equipment, and personnel, and financing of major health care programs. Unless the trend at the federal level is reversed, such a dichotomy will become increasingly anachronistic. Only in terms of the undesirability of a large accumulation of power at any level of government is such a dichotomy attractive. From a rational standpoint it makes little sense. Of note is the fact that some national health insurance legislation proposes to reduce the dichotomy, e.g., federal control of physician licensing.

ACCOUNTABILITY AND QUALITY ASSURANCE

To date, public accountability for most hospitals has been a function of their willingness to voluntarily respond to the community (Moore; Phillips). Information on the extent of this responsiveness is very sketchy. Most charges of unresponsiveness have come from metropolitan areas—where the hospital's neighborhood and constituency changed. Some hospitals have instituted consumer advisory groups; others have included consumer representatives on their governing authorities (Metsch and Veney 1973, 1974). There is little doubt, however, that public financing will carry with it public accountability. As evidence of this, recent federal planning legislation has provided for consumer control of agency boards (Chalk and Mott; Hochbaum). Whether the taxpaying constituency or the service constituency is that to which the hospital will be held accountable has yet to be determined. Historically, by analogy to other programs, it is likely to be the taxpaying constituency.

Increasing costs will probably cause hospitals to attempt new means of interinstitutional cooperation, e.g., joint facilities and shared services (Brown; Owen). Multi-hospital systems, mergers, and contract management are other innovations which offer potential for cost savings and increased effectiveness (Brown and Money; Schoenhard; Shirley; Treat). A leader in innovation is likely to be investor-owned or managed hospitals (Deans; Rushing). Nothing is as stimulating to cost consciousness and efficiency as the profit motive. Hospitals are unique enterprises; however, few would seriously argue that they are not amenable to considerations of efficiency, effectiveness, and cost consciousness (Curry). In addition to organizational arrangements of new types, hospitals will become involved in new delivery and financing arrangements, e.g., surgicenters, health maintenance organizations (HMOs), and prospective payment plans (Cotton; U.S., DHEW, 1970; Saward; Wallace).

Beyond substantial financial constraints, there will be increasing demands that the quality and content of medical care be scrutinized (Buck; Morse, et al.; McKillop). Third party payors are beginning to stress effective utilization review and medical care evaluation. Federal government took an early lead in this type of effort and will undoubtedly continue to have an interest in proportion to its financial involvement. Establishment of professional standards review organizations (PSROs) to review care provided to certain federal beneficiaries is the most recent step (Cardwell; Simmons). Quality of care constraints will have an impact on administration and medical staffs through the governing authority as the latter is held increasingly accountable for the entire functioning of the facility.

There is no doubt that the trend toward greater external control of hospitals is quickening. Whether this is as a regulated industry, such as railroads, or as a public utility, is not important; de facto regulation or public utility status has already been substantially achieved. These pressures will increase; however, decisions to enact comprehensive, universal, and compulsory national health insurance, with its likely exclusive federal control of financing hospital care, will make the public utility status of hospitals a moot point.

Greater federal economic involvement in financing hospital care will result in efforts to spend public monies wisely—conservation of dollars. And use of federal funds will permit intervention in governance and management to the extent that politicians, bureaucrats, and others charged with managing public monies consider it necessary to achieve societally mandated goals for the hospital system (Gottlieb). Hospitals continue to be a distinct and complex service industry, and government control or even ownership cannot change that characteristic. As is not uncommon with policy decisions, government involvement is likely to have a number of unintended consequences and unmeasurable results—or at the very least disputed results of policy decisions and implementations. In terms of the long run, one must ask whether the voluntary and investor-owned hospital systems are compatible with large scale federal intervention in the health care field.

BIBLIOGRAPHY

Alford, Robert R. *Health Care Politics*. Chicago: The University of Chicago Press, 1975.
Allen, Rex Whitaker, and Von Karolyi, Ilona. *Hospital Planning Handbook*. New York: John Wiley and Sons, 1976.
Annas, George J. *The Rights of Hospital Patients*. New York: Dutton (Sunrise Book), 1976.
Breckon, Donald J. "Highlights in the Evolution of Hospital-Based Patient Education Programs." *Journal of Allied Health* 5(Summer): 35-39, 1976.
Brown, Montague. "Current Trends in Cooperative Health Care Ventures." *Hospitals* 48(1 June): 40-44, 1974.
Brown, Montague, and Money, William H. "The Promise of Multihospital Management." *Hospital Progress* 56(August): 36-42, 1975.
Buck, Charles Jr. "Terms and Trends in Quality Assurance." *Trustee* 28 (September): 32-34 1975.
Burns, Eveline. *Health Services for Tomorrow: Trends and Issues*. New York: Dunellen Publishing Co., 1973.
Cardwell, Horace. "A Second Look at PSROs." *Trustee* 28(September): 17-18, 1975.
Cater, Douglass, and Lee, Philip R., eds. *Politics of Health*. New York: Medcom Press, 1973.
Chalk, Mady, and Mott, Anthony. "The Board Structure Has to Change!" *Trustee* 28(January): 28-32, 1975.
Collen, Morris F., ed. *Technology and Health Care Systems in the 1980's*. Proceedings of a Conference, 19-21 January, 1972. Washington, D.C.: Department of Health, Education and Welfare Publication (HSM) 73-3016, 1973.
Cotton, Horace. "HMOs Won't Make Americans Live A Day Longer." *Physician's Management* 15(September): 12, 1975.
Creditor, Morton. "The Neighborhood Health Center: Where Does the Hospital Fit?" *American Journal of Public Health* 61(April): 807-13, 1971.
Curry, Wesley. "How Hospitals are Controlling Costs." *Hospitals* 50(16 May): 64-67, 1976.
Deans, John. "Investor-Owned and Not-For-Profit Hospitals Conduct Joint Activities." *Hospitals* 50(16 February): 49-51, 1976.
Dunlop, David W. "Benefit-Cost Analysis: A Review of Its Applicability in Policy Analysis for Delivering Health Services." *Social Science and Medicine* 9(March): 133-39, 1975.

Ellwood, Paul Jr. "Delivery Systems." *Hospitals* 49(1 April): 45-49, 1975.
Epperson, Gordon W., and Juedeman, R.F. "Accounting to the Community." *Hospitals* 49(1 February): 83, 1975.
Gavin, Marshall P. "Consumer Services: Inhospital Reachout." *Hospitals* 49(16 July): 65-67, 1975.
Goates, L. Brent. "A Compelling Public Relations Challenge for American Hospitals." *Hospital and Health Services Administration* 21(Fall): 47-66, 1976.
Gottlieb, Symond. "The Federal Government: Health Care's Not-So-Silent Partner." *Trustee* 29 (September): 22-24, 1976.
Harris, Seymour E. *The Economics of Health Care: Finance and Delivery.* Berkeley, California: McCutchan Publishing Corp., 1975.
Health Services Research Center of the Hospital Research and Educational Trust and Northwestern University. *Multihospital Systems: An Evaluation.* Chicago: Health Services Research Center of the Hospital Research and Educational Trust and Northwestern University, 1975.
Hirshfield, Daniel S. *The Lost Reform; The Campaign for Compulsory Health Insurance in the United States from 1932 to 1943.* Cambridge, Mass.: Harvard University Press, 1970.
Hochbaum, G.M. "Consumer Participation in Health Planning: Toward Conceptual Clarification." *American Journal of Public Health* 59(September): 1698-1705, 1969.
Holloway, Robert G. "Planning for Results and Specific Outcomes." *Hospitals* 50(16 May): 77-82, 1976.
Howard, Jan, and Strauss, Anselm, eds. *Humanizing Health Care.* New York: Wiley and Sons, 1975.
Jones, Wanda J. "Hospitals Should Exercise Role in Shaping Health Policies." *Hospitals* 50(16 June): 119-22, 1976.
Kauffman, John. "Are Hospitals Becoming Public Utilities?" *Trustee* 28(August): 24-25, 1975.
Kinzer, David. "Politics and Health: 21 Things to Look For." *Modern Healthcare* 3(May): 42-44, 1975.
Kissick, William L. "Health-Policy Directions for the 1970's." *New England Journal of Medicine* 282(11 June): 1343-54, 1970.
Kovener, Ronald. "Will Official Regulation Help or Hinder Our Health Care System?" *Hospital Financial Management* 29(May): 41, 1975.
Kress, John R., and Singer, James. *HMO Handbook.* Rockville, Maryland: Aspen Systems Corporation, 1975.
Leininger, Madeleine. "Health Care Delivery Systems for Tomorrow: Possibilities and Guidelines." *Health Care Dimensions* 2(Spring): 83, 1975.
Levin, Tom. *American Health: Professional Privileges vs. Public Need.* New York: Praeger Publications, 1974.
Lindsay, Cotton M., ed. *New Directions in Public Health Care: An Evaluation of Proposals for National Health Insurance.* San Francisco: Institute for Contemporary Studies, 1976.
McKillop, William. "Is High-Quality Care Assessable?" *Hospitals* 49(16 January): 43-47, 1975.
Mechanic, David. "Ideology, Medical Technology, and Health Care Organization in Modern Nations." *American Journal of Public Health* 65(March): 241-47, 1975.
Metsch, Jonathon M., and Veney, James E. "Measuring the Outcome of Consumer Participation." *Journal of Health and Social Behavior* 14(December): 368-74, 1973.
——————."A Model of the Adaptive Behavior of Hospital Administrators to the Mandate to Implement Consumer Participation." *Medical Care* 12(April): 338-50, 1974.
Moore, Carl. "Community Relations." *Hospitals* 49(1 April): 125-28, 1975.
Morse, Edward V.; Gordon, Gerald; and Moch, Michael. "Hospital Costs and Quality of Care: An Organizational Perspective." *Milbank Memorial Fund Quarterly, Health and Society* 52:315-46, 1974.
Mueller, William J. "Hospital Financial Management." *Financial Management* 1(Spring): 58-62, 1972.

Myers, Beverlee A., and Wilson, Vernon E. "Health Care Policy Issues in the 1970's." *Health Services Reports* 87(December): 879-85, 1972.

National Health Council, Inc. *Congress and Health: An Introduction to the Legislative Process and Its Key Participants.* New York: National Health Council, 1976.

Owen, Jack. "Wide-Range Sharing for Two Hospitals." *Hospitals* 48(1 June): 105-7, 1974.

Peters, Douglas S. "Peer Participation in Hospital Department Review." *Hospital Administration* 20(Spring): 8-15, 1975.

Phillips, Donald. "Hospitals vs. Communities: The Grant Hospital Experience." *Trustee* 28(July): 30-34, 1975.

Phillips, Donald, and Sprague, Joseph. "Hospital Regulations Reach a Collective Critical Mass" Part 1 *Hospitals* 50(16 July): 63-68; and Part 2 *Hospitals* 50(1 August): 78-82, 1976.

——————."Regulation: Can Hospitals Tame the Paper Work Monster?" Part 1 *Trustee* 29(July): 16-19; and Part 2 *Trustee* 29(August): 23-26, 1976.

Rhein, Reginald W. Jr. "HMOs: Threat or Opportunity." Conference on Quality Assurance of Medical Care, St. Louis Mo. *Medical World News* 16(27 January): 53-60, 1975.

Roseman, Cyril. "Problems and Prospects for Comprehensive Health Planning." *American Journal of Public Health* 62(January): 16-19, 1972.

Rushing, William. "Differences in Profit and Nonprofit Organizations: A Study of Effectiveness and Efficiency in General Short-Stay Hospitals." *Administrative Science Quarterly* 19(December): 474-84, 1974.

Saward, Ernest. "The Economic Argument for HMOs." *Hospital Medical Staff* 4(January): 18-24, 1975.

Schoenhard, William Jr. "Growth Potential of Hospital Management Corporations: An Analysis." *Hospital Progress* 56(July): 72-75, 1975.

Shirley, Robert C. "Analysis of Employee and Physician Attitudes Toward Hospital Merger." *Academy of Management Journal* 16(September): 465-480, 1973.

Simmons, Henry E. "PSRO Today: The Program's Viewpoint." *New England Journal of Medicine* 292(13 February):365-366, 1975.

Somers, Anne R. "If the Hospitals Won't Lead the Way to Health Care Reforms, The Reforms May Lead Away from the Hospital." *Modern Hospital* 121(August): 65-68, 1973.

Tetelman, Alice. "Public Hospitals-Critical or Recovering?" *Health Services Reports* 88(April): 295-304, 1973.

Torrens, Paul R. "Health Information Systems: The Wave of the Future or a Wave at the Past?" *Medical Record News* 46(February): 10-15, 1975.

Treat, Thomas. "The Performance of Merging Hospitals." *Medical Care* 14(March): 199-209, 1976.

U.S., Department of Health, Education, and Welfare, Health Resources Administration, Regional Medical Programs Service. *Quality Assurance of Medical Care.* Rockville, Maryland: Regional Medical Programs Service, Monograph, February, 1973.

U.S. Department of Health, Education, and Welfare, Health Services and Mental Health Administration. *Health Maintenance Organizations—The Basic Facts.* Rockville, Maryland: Department of Health, Education, and Welfare, 1970.

Wallace, Samuel. "HMOs Don't Just Happen." *Hospitals* 48(1 June): 87-90, 1974.

Walls, Edward L. Jr. "Hospital Dependency on Long-Term Debt." *Financial Management* 1(Spring): 42-47, 1972.

Whiting, Roger N. "Suggested Organizational Changes for the Hospital Industry." *Health Services Reports* 88(October): 743-49, 1973.

Wigley, Richard, and Cook, James R. *Community Health: Concepts and Issues.* New York: D. Van Nostrand Co., 1975.

Yoeli, Meir. "A Century of Advances in the Health Sciences: The Global View." *American Journal of Medical Sciences* 270(Nov.-Dec.): 508-13, 1975.

FOOTNOTES

[1] Committee on the Costs of Medical Care, *Medical Care for the American People,* Final Report adopted October 31, 1932 (Chicago: University of Chicago Press, 1932). Reprinted by U.S., Department of Health, Education, and Welfare, Public Health Service (Washington, D.C.: Government Printing Office, 1970).

[2] Gilman Ostrander, *The Rights of Man in America, 1606-1861* (Columbia: University of Missouri Press, 1960), p. 88.

[3] Dennis Lloyd, *The Idea of Law* (Baltimore: Penguin Books, 1970), p. 84.

[4] Max Farrand, ed., *The Records of the Federal Convention of 1787,* vol. 2 (New Haven: Yale University Press, 1911 and 1937), pp. 322, 325.

[5] Max Farrand, *The Framing of the Constitution of the United States* (New Haven: Yale University Press, 1913), p. 202.

[6] Farrand, *Records of the Federal Convention.*

[7] Farrand, *Framing of the Constitution.*

[8] Albert Gallatin, Speech in the U.S. House of Representatives, June 19, 1798, *Records of the Federal Convention,* ed. Max Farrand, vol. 3, p. 379.

[9] Farrand, *Records of the Federal Convention,* vol. 5, pp. 352-65.

[10] James A. Tobey, "Public Health and the Police Power," *New York University Law Review* 4 (1927):126.

[11] Chilperic Edwards, *The Hammurabi Code* (London: Watts and Co., 1921).

[12] James A. Tobey, *Public Health Law* (New York: The Commonwealth Fund, 1947), pp. 9-10.

[13] *Gibbons v. Ogden,* 22 U.S. 1 (1824). In this first commerce clause case to go to the Court, it was determined that congressional power to regulate commerce is unlimited except as prescribed by the Constitution.

[14] Act of August 13, 1946, ch. 958, 60 Stat. 1040-41.

Responsibility

Ray R. Eppert in Selection 33, "A TRUSTEE VIEWS THE VOLUNTARY HOSPITAL SYSTEM," discusses the voluntary, not-for-profit segment of the hospital industry—still the largest in terms of numbers of facilities and numbers of beds. He emphasizes the importance of the organization and future role of hospital trustees. In Selection 34, "THE SOCIAL RESPONSIBILITY OF GENERAL HOSPITALS," Bright M. Dornblaser addresses a timely topic—the social dimensions of hospitals as viewed within the context of their medical activities. Emphasis is placed on the hospital as a key social control point and questions about the continued quality of care are raised.

33.
A Trustee Views the Voluntary Hospital System

RAY R. EPPERT *

Ray R. Eppert was formerly Chief Executive Officer and Board Chairman of Burroughs Corporation and is currently Vice-Chairman of Harper Hospital in Detroit, Michigan.

Last March, it was my privilege to be one of the American Hospital Association's witnesses on Public Law 89-97 (Medicare) at hearings in Washington, D.C., before the Ways and Means Committee of the House of Representatives. I was testifying as a hospital trustee in behalf of the voluntary hospital system.

What do we really mean when we speak of the voluntary hospital system? Several years ago, a committee of the American Hospital Association took a hard look at the nature of the system and defined it very well. In the light of current developments, it is important that we keep this definition fresh in our minds. The committee said that the distinguishing feature of our hospital system is "its dependence in large part upon the voluntary principle—that principle that emphasizes the individual rather than the crowd; that stresses freedom of choice rather than compulsion; flexibility rather than rigidity; quality rather than quantity; that provides a place for charity as well as duty; that is in essence freedom, and, in sum, the aggregate of free choices made by individuals through all other means than increasing the powers of government, which involves the use of involuntary taxing and police powers."[1] The statement went on to say that this voluntary principle code is most manifest and society is best served when the following criteria are most fully met:

1. The individual hospital has autonomy and local nongovernmental control.
2. The hospital is responsible for its own financing and receives its support from those who use it and from those who donate funds or services for its continuation and improvement.
3. The hospital is not operated primarily for profit.

I endorse this statement, including the last point: "The hospital is not operated primarily for profit." Not that I am opposed to for-profit enterprises. As I told the Congressional committee, "I am an advocate of the profit system. I have spent my life working within that system, and I believe I understand and appreciate the broad

[1] Voluntary hospital system: American Hospital Association Board of Trustees statement. *Hospitals, J.A.H.A.* 35:33 Aug. 1, 1961.
*Deceased.

From *Hospitals, J.A.H.A.:* Reprinted, with permission, from *Hospitals, Journal of the American Hospital Association,* (Vol. 42, No. 1, January 1, 1968, pp. 30-36). Copyright 1968 by the American Hospital Association. All rights reserved.

benefits that this country, and all of us as individuals, have derived from its motivation. Yet I seriously doubt that it is possible—or wise—for the health field to depend upon hospitals developed primarily as private for-profit organizations. These proprietary, for-profit institutions serve their communities well, and they provide an essential service; but it would be a mistake to leave the future of hospital care entirely in the hands of such organizations."

VALUE OF NONPROFIT HOSPITALS

I am proud to have been the chairman and chief executive officer of a very large *for-profit corporation*. I am equally proud to be the chairman of a *not-for-profit hospital*. These two statements are not in fundamental conflict.

Just what is it that businessmen dedicated to the profit motive see in nonprofit hospitals? They believe that the free enterprise system is something much broader than the producing of individual and corporate profits. They believe that it provides freedom to operate, freedom of incentives, freedom for change, and freedom to improve the quality of a product. In the operation of a nonprofit hospital, they recognize, as does the AHA statement, these same freedoms. These hospitals provide more than the basic, essential services. They offer their communities high quality care, and they do this not because they have to, but because they want to. Business leaders want the hospital to continue to have this freedom of action not for the sake of profits, but so hospitals can continue to innovate and improve and to keep their services at a high level of quality and efficiency.

But just because I and my fellows in the industrial and business community support and believe in our nonprofit hospital system doesn't mean that we believe in or support an unbusinesslike operation. There has never been a time when it was as necessary as it is now for these hospitals to be conducted in a businesslike fashion and to be able to demonstrate it. Today, hospitals are in the spotlight and that means they are on the spot.

At the present time, some 24 per cent of the patients in the non-profit hospitals are Medicare patients. And if the Medicare reimbursement is inadequate, and it is, it presents a serious threat to our voluntary short-term care institutions. You can't afford to be underpaid for 24 per cent of your business. No one has that kind of margin. Industry doesn't, and the hospital doesn't. Furthermore, any business enterprise that does not have sufficient income so that it can generate adequate retained earnings puts itself in a position of gradual liquidation.

A nonprofit hospital doesn't have retained earnings as such, but the problem is the same in the sense that we must be certain that we are not dissipating our capital. This business of earnings and capital is fundamental to the growth, even the survival, of our voluntary hospital system. I say in all earnestness that inadequate reimbursement, the ignoring of the need of the nonprofit hospital for earnings, could lead to the gradual liquidation of our system. We cannot lose capital faster than our ability to replace it and remain the viable, dynamic institutions that the public expects us to be.

COSTS A NATIONAL CONCERN

Perhaps we have all heard too much talk about costs. The unpleasant truth, however, is that we are going to hear more rather than less because we all know that costs are going to become higher, not lower. The hospital may or may not be the whipping boy, but it certainly is the principal object of the national concern with medical costs.

Whenever I speak of hospital costs, I try to stress the vital fundamental that any cost-cutting and efficiency drive must be performed within the context of maintaining and, if possible, improving patient care. We could cut costs tomorrow just by arbitrarily reducing the quality of the product—that which goes on with the patient while he is in the hospital. We could also reduce our teaching and research. Instead of moving forward in the health field, we could stagnate. It would be cheaper. But our goal, the goal of the board and the medical staff and administration, must be to improve and not to retrogress.

COST AND EFFICIENCY FACTORS

We must seek answers to the problems of cost and increased efficiency, but not at the expense of better service and greater progress in the health field. I doubt that, even in the face of outcries about costs, the public would let us do it. The citizens see the definite evidence of the results of our health care progress and they read about it every day and they like it.

I don't know of anyone who isn't in favor of better health, be he Republican or Democrat. We can be certain that the demand for high quality institutional care and for all the other components of comprehensive health care is going to increase. And so rising costs will keep us, we may be sure, in the spotlight and on the spot.

The not-for-profit health system is going to be called to account and it must be able to respond promptly and adequately. Therefore, it is urgent that we not stand idly by and wait for developments but rather take the initiative to determine what can be done better than we are now doing. How can we better discharge our responsibility and still, so to speak, be in the economic ball park? The time has come when the hospital must look at itself critically, analytically, and objectively.

For a moment, let's look at hospital administration. I think the time has come when the top administrator should be and must be recognized as the chief operating officer of the institution. At Harper Hospital in Detroit we deliberately adopted a corporate format. I am not the president of the board of trustees. I am chairman of the board. The executive who was director of the hospital is now its president and he is on the board of trustees. That doesn't mean that he is dictating policy unilaterally, but it recognizes his proper position, responsibility, and accountability.

The chief operating officer of a hospital requires great executive talent, sometimes more than in business because there is really more coordination of diverse elements and less direct control. For example, in dealing with the medical staff, the president or director or superintendent of a hospital cannot deal with the physicians as though they were subordinates in a manufacturing division or design division of an industrial company. He cannot just implement a procedure. He can't just demand. The top administrator must be more than a fine executive, he must also be a consummate diplomat.

Are there enough top hospital executives? A great deal is being done by the American Hospital Association, but is there a more direct method of upgrading top administrators, not just in title but in breadth of thinking, in knowledge, and in ability to make executive decisions?

ORGANIZATIONAL TECHNIQUES

How many hospitals do formal budgeting? It has been said that a budget is the point of departure, but the budgeting process does encourage operations planning.

Should the hospital have a profit improvement committee, looking at not the dollar profit—there isn't any as such—but at the profit in service to the community, and looking at it from all angles?

Should there be a program improvement committee, one in which the medical staff would play an important role? This would be apart from the joint conference committee, because at the moment I am looking at inside management, and the joint conference committee, quite properly, is made up of some trustees, medical staff, and hospital management.

Should there be an incentives study committee, and what phases of operations should be studied?

How closely are hospitals today measuring the balance between inpatient care and outpatient care?

How many hospitals have looked, from the management and medical standpoint, at the whole gamut of hospital-related medical services? Understandably enough, we tend to have an inhospital fixation. But there are health profits to be made in other ways and a soundly organized and efficiently operated hospital is our best method of realizing these advances.

Although it may not be too productive to seek pat comparisons between industry and the hospital, that is no excuse for ignoring some approximate resemblances. The balance sheet of a hospital is not like that of a for-profit corporation. Its principal asset, the bed count, is not shown. The bed count does not necessarily determine the quality of the institution. The point I strive to make is that good financial practice calls for recognizing the importance of "turnover" of our assets, whether they be food, drugs, accounts receivable, or beds.

A tissue committee tells us whether a particular operation was really necessary. Are we auditing our bed utilization factor similarly? I recognize that the primary purpose of a tissue committee and the primary purpose of the medical audit and of bed utilization review is to enhance quality of care. In this paper, I am looking at the hospital performance from the business standpoint and there is an undeniable and important fiscal factor in proper utilization. When a patient convalesces in an acute hospital bed rather than in an extended care facility bed or at home, it might be considered an improper use of the principal hospital asset. And the better the bed, and the better the hospital, the bigger the asset and, therefore, the greater the waste.

Proper bed patient turnover ensures that our invested capital serves the maximum number of people. Efficient utilization performance may permit the necessary price increases and at the same time effect a reduction in total cost to the patient. Proper bed utilization is not a program of downgrading the end health result produced. It is good for the patient, good for the doctor, and good for the hospital.

CONTROL BY THE MEDICAL STAFF

In the hospital, the conservation of this asset is not merely an executive decision. The true control in the hospital doesn't lie with the executive alone, it lies with the physician. It is the medical staff that is, in a very real sense, the marketing organization of the hospital. They don't say "come on in and try our beds," but the doctor is the input and he is also the output. He is the one who signs the patient out to home or to the extended care facility. No one is asking the physician to subordinate his professional judgment as to what is medically good for the patient to economic considerations. But it is the responsibility of the hospital, and, therefore, of administration, to make the physicians aware of their stake in this matter. The doctor must make the best possible use of this frightfully expensive instrument, the hospital, that we have put at his disposal. This calls for wholehearted cooperation with the hospital in attempts to do those things that will improve efficiency without impairing in any way the doctor's professional prerogative or the quality of the care rendered to his patient.

Nothing is more important to hospital management than people. But is hospital management managing people properly? Does the hospital have a clear, concise set of rules and procedures? Are they enforced? Are they in writing? Are they understood? Wages represent some two-thirds of the hospital costs. We must, therefore, ask ourselves: Are we doing everything we can from the standpoint of methods, procedures, and time studies to ensure maximum productivity without any loss of good patient care?

WAGE FACTOR IN POLICY

There was a time when wages were so low in hospitals that the employment scale had to be downgraded. You didn't have to tell those workers they were being underpaid. They knew it. And there was not the same feeling, probably, of performance, of giving a good day's work for a good day's pay. Now, things have changed. Hospital wages are rising. Have we really taken a good look at our personnel department, our personnel management and practices since this wage movement started coming closer to the community wage level? Or are we still receiving the same attitude that we used to get from employees and which we accepted because we were paying them less than that which would ensure maximum performance? Certainly, with rising wages, management has more latitude and more right and more obligation to insist upon high performance from personnel. This takes us right back to job descriptions and accountability. What do we expect? Do we really know? Let's not criticize our employees if they don't fully understand what they are expected to do, what constitutes a day's work, what is the most efficient way of performing their particular job, and their individual accountability.

COMPREHENSIVE PLANS NEEDED

It seems quite obvious even to one who is not involved in a direct way in the day-to-day operation of a hospital that the spotlight I mentioned earlier will focus its sharpest beams on how well the hospitals behave from the standpoint of sensible planning. This is as it should be, because when we talk about comprehensive health facilities, we cannot escape the necessity for good, efficient planning. I believe that the communities that purchase and use our services directly or indirectly through governments and third-party payers are going to insist on a form of policing. This may take the legislative route, as it did in New York, or it can take the voluntary route as it did in Detroit. But regardless of the device, it must have teeth. In Detroit, sanctions are applied through a united capital fund drive for hospitals. Every five years we have a capital fund drive for the social service agencies involved in our united fund and for the hospitals. The large prospective donors—corporations, for example—are exempt from further contributions during that five-year period. Thus, any hospital that attempts to raise capital funds without going through a regular procedure requiring documentation of need by the Greater Detroit Area Hospital Council doesn't have a mass market in which to raise capital funds.

We would still need areawide planning even if there were no insistence on it as a method of assuring hospital cost effectiveness because it is the only way we can achieve the proper type, the proper size, and the proper mixture of institutions. To use the language of business again, areawide planning is really sophisticated, community-wide market analysis and product planning for better health. It provides us with a means of product innovation, product improvement, a way of assimilating the research results that are pouring in on us from every side. I know of no more dynamic industry than the health industry. I know of none that requires more innovation, more product planning, more product change, more tooling for new production than the health complex. This is the aspect of areawide planning that is often overlooked. We are too inclined to look upon this technique simply as a way of preventing us from doing those things that we shouldn't do, rather than telling us the things we should do and ways of doing them better.

Forces are at work against areawide planning and I think we all know them: the administrator who believes there is a direct relationship between the size of his institution and the size of his paycheck and his prestige; the physician who discourages a patient transfer to an extended care facility because it is a few blocks or a few miles away and personal time is involved; the trustee who wants to create a veritable monopoly, who doesn't stop to determine this institution's proper role in the community, and then stick to it. Some trustees can become quite impatient, almost unbalanced, when they start thinking in terms of the great hospital they happen to be connected with. They lose perspective.

I have already said a few things about management and the medical staff from the viewpoint of a trustee wearing a businessman's hat. Now I would like to look at the hospital as a businessman wearing a trustee's hat and examine somewhat more searchingly the trustee in this complex enterprise of ours. I think the time is past when the hospital will take a trustee, or be willing to take a trustee, simply because he has a good name to put on a letterhead or because it's a chance to pick up some endowment money. If you are building a business, you would not elect a director to the board simply because he might make a voluntary contribution as a dividend payment to the stockholders. You want mature judgment on the board, not a promissory note for some future legacy.

DUTIES OF TRUSTEES

We have formal training programs for administrators and, everyone knows, it takes an increasingly long time to educate a doctor. But do we fall short when it comes to the education of the trustee? Can we honestly say that all trustees, even a majority of them, truly understand their job so that they can provide the proper—and I emphasize the word proper—backing for good administration, in such a way that their actions will also ensure the best possible institutional results?

You can have a fine administration, you can have a fine medical staff, but you can quickly get the hospital into serious trouble if the board is made up of well--intentioned but poorly informed trustees who treat the hospital as sort of a prestigious avocation and tend to make snap decisions without the kind of evaluative study they would bring to their own business board on important issues.

Actually, the hospital is just about the worst place in the world to make snap decisions because only too often that which has been done is irreversible. Are we being fair to the trustee when we put him in a position of assuming such great responsibility without proper preparation? Do we need something more direct than we have for the education and training of trustees? Most of them are sophisticated and successful men, and it may seem gratuitous to be talking about training and education for them, but trustees do need training and education. No man likes to expose his ignorance, especially when he has made his mark in his own world, and unless someone takes the initiative to inform and educate him to the full measure of his responsibility, he will never fully appreciate what a really splendid thing it is to be a working trustee of a hospital.

SYSTEM'S GREATEST STRENGTH

The more than, 30,000 trustees—the figure may be 50,000—in our voluntary hospital system are that system's greatest strength, but often they do not do the job they could do for their individual institution and they certainly are not doing the massive job they could do for the nonprofit hospitals of this country as a group. It isn't because they don't want to. I believe it is because too many do not have a true understanding and knowledge of how and why a hospital is a different kind of enterprise, of the problems of administration, of the problems of the medical staff, and the physician's separate and special personality. So we often deny the trustee a chance to adjust himself to the fullest to the hospital enterprise.

Often trustees serve on the boards of many companies and they know that they cannot serve as a director in the same way on any two boards because the purposes of one company differ from the purposes of another. In this corporate role, the trustee recognizes that he must understand the business before he can be a good director for the company. Now, I ask, is this recognition of the need for understanding less important when we're dealing with human life? A trustee has a responsibility to be more than just pleased with his membership on the board of an important hospital. He has a personal responsibility to understand enough about the operation so that he can be certain he is contributing to the best of his ability to the decisions that are made.

There is a radical difference between a corporate director and a hospital trustee. The board, in the case of a corporation, a business, or even a for-profit hospital, can measure the competence and performance of management on the basis of profit and loss results. If revenues and earnings are increasing, if dividends are increasing and retained earnings are satisfactory, the corporate director logically assumes that things are pretty much in gear. Those same yardsticks do not exist for a trustee of a voluntary nonprofit hospital to measure either the status of the institution or the performance of management. A greater depth of knowledge of operations is necessary. I'm certainly not suggesting that trustees get into operations or interfere in any way with management other than in a support and leadership role. But it should be an intelligent support and leadership role. There probably are some hospital administrators who do not want a too well-informed board or shirk their part in trustee training and education. Maybe the administrator believes it would downgrade his position or possibly he may even believe that he wouldn't be competent to deal with a better informed board. A really good executive believes just the opposite. He knows, and the good hospital trustee knows, that the only meaningful audit the board member can make of the hospital comes through knowing enough to be able to gauge the programs that come up for consideration, to evaluate the discussions and the pertinency of the points the administrator is making. The trustee cannot do it by snooping. Trustees should not bypass administration, especially in matters of medical staff relationships. The trustee who listens too much or talks too much with members of the medical staff other than through the formal joint conference arrangement is asking for trouble for himself, the administration, and the hospital.

JOINT CONFERENCE COMMITTEE

The joint conference committee is the proper method of communication among trustees, management, and the medical staff. There are physicians who believe that the doctor ought to be an actual member of the board. I, for one, believe that the physician who represents the medical staff at the board meetings—in the case of Harper Hospital it is the chief of the medical staff—is in a stronger position than one with a vote on the board. If I were a physician, I wouldn't want to be a voting trustee and certainly if I were the chief of staff, I would not want the medical staff represented by anyone but myself. The chief of staff is the link to the medical executive committee, and he is the proper spokesman for the staff at meetings of the board. That role should be given to no one else.

I want to emphasize that by and large, our hospitals and our people have been well served by governing boards across the breadth and length of this land and throughout the history of the whole voluntary movement. But the point I want to underscore is that, to a far greater degree than ever before, hospitals are going to be under the scrutiny of outside agencies, and what was sufficient in the past may not be good enough for the future.

At the local hospital level we can point to many great trustee accomplishments. I do not think we can do so on nearly the same scale at the national level. There are many trustees who are not yet aware of the impact that government now has and will have on the future of not-for-profit hospitals.

I do not believe that trustees and their hospitals fully realize the great power of trustee collective strength for good if this potential were fully mobilized. A list of all the trustees of nonprofit hospitals would be a veritable Who's Who in America. No single organization would even compare with it. Amplified properly and constructively through organization, that voice cannot be ignored.

The organization necessary to bring the amplification of our trustee voice for the preservation and enhancement of the values of our voluntary system is, I believe, the American Hospital Association, and to my mind this is one of its most important tasks. Almost all voluntary nonprofit hospitals are members of the Association. While it is the hospital's chief operating executive who participates most actively in Association affairs, we should remember that each trustee of a member institution can be considered an ex officio member of the American Hospital Association. I know the difficulties that face the Association in developing such an action program, but the importance of doing so cannot be ignored.

TRUSTEES' ACTIVITIES

In one of the Association's own reports,[2] it is stated that "the Association should encourage hospitals to involve trustees in activities beyond the traditional emphasis on finances and internal management, and to urge them to take a vigorous role in pressing external hospital problems such as areawide planning and relationships with government." The report goes on to say that "If the Association is to grow in usefulness, it must adapt to changes in hospitals and their environment. Such important changes are occurring so steadily that it is imperative that the Association's objectives and programs be broadened to meet the enlarged definition of the hospital's responsibility."

Never have changes so important to our hospitals been occurring more often than at present. Never has it been more important for the American Hospital Association to give urgent priority to the task of mobilizing the trustees of our nation, of marshaling the vast resources they represent in talent and accomplishment. Properly oriented and informed, the trustees will respond enthusiastically.

Our voluntary not-for-profit hospital system is one of America's most precious assets. That system must now welcome and meet the challenge of our national determination to achieve ever higher health standards for all our citizens. They must give leadership in these programs because we know, and I think Washington knows, that success at the national level can only be achieved through the continuing success of our voluntary nonprofit hospitals, which represent 75 per cent of the nation's short-term care hospital investments and facilities. Without them there could be no national program. It's just that simple.

The voluntary way is the American way, and I am very certain that the new health challenges will be accepted, not as insoluble problems, but rather as new opportunities to quicken our pace of forward progress. Our indicated action calendar is moving very fast. It is time to mobilize our boards. Suggesting this mobilization of trustees does not mean that I am advocating the formation of a pressure lobby. Rather, I am recommending the creation of a well-informed, influential, vigilant, voluntary army, dedicated to achieving the maximum advances in physical health and determined to maintain concurrently our vital institutional economic health, without which we will surely fail. This is a trustee responsibility that cannot be subcontracted or ignored.

[2] American Hospital Association, *Statement on the Changing Hospital* (Chicago: the Association, 1965).

34.
The Social Responsibility of General Hospitals

BRIGHT M. DORNBLASER

Bright M. Dornblaser, is Director of the Graduate Program in Hospital Administration at the University of Minnesota.

The hospital field is under pressures from society to expand its missions, or to significantly alter how and where its missions are performed. What is the appropriate response?

OBJECTIVES

We recognize that the basic objective of the hospital as a social institution is to improve the quality of living—while working for life itself.

We further recognize that we can sharpen our ideas of ends of health care institutions from the honing action of experience in applying ideas within the context of the general hospital, its problems and realities. This is particularly so if cybernetics applies, if there is a feedback mechanism to the university or other sources of ideas which are being tested through application.

On the basis of experience, what should be the response to the question, "what is the mission of the hospital beyond beds and out-patient services?"

THESIS AND ANTITHESIS

One quick, if perhaps unpopular, answer to this question is "None!" The underlying rationale is that the hospital has more than enough to do to perform its medical care mission well, and "Whatever we undertake to do, we must do supremely well."

This position is, of course, the antithesis of a thesis with common currency today: That the quality of personal health care services for the middle class people now receiving such services is adequate; that the important unmet needs now are social; that hospitals have demonstrated a capacity to serve well; that they should expand their scope of service in response to social need; and that they are socially irresponsible if they do not. Is this thesis correct? Should the hospital become the hub rather than a medical care spoke of the health care wheel?

Reprinted by permission from *Hospital Administration* (currently *Hospital and Health Services Administration*): Quarterly Journal of the American College of Hospital Administrators, Chicago, Vol. 14 (Spring, 1969), pp. 6-17. Copyright 1969 by the American College of Hospital Administrators. All rights reserved.

MEDICAL CARE MISSION

Some traditionalists might respond by saying that to expand the general hospital's missions would jeopardize the quality of medical care. Our concentration, they believe, should continue on the quality of care provided to the individual patient who requests personal health services. The problems of continuing to provide care at the level of quality perceived possible by the producers of care are extensive, they are burdensome, and they are continuing. Subverting a specialized interest and skill to a more generalized concern, they feel, will exact too high a social price.

Proponents of this position suggest that the explosion of knowledge of the medical sciences and technology—with increased costs and shortages of dollars and competent manpower—can consume all the skilled health manpower and the fiscal, organizational, and managerial resources now available. These resources are subject to urgent demands today for improved efficiency, which suggests considerable change is manifest even within the medical model.

WRESTLING WITH SOCIAL ASSIGNMENTS

Those pressing for increased efficiency state that quality of care to the individual is not enough, that medical care excellence is insufficient—the least hospital people must admit is their obligation also to serve the community with efficiency, so that the highest benefits can be obtained for the medical care dollars expended.

It is hard to deny the reasonableness of this position.

This argument will be reinforced by management incentives—a summarizing test of management.

By one means or another, hospital management will be stimulated to "reduce" cost by increasing efficiency:

Through higher productivity, e.g., through establishing group practice and use of full-time physicians;
Through trade-offs of less skilled health manpower for the more skilled;
Through trade-offs of less costly programs for the more costly;
Through control of the construction of facilities, costly to construct and still more costly to operate.

The hospital will be a key social control point, even if choosing to remain in the medical care mode. As such, it will receive inexorable pressure in the name of efficiency to make significant and traumatic changes in the ways in which the accepted medical model missions are executed. Wrestling with these socially loaded "bear-by-the-tail" social assignments is a first full-time job. At this point we might identify with the farmer who protested to the Farm Bureau representative who wanted to instruct him on improved agriculture methods: "I ain't farming half as well as I know how yet!"

From these viewpoints we might well conclude that the hospital's first responsibility for service continues to be found in the medical model: Resources will be strained in order to continue executing these unique service responsibilities. Hospital representatives should be the leading advocates of continuing to perform them at a quality level. Furthermore, it is essential that hospital spokesmen not let others—who are clamoring for the general hospital to expand its mission—assume the continuance of past accomplishments, if added responsibilities are accepted.

SOCIAL MODEL VS. MEDICAL MODEL

It is the view of the general hospital mission from the perspective of a social model which contributes to the demands for increased service. These accelerated demands, of course, reflect rising public expectations. They reflect a concern for the well, as well as the ill. Furthermore, they reflect a belief that the poor should have the opportunity and be encouraged to use the health care system. Drawing from the models of the past, the hospital is today expected to be more than the haven or *hospitia* for the wayfarers climbing over the snow-covered passes of life. In addition, it is expected to send out the human equivalent of the St. Bernard dogs, to seek actively those who may be in need. The president of the University of Minnesota has coined the word "communiversity" to express this sense of social responsibility in terms of the university.

Assuming hospital efficiency will be increased, how will the "saving" from increased efficiency be used? To reduce taxes, unlikely. To increase medical care benefits, perhaps. To increase social model benefits, more likely.

What are these social model benefits?

FULFILLING SOCIAL DEMANDS

Basically, these benefits are intended to give substance to the accepted principle that health care is a right rather than a privilege.

We recognize this principle is more fiction than truth for perhaps 40 million Americans. We recognize, further, that those deprived of health services have advocates chanting, "we shall overcome."

The problems identified with our present health care non-system, which apply in varying degrees to all people presently served by our general hospitals, are familiar. They include:

1. Absence of program appropriateness, availability, accessibility, acceptability.
2. Absence of comprehensive care, of continuity of care.

From a social viewpoint, patient advocates state these deficits are intolerable, that they can be rectified if there is a will to do so, that they can be rectified without penalty if improvements in efficiency are made.

Patient advocates say, further, that the human costs gaps in health care services should be closed regardless of gains in efficiencies, despite the possible penalties of requiring a higher allocation of our gross national product, or of diminishing the quality of health care to our middle class society.

Patient advocates further assert that the general hospital has special capability to perform well the added health care missions of a social model, such as programs of "preventicare" and ghetto care. These characteristics and abilities include the needed philosophy of care, and the nucleus of the key health professionals needed to plan and execute such programs. It is natural that society, recognizing these strengths, and recognizing a heritage of a job well done, is asking hospitals to assume expanded missions of service to the community.

A second full-time job lies in fulfilling these social demands: To expand, relocate, and modify the manner of performance of general hospital missions.

OTHER SOCIAL MISSIONS

There are still other social missions which hospitals are asked to undertake in serving the community. They should be assumed, if the hospital as a social institution is going to advance the society of which it is a part as fully as possible. Lists of these needs are readily available from numerous sources. However, the Commission on Civil Disorders provides a convenient catalogue. Such pressing needs as eliminating unemployment and underemployment, improving inadequate education, and reducing disrespectful white attitudes are examples of monumental problems which general hospitals genuinely interested in serving their communities can help resolve. The difficult social demands in these areas require not so much in the way of finances, knowledge, or skills, as in attitudes.

CONCERN FOR HUMAN VALUES

Hospitals are being asked to provide their services in a human as well as humane fashion. While there are some penalties attendant in developing programs in response to social needs of this type—as against only those which reflect the health needs of our medical model, the cost/benefit ratio is probably highly favorable.

Society needs individuals with a concern for human values, and for social health, which lie beyond a concern for individual personal health. It is to be hoped, at least, that the humanitarian-oriented health field will prove a repository for human beings interested in the human being. This is particularly requisite when this end requires primarily a change of attitude. This can be considered a third major job of hospitals today.

It would seem that a possible responsibility of the hospital is to serve as a hub of the health care wheel, and in addition, to form part of the axle joining the health care wheel to the social welfare wheel. Indeed we have come a long way from our mission of service to the community solely as a medical care spoke of the health care wheel.

Some hospitals are accepting these responsibilities today; others very likely will tomorrow. Many, if not most, however, without questioning the statements of unmet need, may well challenge the assumption that hospitals should meet them.

This position questions the timing and asks for a social cost/benefit study of alternatives. It recognizes the spirit of compehensive health planning which pervades our land today asks, and even insists, that we examine alternatives in our planning process.

HEALTH CARE AS A RIGHT

Such study is needed. As one example, the costs of providing health care as a right to all, as some are privileged to know it today, is estimated as ranging on a gross basis as from $125 to $250 per person, for from 40 million to 200 million persons. Clearly, definitive study is needed of the economic consequences of implementing quickly and fully our stated natural health policy that health care is a right to all, rather than a privilege for the middle class of today. We should challenge the proclivity of some to promise benefits without resources to make them viable, except to ask those who have enjoyed benefits in the past to share them on the level of a greater common denominator. We should point out the problems of the "expectation gap" which are created by promises unfulfilled.

Clearly, the implications for health manpower requirements also need definition. The potential costs—or penalties, depending on our viewpoint—are also potentially large. Within this context, general hospitals can legitimately challenge the demands by public advocates by asking them to demonstrate the effective demand for health services from a large portion of the poor. For example, a stated need for improved health care service is conspicuously absent from the *Report of the National Commission on Civil Disorders,* which lists the twelve social problems identified as most important by the black community.

Further, it appears reasonable to challenge whether expenditure of funds to encourage effective demand for personal health services would provide the highest cost/benefit payoff. Environmental health expenditures, for example, might well have a higher payoff, socially and politically, as well as from a health viewpoint. So while allocation of savings from efficiencies to social model health programs is likely, the timing, appropriateness, and degree can be legitimately questioned.

We are entering an era when these now unanswered questions of cost/benefit relationships for personal health care services are of even greater importance. This is an era where personal health care services, or elements of such service, are increasingly going to be considered a responsibility rather than a right. A compelling case can be made for this principle. A proposal has been made that this principle be reflected in the health program in Minnesota's "Experimental City" by calling for compulsory annual multiphasic screening examinations. This requirement may well increase the consumers' effective demand upon providers of care to add or expand services, or both.

SYNTHESIS

The demand upon the providers of care from the social model for increased quantity of care could be the straw that bends the quality care back of the medical model camel. Public advocates of the social model may prove stronger than the champions of the medical model. Selected health care providers should provide leadership, in a response to conflicting demands, by demonstration and research.

The general hospital is the health care cutting edge on the interface between social science and evolving technology. Society can expect hospitals to be vitally concerned with the development and use of the knowledge, one of the most fundamental of social commodities. It is only through the heuristic application of new knowledge that it gains ultimate social significance.

Selected general hospital leadership needs to demonstrate the equality of right to health care by finding ways to make it viable, while recognizing the penalties of broadly promulgating one alternative before planning others and examining them comprehensively. We do need, and should encourage and support, social model demonstrations such as may be found in Roxbury and Columbia Point in Boston, in the Grovenure program in New York City, in the Watts area of Los Angeles, and others. This is not the same, however, as asking all hospitals, as they are presently constituted, to do likewise.

The current focus of attention on the appropriate future mission of the general hospital is basically a matter of social organization. Demonstration and research into different organization models for the delivery of health care therefore is particularly pertinent. This approach offers hope for the development of an organizational base to mount programs which synthesize the conflicting demands of our medical and social health care models.

It is not a question of the appropriateness of goals and objectives—what the consumers or their advocates want, they will, like Lola, get. Consumer power as expressed through the political system does and will prevail. The question is the degree to which existing social organizations such as the general hospital will provide the means to the ends—to the evolving social objectives. It is a social organization question which asks:

1. whether existing organizations, like the general hospital, will assume new program responsibilities, or whether new social organizations should be established which will be both more willing and able to do so.
2. whether new organizations should be established to manage the health care system—removing and centralizing some decision-making authority now held by the service organizations, i.e., hospitals.
3. whether new organizations should be established to perform existing programs to meet newly emphasized performance standards better than do existing organizations.

Hospitals, as we have seen, have a reasonable and perhaps even legitimate option of rejecting the social model to better serve the heavy demands of the medical model. Doing so efficiently releases resources to support other organizations endeavoring to meet the social model performance criteria for health care programs.

The general hospital has a further option within this context. It can choose to utilize programs developed by other community health care organizations, e.g., long term care, public health, Office of Economic Opportunity, model city organizations, rather than to plan and execute such programs within the general hospital organizational framework.

THE HOSPITAL'S OPTION

If general hospitals individually or collectively provide leadership in the planning and organizing of health services, if not in the actual performance of them, they can in this organizational sense become the community health center which is the self-established model widely held by hospitals today. Whether other health service organizations would grant such authority to hospitals is of course a question.

Should general hospitals select these options, they should recognize they are accepting a mission as a medical care spoke, rather than the hub of the health care wheel. Other organizations will be needed to serve as other spokes of our health care wheel, and may have hub organizational responsibilities as well. Government has filled service, coordinative and directive needs of society in the past, when not provided by the private sector, and is one viable alternative for doing so again.

Hospitals should have no complaints if society forms other organizations to perform additional missions which hospitals elect to forego. Conversely, society should not be critical of hospitals for electing to be the public advocates of quality performance of certain health functions that have and will need considerable support if they are to continue to be provided on a quality basis.

Hospitals have still another option: To form vertically integrated "health utilities" in which they could perform their specialized function. Other organizational sub-units of the health utility could plan and execute the health missions demanded and needed by our social model. These missions possibly could include responsibility for selected environmental health or welfare programs. The utilities could well be responsible for developing or assembling associated prepayment programs.

This organizational alternative to planning and executing expanding health missions is to be preferred, in the author's judgment. It provides the scale to accomplish both medical and social missions, permits the advantages of specialization while reducing the organizational fragmentation of our health care non-system, and lowers the need for centralization of program planning and execution under governmental auspices.

These organizations could form the needed bridge between programs for the middle class and the urban and rural poor; permit a "fresh start" towards the changes needed for efficiency; and ease the pressure on the hospital to reduce quality in order to reduce high unit cost.

The health utility would provide an organizational symbol for the change of role of the central personal health care delivery organization. It could assist the assembly of managerial talent and staff resources needed for improvement in both efficiency and effectiveness. It would permit the continuance of specialized functional interest and expertise in humanly compatible organizational sub-units.

"CORNER GROCERY STORE" ORIENTATION

The health utility with associated franchisement implies increased formal community responsibility and accountability, allocation of tax resources now reserved to governmental agencies, and centralization from a local perspective (but potential decentralization from regional and state governmental perspectives, and quasi-independence from their bureaucracies).

This organizational "tool up" may well be an essential foundation for the service and educational missions now being effectively demanded.

It is difficult to be sanguine that this organizational alternative will be adopted, except perhaps in such places as Minnesota's Experimental City, where it has been proposed. The existing hospital field still exhibits much of the "corner grocery store" orientation, in a chain store age. However, there are some hopeful signs. On this basis, as well as need, this alternative then is reasonable when endeavoring to define the general hospitals' future mission in service to the community.

FOCAL POINT FOR SOCIAL CONTROL

Regardless of the scope of the future mission, or the organizational context within which hospitals will operate, they will be a focal point for social control. The control will be concerned with both costs (efficiency) and benefits (effectiveness). The hospital's future missions will reflect judgments on costs and benefits, which in turn will reflect the criteria or standards used in making such judgments. The conclusions may well be expressed in franchisement of services. If hospital leadership wishes to have some control over the destiny of hospitals, for the quality and scope of hospital future missions, they need to be experts in the appropriateness of such standards.

This again will require a willingness to engage in collective effort. This could well be one of the most central and crucial missions of the general hospital in service to the community.

CONCLUSION

Society is demanding that further health missions be performed. Hospitals can legitimately consider their acceptance as alternatives, or their rejection so as to serve with excellence the continuing missions of the medical model. A preferred alternative is to develop health utilities. Such organizations could meet social needs for an expanded scope of service, while preserving the capability to perform on a quality, in-depth basis, the medical care functions which will need this concern in the future, as in the past.

Changes in the way existing health missions are performed, so as to increase efficiencies, can be anticipated. Allocation of the benefits of increased efficiency to expanded health/social missions can be expected. Both existing and expanded missions need to be performed with the social needs of minority groups in mind. Demonstration and research projects by selected general hospitals should show the way by synthesizing a response to the medical and social models. Translating the findings into standards of performance, for guidance of public expectations and decisions, is a basic mission.

Assiduous definition by public advocates of gaps in the meeting of health care needs should join with sedulous recognition of the "tooling up" effort needed to overcome these needs. The absence of qualified professional manpower is but one example of a long term obstacle even if organizational and financial problems can be overcome. Economic and social cures should be promised and delivered as carefully as medical cures. Full participation by the leadership of the hospital field can be vital to this end.

It is an endeavor worthy of the devotion of the talents and energies of the management of our nation's hospitals. Commitment of this capability with vision, imagination, drive, and resourcefulness will provide the managerial leadership demanded and needed by our times.

Planning and Programs

Three selections are included which cover the spectrum of forces and influences of hospitals. Selection 35, "EFFECTIVE PLANNING COMMITTEES FOR HOSPITALS" by James B. Webber and Martha A. Dula, describes the internal planning activities which hospitals are being encouraged and required to take. Tables showing changes in basic concepts of hospital planning and the reasons for the changes are presented. Models for effective committee environmental analysis and planning as well as implementation are proposed. Selection 36, "PROSPECTIVE RATE SETTING: CONCEPT AND PRACTICE" by William L. Dowling, discusses the issues surrounding a new payment scheme which proposes a means of cost control by providing incentives for cost containment. This mechanism is currently used by a number of third-party payors and is being investigated by others. Such measures are additional steps in moving control outside hospitals. The impact of professional standards review organizations (PSROs) is discussed by Kurt Darr in Selection 37, "INSTITUTIONAL PROVIDERS AND THE PROFESSIONAL STANDARDS REVIEW ORGANIZATION." This federally initiated and financed program is primarily directed at cost control and secondarily at quality of care; hospitals are being forced to do what it is argued they should have been doing before this federal government initiative. Clearly, it carries the hospital's loss of independence a substantial step further.

35.
Effective Planning Committees for Hospitals

JAMES B. WEBBER AND MARTHA A. DULA

James B. Webber, M.B.A., is a management consultant specializing in health planning.

Martha A. Dula, M.A., is a management consultant with the Cambridge Research Institute, Cambridge, Massachusetts.

Reviewing the progress of a three-hour long-range planning committee meeting, the haggard chief surgeon lamented, "It takes too long." The representative of the trustees, a prominent businessman who had rushed from his office at 4:30 p.m. to sit through the meeting, agreed, "There must be a better way." And the director of the hospital unhappily reminded both men, "But we're required to have a long-range planning committee, and we're required to have monthly meetings."

Partly for statutory reasons, the long-range planning committee exists in most hospitals today—perhaps in as many as 77 percent.[1] But the majority seem to be singularly ineffective bodies: they make no decisions, they solve no problems, and they do not seem to get anything done.

Still, pressure on hospitals to form long-range planning committees (hereafter, called simply "Committees" or "the Committee") continues to come from various sources. In their 1970 announcement of standards, for example, the Joint Commission on Accreditation of Hospitals stipulated that the governing boards of all hospitals seeking accreditation must show evidence of long-range planning. They further recommended that the hospital appoint a separate planning body or a Committee to develop a plan for the hospital.

The formation of such a Committee for a hospital has been seconded in recent years by hospital insurers, hospital associations and state planning agencies, and state laws. Massachusetts, for example, is developing new rules and regulations for licensure that may include mandatory Committees; such regulations may be unnecessary, however, since most hospitals already have such Committees or are in the process of forming them.

The Committee has been defined as a hospital's "primary source of direction concerning the future allocation of resources, including money, manpower, facilities and

---

Reprinted by permission from the *Harvard Business Review*, (May-June, 1974, pp. 133-142). Copyright 1974 by the President and Fellows of Harvard College; all rights reserved.

services."[2] But its actual functioning varies from hospital to hospital. Some have actually used the Committees for strategic planning—others, as forums for identifying problems. There is, in fact, considerable disagreement about the role the Committee should play in decision-making, goal-setting, implementation, and so on.

This disagreement reflects the intricate, changing nature of the hospital and its planning needs. To clarify some of the issues of this debate, let us look at Hospital A's Committee as it was five years earlier and again in the fall of 1973.

Shortly after its creation in January 1968, this Committee surveyed the hospital's needs and reported a list of priorities to the executive committee, implicitly assuming a relatively static outside environment and community. The first two priorities were construction of adequate facilities for the nursing school and replacement of the older hospital buildings. Parking was also listed as a high priority item. Together, these formed the agenda for stage 1 of the hospital's modernization program. An architect was hired to develop a master plan to meet these priorities, and by March 1969, the nursing school had been completed, at a cost of $350,000. The total plan required an expenditure of $7,500,000.

By 1972, Hospital A's nonconforming facilities were beginning to threaten its accreditation, wards were overcrowded, and parking problems severe. The Committee was reconvened to implement stage 2 of the architect's master plan: renovation of the nonconforming facilities and construction of a satellite facility in an adjoining town which the hospital had historically served, to relieve the pressure on the main plant.

In the meantime, the state hospital association had sponsored a "certificate of need" bill, signed into law July 18, 1972, which required approval by the Department of Public Health for any hospital construction project in the state costing over $100,000. Shortly after this legislation was passed, another hospital—a nationally known institution—was granted a certificate of need to relocate its entire facility within the area served by Hospital A. And Hospital A's preliminary feasibility study had proved that it could only expect to raise $5 million for its second-stage development activities under the then-current Phase III economic controls and the newly announced Phase IV controls.

Thus, Hospital A was left in a terrible quandary: The public as a whole was demanding high-quality health care as a basic right of all people. Pressure was being applied to politicians to improve its availability; in response the politicians were setting up more stringent regulations, and agencies to administer these regulations. And even as the regulative nooses were tightening, this hospital found itself facing strong, new competition—at a time when it could not possibly fund even its own renovation.

The planning its Committee had done in 1968 was no longer adequate or viable; but it was only during the past year, when its members were forced to face their total predicament and search for workable, long-range options, that they began to understand the complexities of today's hospital planning and the shortcomings of their Committee's prior efforts.

There is nothing unusual or atypical in this story—indeed, it merely points out the besetting problem of the health care system today. Hospitals need far more than the kind of facilities planning that sufficed until a few years ago; the Committee that contents itself with functioning as a traditional building committee is inevitably shortchanging the hospital in its grave need for broad-scope planning.

EMERGENCE OF THE GROUND RULES

Exhibit 1 diagrams the ways in which the assumptions and premises of long-range planning for hospitals have changed over the past five years.

As the exhibit shows, long-range planning was a nebulous and ill-formed concept for hospitals five years ago—they really did not have a clear idea of what a Committee could or should do for them, and hence did not know what function to assign it. Everyone seemed to agree that long-range planning was good, and that a Committee was a good means of promoting involvement and participation in hospital planning, but no one seemed to know how to plan for the long range or how to involve people in the planning process.

The Committees themselves certainly did not know what they were supposed to be doing or how to function. They had no sense of structure or purpose. As a result, some were caught up in a goal-setting syndrome; the Committee at Hospital A, for example, functioned in the beginning as a goal-setting body by reporting a list of facilities priorities to the executive committee after surveying the hospital's needs.

This Committee's meetings tended to be brainstorming sessions—endless discussions of ideas and definitions without any systematic past, present, or future data. Searching self-examinations on the validity of the hospital's real needs and goals were almost nonexistent; realistic considerations of the needs of the outside community were totally nonexistent. Since the Committee's members usually felt no real sense of identity with nearby hospitals or other health centers, they did not make any attempts to coordinate their overall planning with these other institutions.

In Committees of this kind, members become frustrated because the process takes so long and because they have nothing tangible to show for their efforts. Attendance drops off. The hospital loses confidence in the Committee's ability to deal with the problems of planning. Environmental trends pass by unnoticed, and activities and forces that are inexorably changing the nature of the institution grind on unperceived. And often the very creation of the Committee has destroyed what momentum the hospital has developed, by postponing debate on new proposals for services until after the Committee has gone through the exercise of setting the hospital's goals.

ENVIRONMENTAL ANALYSIS AND PLANNING

A Committee can function effectively if it can lift itself out of the goal-setting syndrome and if it defines its role clearly and realistically in terms of the new and dynamic relationships that are developing between the hospital and its environment.

Exhibit I
The Evolution of Concepts for Long-Range Hospital Planning

	Basic concepts of the hospital five years ago	Basic concepts today	Reason for the change
Environmental	An institution comfortable in its established role	An institution whose role is increasingly challenged	External forces are changing the premise for survival in the future
	Provider of acute care	Center for comprehensive care integrated within a much larger health system	Hospitals are the focus of the demand for comprehensive care
	A self-determinate institution independent of its environment	An institution intimately linked with and dependent on its environment	Environmental forces—regulations, politics, economics, technology, and social expectations—have evolved rapidly
	Growth is the name of the game, in a rapidly growing market for hospital beds	Survival is the name of the game, in a mature market for hospital beds	The bedding surge created by the advent of Medicaid and Medicare is over, and overbedding is inducing regulative restrictions
	An institution that had no competition	An institution struggling to maintain patient referrals and service offerings under competitive restraints	The rapid growth of the 1960s has been restrained by regulatory emphasis on regionalization, consolidation, and zero growth
	All costs fully reimbursable	Cost containment	Growing public concern over spiralling health-care costs has been expressed in measures such as (a) prospective budgeting under third-party contracts and (b) narrowing definition of allowable costs under Medicaid

366

Institutional

Slavish adherence to architect's master plans, many of which were outdated	Long-range plans developed in a systematic way, as the basis for architect's master plans	Systematic thought and analysis must now precede plans for facilities development
Concentration on facilities as the key area to be planned	Planning that includes services to be offered, patient groups to be served, and interinstitutional relationships to be developed	Regulators demand to know how any one proposal for a new service or facility fits into an overall scheme
One-shot, episodic planning activities	Continuous planning activities	The pace of change demands adaptation and a continuing learning capability
Planning inputs gathered from the power centers of the hospital	The source of planning inputs expanded to include consumer, regulatory, and community bodies	Outsiders are effectively demanding a role in the planning effort
Closed, secretive planning and decision making, internally oriented	Open discussion, cards-on-the-table planning and decision making, externally oriented	The best brainpower of all concerned is needed to arrive at plans suited to the demands of the environment
Reactive planning, where the hospital waited for problems to arise	Proactive planning, where the hospital anticipates problems and seeks opportunities	The need to compete for scarce resources and referral bases has become crucial to survival

Environmental analysis and planning provides a clearcut framework for the Committee to define its role within the institution and for it to outline appropriate and specific tasks for itself within that role.

Exhibit II shows how a Committee can use the steps of environmental analysis and planning to perform its function. The Committee should first collect information about institutional relationships, fiscal policy, and so on from the trustees; information about management policy, economic feasibility, and reimbursement policy from the hospital administration; information about medical trends from the staff; and information about community needs from the community. Then it can subject this information to the four kinds of analyses required by the discipline of formal environmental analysis and planning—external, internal, issue, and alternative analyses—drawing on the people who supply the information in the first place and the people who will be affected by its recommendations. This kind of activity produces better bases for decision-making, helps ensure the acceptance of the decisions, and drums up general support for implementing change.

External Analysis

As we have implied, environmental analysis and planning is an outside-in approach. This process requires that the Committee begins by analyzing the needs of the external world, rather than begin with the internal goals of the hospital. This approach challenges the hospital's traditional modus operandi: up until now hospitals have not acted with, but rather reacted to, forces in the external world.

Characteristically, they have fought regulators on ideological grounds and, as private institutions, have been resentful of any intrusion on their total autonomy. It is true that the interests of official advisory and regulatory forces are quite often at odds with those of the hospital. To that extent, hospital planning today is a political process, and any Committee must be prepared for that fact.

One hospital that wanted to build a doctors' office building was not permitted to do so, partly because such organizations as the Association of Retired Persons raised objections which the hospital was not prepared to counter. The hospital had begun with a goal statement, "We need this building because it will facilitate health care and attract young doctors." However, the plan was sharply criticized because the location of the proposed building was highly inaccessible to elderly people and because the hospital had not explored alternatives to this particular use of its land. And, in fact, this hospital had not recognized that it would find itself desperate for land for further expansion in another five to ten years.

In the face of these forces, hospitals and their Committees are becoming understandably paranoid and reactionary. But if the Committees begin focusing on the basics of the problems involved and on the pressures impinging on the regulators (such as the consumer outrage over the high cost of health care), and stop focusing on the mere symptoms of these pressures (such as cost-containment measures established by the regulators), then they can anticipate the regulators and perhaps even help fashion appropriate responses to these pressures for change.

Exhibit II

How the Committee Can Use Environmental Analysis and Planning

Drawing data from the groups concerned,	in the areas of special relevance,	the committee works to perform	analyses and first-cut planning	to provide guidelines on specific topics	for the groups concerned
Trustees	Institutional relationships	Gathers input and performs analyses	External analysis	Recommendations for decision making and goal setting	Trustees
	Fiscal policy	Plans and implements decisions	Internal analysis	Education	
	Community needs		Issue analysis		
Administration	Management policy		Alternative analysis	Education	Administration
	Economic feasibility		Implementation and planning	Start of implementation	
	Reimbursement policy				
Medical staff	Medical practice			Support for change	Medical staff
	Technology			Education	
	Referral relationships			Economic realities	
Community representatives	Community wants			Education	Community representatives
	Community needs			Feasibility of responding to needs and wants	

Hence a Committee should establish environmental scanning as a part of its administrative function. The findings, particularly as they affect the future role of the institution, should be widely publicized. By drawing out the implications of trends and forces in the external world, the members develop an objective base on which the medical, trustee, and administrative groups in the hospital can discover and pursue their mutual interests in maintaining and enhancing their institution.

One Committee delegated the scanning task to a three-man subcommittee. The administrator on this subcommittee monitored and collected information from hospital journals, the state hospital association, and the regional planning authorities. The doctor reported on trends detailed in medical journals and discussed in medical society meetings. The trustee, a businessman with contacts throughout the city, tracked the plans of other institutions and watched trends in funding. After four months the information collected was summarized in a binder of memos and clippings. This constituted an impressive and useful first stab at external analysis.

Internal Analysis

Once it fully understands the forces at work in the external environment, the Committee is a natural vehicle for conducting internal analyses of the hospital. First, it can examine services and facilities in terms of the unmet needs of the community and realistically evaluate demands and pressures for better utilization and cost containment. It can then arbitrate among the various interest groups and factions within the hospital, identifying the real problems and making informal recommendations among alternatives.

Second, it should build a systematic data base that describes the institution as it stands at present, the ways in which it has arrived at its present condition, and its likely future condition if it continues as it has in the past. Some existing information and formats will be useful for this purpose; other data might be gathered by open-ended questioning processes, written or verbal. (These processes can also help to inform personnel about what kinds of actions they can realistically expect from their committee, and induce a feeling that planning is an open field in which all data and proposals are welcomed.)

One Committee compiled a statistical handbook for its internal analyses. This handbook, accumulating data from the preceding 20 years, was put together by an administrative intern on a six-month project basis. Individual sections covered trends in patient origins and characteristics by services used, facilities and space utilization, distribution of ages and specialties of the medical staff, changes in length of patient stay over time, income and expenses, and reimbursement.

Issue Analysis

In short, a Committee today must take an objective look at the outside world to determine what changes have occurred and are occurring that will affect the hospital as an organization. Then it must determine where the hospital is, how it got there, and where it wants to go. Through this external/internal analysis, the Committee will identify particular issues that the hospital must address.

Many hospitals, for example, are now facing the "bed issue." They must decide, given the over-bedding in some areas, whether it is desirable or feasible for them to increase their own number of beds. For example, one metropolitan area now has too many beds. The regulators, therefore, are turning down applications for certificates of need to hospitals requesting permission to add more beds. The Committee of a town-owned, community hospital on the outskirts of the central city, however, knows that the population of the community served by the hospital is growing dramatically and that this growth will demand more hospital beds. The hospital has the shell space for more beds. The issue clearly facing this Committee and the trustees is this: "Given the regulatory trend, how can we serve our town?"

Maternity services are also becoming an issue for hospitals.

On the external side, in many communities declining birthrates and increasing life spans have caused a decrease of 70 percent or more in the utilization of maternity beds. Since these beds cannot be used for other patients, the low utilization rates of this service detract considerably from the hospital's overall utilization rates, a circumstance that the regulatory forces are pressuring the hospitals to correct. Still, the community often becomes angry at any hint that a maternity service will be discontinued.

On the internal side, staff obstetricians are not overjoyed at the prospect of the service being discontinued. However, administrators must now think in terms of cost containment, and how low utilization rates affect revenue.

Another issue which is certainly being debated now is consolidation: Should hospitals merge in order to provide services more efficiently? Regulators are supporting and trying to effect consolidation of underutilized services and facilities, to serve public health-care needs better and more economically. So far, they can only induce consolidation through the back door, by denying certificates of need and encouraging hospitals to negotiate with one another. But hospitals are accustomed to their traditional character as autonomous institutions. Committees can serve their hospitals quite well by researching the issue of consolidation and making recommendations to the trustees, *before* the regulators take the initiative.

Obviously, many issues will emerge in the Committee, some of which will be resolved and others not, whether because of time or other constraints. In fact, so many issues will emerge from the interaction of external and internal needs that the Committee will have to be selective. Basically, members should choose the issues that will help define and determine the basic nature and direction of the hospital—the elements, in other words, that most affect and contribute to the long-range plan.

The secretary of one Committee has developed a means of keeping track of issues and alternatives as the work of the group has progressed. She has kept a running log on each issue that has emerged and on each alternative solution that has been presented. After six months, the Committee has not only a compendium of the issues and alternatives facing the hospital, but also some visible evidence of its own progress. Additionally, it is learning how to select suitable issues for further investigation.

Alternative Analysis

Developing solutions to the various issues builds the fabric of basic alternatives available to the hospital to be debated by the Committee. After the steps of external analysis, internal analysis, and issue analysis, the Committee is ready to deal with the big questions that relate to the hospital's long-range future. Some hospitals may have to decide whether they should become community hospitals offering more general services, or become more specialized or specialty-referral hospitals. The issue of merger or consolidation may be a major alternative for some. And since alternatives are courses of direction, "continuing as is" is a legitimate alternative that all hospitals must seriously consider.

For example, a major metropolitan hospital had to consider all these alternatives. The city was demanding that the hospital become more community-oriented. The expected relocation of a major clinic to another area threatened to disrupt the hospital's referral base. The environmental analysis and planning process outlined the pros and cons of each of the alternatives; after due deliberation the Committee concluded that the hospital should become more of a specialty-referral institution, and so the trustees set in motion a series of plans to carry it in this direction.

IMPLEMENTATION AND PLANNING

Exhibit II outlines some of the appropriate outcomes of a Committee's deliberations. Note the position of "Recommendations for decision-making and goal setting." Environmental analysis and planning forces both these activities into their proper place—*after* the basic institutional alternatives that have emerged from the process have been evaluated. In other words, after the Committee has recommended the best alternatives available, and after the hospital has decided among them, the hospital is then ready to set goals within a long-range plan.

Another very appropriate task for a Committee to undertake is education. It can do great service to the hospital by first bringing all its own members up-to-date and then by transferring this knowledge and understanding to the members of the hospital at large. The essential task here is to communicate (1) an integrated perception of the outside world, (2) a sense of competence in dealing with the issues, and (3) the urgency of resolving the issues to get action. It may be that in its first year the Committee will spend most of its time just getting the external-analysis subcommittee working smoothly on particular projects.

Education is one area where a Committee may find itself bearing too heavy a burden. One Committee we know has become so sophisticated in planning that it now finds itself two years ahead of the rest of the organization—it has literally outdistanced the hospital. This is something of a hazard, particularly in a large hospital. This Committee will now have to extend its task as educator greatly.

A Committee may also be able to serve as a support system for change. Any change is a wrench, particularly if the changes are of a deep and profound nature, as in health care. These changes are causing a terrible dislocation. Although some Committees find governing bodies resistant to change, more find that the major source of resistance is the medical staff, many of whom are independent professionals and still behave as if the hospital were their workshop. They fail to recognize that the hospital itself is a medical practitioner.

Getting a Committee Started

A Committee will work as an effective planning vehicle only if its role is tailored to the hospital's particular planning needs. The Committee of any given hospital is usually performing several tasks at any given time, and the assortment will change as the hospital's planning evolves and advances toward objectives. It should be aware of its current tasks and of how it wants or expects its activities to evolve over the next few years.

Exhibit III traces the evolution of one Committee's activities in a medium-sized hospital from start-up to a point two years later. Initially a great deal of attention was given to external analysis; this emphasis was gradually displaced by an effort to understand the hospital itself in a systematic way; issues emerged and were dealt with by defining alternatives; and, finally, the Committee shifted its emphasis to implementing the alternative course of action chosen for the hospital.

One of the most crucial factors in establishing an effective Committee is appointing the right members. They should, first of all, be selected in terms of the role the Committee is expected to perform within the hospital. If it is expected to function as a real planning body, it needs planning expertise; if it is expected to affect decision-making, it will have to be composed, at least in part, of decision-makers; and so on. This implies, accurately, that key people in the hospital must be appointed to the Committee. The Committee of one rather complex urban hospital is composed of several key trustees, including the president of the board, the administrator of the hospital, the chiefs of service, and so on.

So far as doctors on the Committee are concerned, the most progressive ones are very often the older ones. Young doctors are involved with developing a practice; middle-aged doctors are often preoccupied with their practices and thus feel threatened by changes. But older doctors with established practices can afford to be statesmanlike. Mistakenly, some hospitals do not want older doctors on their Committees because they feel that by the time the future is here, the older doctors will not be, and hence it is irresponsible to appoint them to the Committee. Such thinking eliminates a lot of useful experience, wisdom, and interest from the planning process.

On the external side, Committees are being required more and more frequently to

Exhibit III
Evolution of Committee Activities Over Time

Activity	Example of topics to be considered	Relative time spent at sequential stages (in percent)			
		Start-up	+6 months	+1 year	+2 years
External analysis	National trends	50	30	20	20
	Changes in the demography of referral base				
	Outlook for regulation				
	Competition				
Internal analysis	Patient origin	30	40	10	10
	Changes in medical staff specialties				
	Projected space needs				
	Relationships with medical schools				
Issue analysis	Services to be offered in the future	20	30	30	10
	The hospital's role in comprehensive health care				
Alternative analysis	Continue as is	0	0	30	10
	Become more specialized				
	Become less specialized				
	Develop a health maintenance orjganization				
Implementation and planning	The hospital's ability to accept change	0	0	10	50
	The steps necessary to carry out the direction chosen				

accept members from the community, even though they have been slow to do so. It is important to do this early; if it is difficult to educate the hospital, think how much more difficult it is to educate Committee members from the outside community, and the community itself. Here again, the Committee's effectiveness can be improved if it acts to deal with forces, rather than reacts to regulations.

True, it is hard to find appropriate community representatives. One suburban hospital resolved this problem by listing possible classes of community representatives: abutters, consumer advocate leaders, patients, nonpatients, local government personnel, trustees and corporation members, and Comprehensive Health Planning Agency staff members. In making the final selection, the chief administrator used as criteria what he felt were the three key issues facing the hospital. He chose abutters, because new buildings would probably have to be built; he chose a consumer advocate for the elderly, since the town population was growing older; and he chose two corporate executives who were active in the community.

But the Committee cannot be too large if it is to do real planning—probably no larger than 12 members. There are too many sensitive issues to discuss, such as medical-financial relationships, for a larger Committee to be effective. However, it can involve more people in the planning process through subcommittees and the use of such tactical devices as spot surveys to assemble information and trace attitude changes. It can also assign issue analysis to subcommittees for recommended solutions. By including non-Committee members as participants in the subcommittees and by rotating the memberships, the depth and validity of its overall work can be increased.

For example, if members are switched between the building committee and the Committee, these committee members begin to see the connection between planning on the one hand, and facility development and maintenance on the other. This is beneficial because the capital budgeting process is one of the last things ever to come under control of the planning process in any organization; this is especially true in hospitals. Hospitals are accustomed to facilities planning—they are geared for it, they have people experienced in it, and they have architects and contractors. They are expert at building buildings. But they have often been building the wrong things because they could not see the connection between planning and plant. Membership rotation can heal this situation. Obviously rotation has other educational effects as well.

A Committee's effectiveness can also be improved by upgrading the quality of its meetings. It should be given super staff support—by enthusiastic members of the administration who can help think out agenda and presentations. Meetings can be sparked with guest appearances. The frequency of the meetings can be varied—for example, when the Committee has an exciting task, the number of meetings can be increased. After a major accomplishment, the members can be rewarded with some "time off." Occasionally a fun meeting can be planned around a learning event or even a dramatic event. Off-site seminars can be arranged for specific updating and educational activities. Meetings can be held in the morning, when people are fresh. And, since many Committees have found that the most important action occurs between, not at, meetings, one-to-one interchanges can be stimulated, both to build bridges and to effect compromises.

To accomplish all its tasks, the Committee must have some emotional support itself. To give members a sense of pace and accomplishment, spot surveys on progress should be administered every few meetings. Members will be surprised, gratified, and encouraged by their progress. When issues are resolved, the results should be put in writing. Then the Committee can say, for example, "Here is our position paper on community service," and the members will not have to deal with the same problem next year.

Perspective on Operations

The environmental analysis and planning process will provide the type of long-range planning that regulators are demanding. The hospital itself will benefit from the process because its trustees will be able to take rational initiatives in planning, rather than make fragmented decisions in reaction to increasing regulation.

Further, if it goes through the steps of environmental analysis and planning, the Committee will be the most knowledgeable body in the hospital, and it will be able to transfer this knowledge to the rest of the hospital and perhaps the outside community as well. If it has included representatives from all parties—the administration, the medical staff, and the outside community—and if it has collected information from all the groups who will be affected by its results, a certain degree of education will occur naturally, and an air of openness, which is demanded in hospital planning today, will be developed. And the path will be smoothed for change.

Finally, the members themselves will feel less frustrated because they will have a sense of direction; they will not get caught up in unfocused, time-consuming discussions and exercises, and will be more likely to produce results. The hospital's planning as a whole will then become more effective because the institution will not be looking to the Committee to set goals prematurely, or to perform other unrealistic tasks.

Author's note: The authors wish to acknowledge their debt to John D. Glover, Lovett - Learned Professor of Business Administration at the Harvard Business School, for his work on environmental analysis and planning.

FOOTNOTES

[1] Martin S. Perlin, "Current Practices in Long-Range Planning," *Hospitals,* September 1, 1972, p. 62.
[2] Health Planning Council for Greater Boston, *A Guide to Comprehensive Health Planning for Hospitals* (Boston, 1971), p. 6.

36.

Prospective Rate Setting: Concept and Practice

WILLIAM L. DOWLING

William L. Dowling, Ph.D., is Associate Professor and Director - Graduate Program in Health Services Administration and Planning - School of Public Health and Community Medicine - the University of Washington.

WHAT IS PROSPECTIVE RATE SETTING?

Prospective rate setting is a cost containment strategy wherein an external authority establishes the prices that providers are allowed to charge and/or that third parties are required to pay for specified services in advance of the period in which the services are actually provided. To the extent that patients and third parties do in fact pay the prospectively set rates, prospective rate setting might more appropriately be called prospective rate payment, or just prospective payment. The key difference between prospective payment (or prospective reimbursement as it is often called) and conventional forms of reimbursement is that providers are not paid the costs they actually incur in providing the services being paid for, nor are they free to unilaterally adjust their charges to cover these costs; rather, providers are paid at rates set in advance of and considered fixed for the pertinent period (typically a year). Although costs are not constrained directly under prospective payment, it is assumed that the constraint on revenue imposed by fixing provider charges and/or third party payment rates in advance of the prospective year will cause providers to contain their costs during that year in order to avoid losses (or earn surpluses).

Prospective rate setting differs from retrospective cost reimbursement in that payment rates are specified in advance rather than determined after the fact and are not based on costs actually incurred during the prospective year. Prospective rate setting differs from institutional rate setting in that an external authority is involved and has the final say regarding rates. Providers are not free to set their rates initially or to change them during the prospective year, without going through some sort of review and approval process. Prospective payment systems are designed to introduce market-

---

Reprinted by permission, from Dowling, W.: "Prospective Rate Setting: Concept and Practice," *Topics in Health Care Financing,* Vol. 3, No. 2, pp. 7-37, 1976. Copyright 1976. All rights reserved.

place-like financial incentives into the provider sector. Providers face firm fixed prices for their services. If they are able to keep their costs below these prices, they will make a surplus; if not, they will suffer a loss. Thus, providers are definitely at risk.

The basic elements of prospective rate setting, then, are simple:

1. An external authority is empowered (by statute, market power, or voluntary compliance by providers) to set provider charges and/or third party payment rates.

2. Rates are set in advance of the prospective year during which they apply and are considered fixed for the year (except for major, uncontrollable, unpredictable occurrences).

3. Patients and/or third parties pay the prospective rates rather than the costs actually incurred by providers during the year (or charges adjusted to cover these costs).

4. Providers are at risk for losses or surpluses.

A particular prospective rate-setting system may only approximate these elements in actual practice. For example, a rate-setting agency or program may see itself as "reviewing and approving" rather than "setting" provider rates; that is, the stringency of the rate-determination process and the range of factors considered can vary greatly. The prospectively set rates may be paid only by self-pay patients, or by Blue Cross, or Medicaid, or all three; that is, the applicability of the rates can vary. The prospectively set rates may be adjusted automatically for specified factors like the actual case mix, inflation, volume, etc., experienced by providers during the prospective year, or adjustments may be made so readily upon provider request at the end of the prospective year that most of the risk associated with advance rate setting is eliminated. Or, what amounts to the same thing, any losses or surpluses providers make may be compensated for or taken away in the following year's rates. Hence, the term "prospective" must be applied with care to any particular rate-setting system, depending on how closely it approaches the "spirit" as well as the "letter" of the concept of prospectivity.

WHY PROSPECTIVE RATE SETTING?

Prospective rate setting evolved in response to the dramatic and persistent rise in hospital costs that began in the mid-1960s. It was then (and continues to be) widely believed that the cost inflation problem can be traced to an absence of cost containment incentives in the prevailing methods of paying hospitals—the payment of costs (determined retrospectively) and the payment of billed charges (set unilaterally by institutions themselves). Prospective rate setting was seen both as a means of exerting more external influence over hospital activities and plans, and as a means of building cost containment constraints and/or incentives into hospital payment. All prospective rate-setting systems claim cost containment as a primary objective. State rate-setting laws, for example, typically assign an agency or commission the job of assuring that hospital rates reflect "the costs of efficient production of services" or "the economy-wide inflation rate," or that they are, simply, "reasonable." The range of cost-influencing factors considered in judging the reasonableness of rates varies greatly, however. Some rate-setting systems focus on per unit costs, emphasizing efficiency or productivity; others look more broadly at aggregate hospital costs, emphasizing efficiency and utilization; others look even more broadly at aggregate system costs, emphasizing efficiency, utilization, and the supply of beds, facilities, and services. In general, rate-setting agencies and programs also recognize the need to preserve the ability of hospitals to provide quality care and to remain financially viable.

In a number of states, hospitals acted through their associations to encourage the development of prospective rate setting systems, hoping that impartial rate-setting authorities would come to agree with them that the cost inflation problem was largely attributable to factors beyond their control. These authorities might help explain this to the public and might even serve as advocates for hospitals with regard to certain of their financial problems. In addition, hospitals hoped that all third parties would be willing to pay rates set by independent rate-setting agencies or programs, thereby ending the imposition by the different third parties of arbitrary cost or rate ceilings, different definitions of allowable costs, and different reimbursement practices. This, in turn, would help hospitals achieve the goal of "equal payment for equal services" and end the practice of shifting costs not reimbursed by third parties to self-pay patients. Both hospitals and third parties believed they would benefit from the financial predictability prospective rate setting makes possible.

MANAGEMENT IMPLICATIONS

Proponents of prospective rate setting believe that the financial incentives inherent in this approach to payment (i.e., the possibility of a loss or surplus) will cause providers[1] to give costs more weight in decision making with regard to current operations and future plans. Prospective rate setting makes it essential for hospitals to budget accurately and effectively justify their anticipated expenditures for the coming year, since prospective rates are generally based in some way on a budget review. Even in rate-setting systems where budgets are not used in rate setting (e.g., those in which a formula is used to project historical costs into prospective rates), budgets are fundamental to rate appeals and end-of-year reviews. In addition to providing a way to demonstrate a hospital's financial requirements, accurate budgeting becomes critical for self protection. If costs increase more than anticipated in a hospital's budget, its prospective rates may not generate sufficient revenue to cover its costs. Hence, prospective rate setting should lead to better budgeting practices.

Demonstrate Need

Prospective rate setting also makes it essential for hospitals to demonstrate the need for any new facilities and services to be added during the prospective year and to forecast accurately the additional costs associated with them, since this is the first step in attempting to assure that prospective rates cover the costs of new services. Detailed capital and program cost studies are commonly required to demonstrate the need for requested rates. However, even in rate-setting systems where rates are not based directly on the costing-out of specific programs and services (e.g., in formula schemes), accurate cost studies are important as a basis for appeals, or (where a hospital fails to obtain approval for what it requests) as a basis for internal decisions regarding planning priorities and trade-offs. For example, management might be forced to ask: "If we can count on only so much revenue given our prospective rates, is it more important to provide service x or service y given the costs and benefits of each?" Under stringent prospective payment systems, program budgeting may advance rapidly to a state where alternative program possibilities can be examined by means of budget models to estimate their cost and revenue implications before implementation decisions are made. Capital and program plans may also come to be used in prospective rate-setting systems as a basis for decisions regarding how much "growth and development" to allow hospitals to enable them to accumulate the capital reserves that would be needed in future years to implement their long-range plans. For these reasons, prospective rate setting should lead to better capital and program planning.

Cost Controls

Prospective rate setting also makes it essential to understand the cost implications of the quantity, quality, intensity, and scope of services offered, and to closely monitor these aspects of operation. Under stringent prospective payment systems, prompt adjustments in these and other cost-influencing factors may have to be made during the prospective year in attempting to control costs to keep them within prospective rates. Hence, prospective rate setting should lead to better cost analysis and cost control techniques. It appears that the amount of influence administrators and financial managers exert in organizational decision-making will continue to grow as a greater premium is placed on their planning and control skills. In addition, the scope of their influence should broaden as tightening financial constraints make it essential to recognize and act on the cost and revenue implications of everything from productivity and purchasing to the case mix of patients treated and the services they receive.

Sophistication

In short, management sophistication will improve substantially under prospective rate setting as it becomes more difficult for high-cost hospitals to bail themselves out by raising rates or by expecting cost reimbursement to cover whatever they spend. In addition, since the laws creating state rate-setting systems and the policies guiding voluntary programs typically call for the setting of rates related to "the costs of efficient production" and typically recognize the need to maintain "financial viability," it can be anticipated that new demands will be placed on accounting and financial

FIGURE 1A. COST-REVENUE-VOLUME RELATIONSHIP

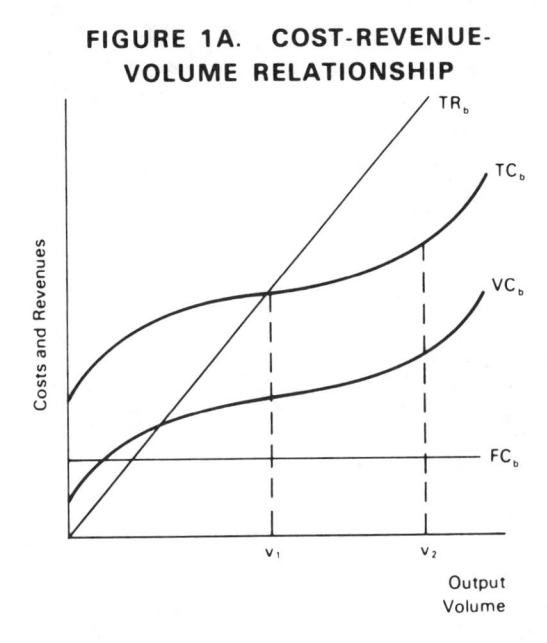

reporting systems to produce the information required to demonstrate "efficiency" and "financial viability." This information will be used more and more in rate setting and in appeals. Parenthetically, financial ratio analysis should emerge as a more important management tool.

ANALYTICS OF PROSPECTIVE RATE SETTING

Cost-Volume-Revenue

The financial incentives and implications of prospective rate setting can be analyzed by means of a conventional break-even model. Figure 1a is a graphic presentation of the cost-revenue-volume relationships for a hypothetical hospital. Output volume is measured along the horizontal axis (in discharges, days, or services) and costs and revenues along the vertical axis. Suppose the hospital's budgeted fixed and variable costs at different possible volumes are shown by the curves FC_b and VC_b, giving

FIGURE 1B. SIMPLIFIED COST-REVENUE-VOLUME RELATIONSHIP

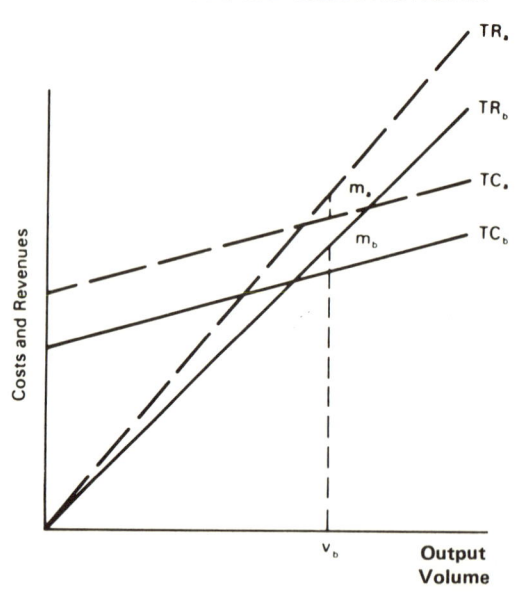

budgeted total costs at different possible volumes of TC_b. Assuming that both self-pay patients and third parties pay fixed charges or rates per unit of service, budgeted total revenue would increase in direct proportion to volume as shown by the straight line TR_b. In actual practice, of course, costs and revenues are only budgeted for some relevant range of volume like $v_1 - v_2$.

Figure 1b is a simplified version of Figure 1a, showing the hospital's TC_b and TR_b approximated by straight lines. In the absence of prospective rate setting or any other constraint on charges, the hospital would presumably set its charges so that TR_b would exceed TC_b by some desired operating margin, m_b, at its expected volume, v_b. If actual volume equals expected volume and the hospital's expectations about costs and revenues are right, the hospital would end the year with an actual operating margin of m_b. If actual costs begin running higher than expected as shown by TC_a, the hospital would presumably increase its charges during the year (again assuming no constraint on rate setting) to a level that would generate total revenue TR_a and operat-

FIGURE 2. RETROSPECTIVE COST REIMBURSEMENT

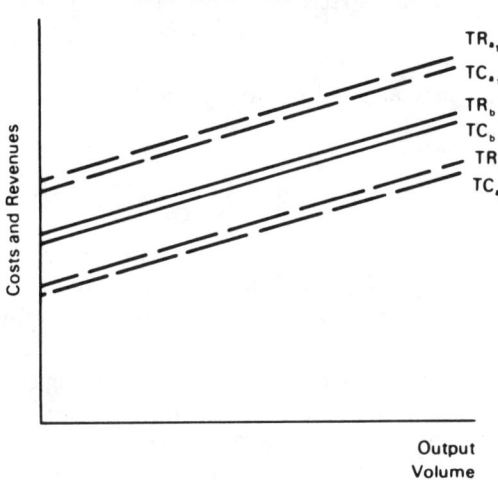

ing margin m_a ($m_a = m_b$). This illustrates why it is felt that billed charges payment systems, in which hospitals are free to increase their charges at will, fail to provide cost containment incentives. Rather than finding ways to prevent costs from increasing more than expected, hospitals can just increase their charges to cover them. From Figure 1b, it can also be seen that if actual volume turns out to be greater than expected volume, the hospital would end up with an operating margin greater than m_a or m_b whether TC_a and TR_a or TC_b and TR_b apply. This illustrates why it is felt that billed charges payment systems encourage increases in utilization. The greater the volume, the greater the operating margin.

Restrospective Reimbursement

Figure 2 illustrates the financial situation of a hypothetical hospital under retrospective cost reimbursement. Abstracting from the realities of nonallowable costs and nonrecognized financial requirements, and assuming for simplicity that all revenue comes in the form of cost reimbursement, this method of payment means that the hospital's revenues would always just equal its costs, whatever they happen to be (i.e., TR and TC would be the same). If actual costs begin running higher than expected as shown by TC_{a_1}, the hospital's revenue would still cover its costs as shown by TR_{a_1}, since payment is based on costs. On the other hand, if the hospital contained its costs to TC_{a_2}, it would only receive revenue TR_{a_2}. This illustrates why cost reimbursement is so often criticized as a scheme under which "whatever a hospital spends, it gets back." Clearly, cost reimbursement fails to provide cost containment incentives; hospitals are neither penalized for cost increases nor rewarded for finding ways to prevent them.

Incentives Contrast

The financial incentives inherent in prospective rate setting contrast sharply with those of the conventional methods of reimbursement. Suppose a prospective rate-setting system sets per case, per day, or per specific services rates for each participating hospital at a level just high enough to generate sufficient revenue to cover the hospital's approved budgeted costs and provide an agreed upon operating margin at the expected output volume. Figure 3 illustrates this situation for a hypothetical hospital. TC_b represents the hospital's approved budgeted costs, TR_{pr} the revenue that the hospital's prospective rates will generate at different output volumes, m_b the agreed upon operating margin, and v_b the expected volume. Note that the hospital's rates are set in advance of the prospective year based on budgeted vs. actual costs, with the hospital's budget first reviewed for reasonableness. Once set, the hospital's rates are considered fixed for the year.

Suppose the hospital's actual costs for the year exceed its approved budgeted costs as shown by TC_{a_1}. Under a prospective payment system, the hospital would suffer a loss equal to 1, since it would not be free to increase its rates. On the other hand, if the hospital is able to contain its costs to TC_{a_2}, it would earn a surplus s, substantially greater than the agreed-to operating margin m_b. In contrast to both billed charges systems (where hospitals are free to set their own charges) and cost reimbursement systems, prospective payment systems provide a penalty for greater than expected cost increases. Higher costs mean financial losses. Thus, once a hospital's prospective rate is set, it faces a strong "negative incentive" to keep its costs below its rate. In contrast to cost reimbursement systems (where containing costs results in less revenue) prospective payment systems provide a "positive incentive" to keep costs down—the possibility of earning a surplus.

It should be noted, however, that it is not clear why a nonprofit hospital would prefer to contain its costs during the prospective year in order to earn a surplus to spend in future years. Why wouldn't it simply spend whatever it wishes each and every year (which a hospital theoretically could do under charges or cost reimbursement)? What is the advantage, in other words, of deferred spending? This is one of the key issues surrounding prospective rate setting. Some observers argue that prospective

FIGURE 3. PROSPECTIVE PAYMENT

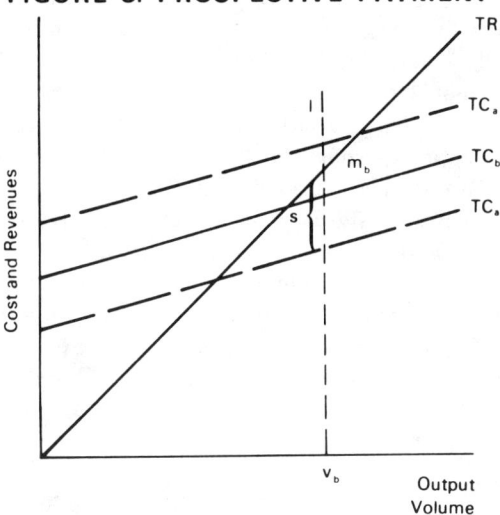

rate setting really offers no positive incentive to hospitals (at least, not to nonprofit hospitals which cannot distribute surpluses to their owners), since by cutting costs to earn a surplus, a hospital is just putting off expenditures it could make during the prospective year while risking lower rates in future years. It does appear that the negative incentive of the possibility of a loss must be present for prospective rate setting to work. However, some observers argue that the positive incentive inherent in prospective rate setting should be emphasized more. Prospective rates should be set so that efficient hospitals can make a surplus. Surpluses so acquired should place hospitals able to make them in an advantageous position with regard to some objectives they value. For example, planning agencies might place more emphasis on the cost of capital in considering competing expansion, modernization, or new service proposals. If several hospitals are seeking approval to add a particular new service, perhaps approval should be given to the one that could finance the project most cheaply as a result of its ability to accumulate enough surplus to obviate the need to borrow and incur debt service expenses.

Efficiency

Whether the planning process is formally structured along these lines, some proponents of prospective rate setting argue that over a period of time efficient hospitals would find it easier than inefficient hospitals to keep their costs below their rates, and would, therefore, be more likely to expand (perhaps using accumulated surpluses). Inefficient hospitals would tend to suffer losses, forcing them to curtail their operations. Thus, there would be a gradual shift from less efficient to more efficient hospitals in the long run. This argument assumes that prospective payment systems can be designed to be sufficiently sensitive to reward efficient hospitals (which may not necessarily have the lowest costs) and penalize inefficient hospitals (which may not have the highest costs). It is not clear, however, that the prospective payment systems currently in operation are sophisticated enough to discriminate between efficient and inefficient hospitals. In large part, the problem is caused by an inability to measure output mix and quality accurately enough to know when a hospital's costs are unjustifiably out of line.

Present Status

At the present time, about 35 prospective rate-setting systems are in operation. Twenty-two Blue Cross Plans operate prospective rate review or rate-setting programs. Most of these involve all hospitals in the plan's region or state, but a few are small experiments involving only a few hospitals. Nine states have enacted rate-setting laws. In four, an independent public utility form of rate-setting commission has been set up; in the other five, rate setting is performed by an existing agency of government, typically the department of health. In three states, state hospital associations operate voluntary rate review programs, and the University of South Carolina operates an experimental program with 16 hospitals.

These prospective rate setting systems are far from uniform. They differ not only with regard to the sponsoring organization, as indicated above, but also with regard to the nature of the prospective rates, the method of rate setting used, the extent to which different third parties actually pay the rates, and other factors.

SPONSORSHIP

The agency or organization sponsoring prospective rate setting may well affect the stringency of the system. Participation by hospitals in Blue Cross and state hospital association programs is generally voluntary, whereas participation in state systems is mandatory; and it is reasonable to expect that programs lacking the authority to require participation are not likely to be as stringent as mandatory systems. Governing boards, given their trusteeship responsibility, cannot be expected to voluntarily subject their hospitals to financial risk. Their duty to protect the financial viability of the institutions simply runs counter to their concept of employing financial risk to encourage cost containment. Only hospitals that believe prospective payment will not detract from the achievement of their goals or the maintenance of their financial viability can be expected to join, given a choice, and any hospital adversely affected can be expected to drop out, if this is possible. Therefore, the impact of voluntary rate-setting systems would likely be less substantial than mandatory systems. This line of reasoning has led many to prefer state sponsored systems.

It should be recognized, however, that prospective rate setting was first pioneered by several Blue Cross plans, and in specific situations, an arm's length but positive relationship with hospitals, expertise, market power, personalities, and a shared concern for cost containment have combined to produce effective Blue Cross programs. In comparison to state agencies, Blue Cross programs tend to be better staffed, more flexible, freer to experiment, freer to negotiate, and less encumbered by regulatory red tape. In the final analysis, however, Blue Cross rate-setting programs are voluntary, and any program seen as too stringent might end up without any takers. In addition, hospitals can always threaten to cancel their Blue Cross contracts, although some plans cover such a large share of the market that such an action is hardly likely. Hospital association sponsored prospective rate-review programs inevitably suffer a credibility problem, although several associations, guided by strong leadership and motivated by the threat of state regulation, have developed extensive budget and rate-review programs.

MANDATORY PROGRAMS

Mandatory rate-setting programs are created by the enactment of state laws empowering an existing state agency such as the state department of health or one created especially for the purpose, such as an independent public utility type rate-setting commission to set rates for hospitals (and in some cases, for nursing facilities and other institutional providers as well). State laws generally require hospitals to provide any data requested by the agency or commission in the format specified. State laws may or may not require the different third parties to pay the approved rates. Hence, there are states in which the rates apply only to patients who pay billed charges with Blue Cross and Medicaid continuing to reimburse costs. In other states, Blue Cross and Medicaid are required to pay the approved rates. No state, of course, has jurisdiction over the Federal Medicare program, but in Maryland, Rhode Island, Washington, and Western Pennsylvania, the Social Security Administration has waived certain of the Medicare reimbursement principles in order to participate in operating prospective payment systems. The question of who pays the prospectively set rates in a particular system is important, of course, because the greater the proportion of a hospital's revenue coming in the form of prospective rate payment, the greater the impact the system is likely to have. In addition, the "equal payment for equal services" goal requires that all patients and third parties pay the prospective rates set by the agency or program, although the issue of how to handle cost differences experienced by hospitals because of differences in third party policies and practices (and hence whether different rates should be permitted) is far from settled.

Of the two state alternatives, the department of health or an independent rate-setting commission, hospitals generally prefer the latter, arguing that a conflict of interest exists when the agency administering the state's Medicaid program and hence purchasing large amounts of hospital services is also empowered to set the rates to be paid for these services. Commissions are also considered freer from political influence than agencies of state government, although in actual practice their budgets are usually determined annually by the legislature. State agencies and independent commissions alike often suffer from underfinancing, understaffing, and inflexible procedures.

ADVANTAGES

Could the advantages of both private and state sponsorship be gained in a rate-setting program cooperatively sponsored by a Blue Cross plan or hospital association and a state agency or commission? This possibility merits further investigation. The authority to set rates and to mandate participation could come from a state law while administration of the program, including the actual budget review and rate setting process, could be carried out by the private organization. The state might finally approve all rates, acting upon the recommendation of the review organization, or it might establish a state-wide ceiling on aggregate costs within which the private organization would be free to work out specific rates for individual hospitals. In New York and Rhode Island, Blue Cross plans operate prospective rate setting programs within the framework of regulations promulgated by the respective states. The plans administer the rate setting process and recommend rates and rate appeal settlements to the appropriate state agency.

PLANNING AND RATE SETTING

Another fundamental issue is whether certification of need, licensure, and other regulatory functions should be placed in the agency that handles rate setting or be kept separate. No state has given all of these powers to an independent rate-setting commission, and although in a number of states where rate setting has been assigned to the department of health, the department carries out the certificate of need and licensure functions as well, there is surprisingly little coordination between them. Reflecting the lack of coherent state (or national) health policies, no state has a truly comprehensive, cohesive regulatory program at this time. In part, this may stem from an unwillingness of states to face up to the effect of their own decisions granting certificates of need, or raising licensure standards, or expanding Medicaid eligibility and services on costs and hence on rates. Examples can be found of states in which the state's Medicaid program is unwilling to pay the prospective rates set by the state's own rate-setting commission as fair and reasonable. It should be noted, however, that some prefer the problems caused by multiple, uncoordinated, often conflicting regulatory and payment programs to the centralization of programs and hence power in a single agency.

Spiraling Cost

Perhaps the most fundamental question is whether the cost spiral can ever be dealt with definitively until financing, planning, licensing, utilization and rate setting programs are linked. Clearly, for example, the scope and sophistication of facilities and services offered by hospitals affect costs, and it is generally agreed that decisions about the appropriateness of existing or new services should be based on both cost and need criteria. It seems only fair, however, that once approvals for new services are given, they carry with them authority to adjust rates to cover the costs of these services. Likewise, costs should be considered in determining the eligibility limits and the services to be provided in programs that finance care for the needy, but once services are promised, they should be paid for. In the final analysis, it is the inevitability of making cost availability-accessibility-quality tradeoff decisions such as these that argues both for coordinating the different financing and regulatory programs that deal with these matters and for placing them in public agencies where such decisions can be legitimized in the public interest.

Coordination

Coordination of planning and rate setting remains an illusive goal, although some steps have been taken. It has become commonplace, for example, to require planning agency approval before the capital costs, and in some cases the operating costs, of new services are figured into payment rates. Another coordination mechanism operating in several states is where the rate-setting agency or commission advises planning agencies regarding the reasonableness of the capital and operating costs as well as the financial feasibility of proposed projects. It has been suggested that the rate-setting agency might even suggest a statewide ceiling on capital expenditures each year, with only the highest priority new services (as determined by planning agencies) implemented up to the point at which the ceiling is reached. Certainly, the rate-setting agency should expect help from planning agencies in encouraging the sharing of services to improve operating efficiency.

It has also been suggested that the powers of rate setting be brought to bear to back up the decisions of planning agencies. For example, if an area is found to be overbedded by the appropriate planning agency, the prospective routine daily service rates for area hospitals could be based on what per diem costs would be at efficient occupancy levels rather than on what they are at actual occupancy levels, thereby forcing the closure of beds or merger of units to avoid financial losses. In Massachusetts and New York, for example, prospective rates are adjusted to penalize hospitals with obstetrics units operating under 60 percent occupancy, pediatrics units under 70 percent, and medical-surgical units under 80 percent. This approach could be taken to force the phase-out of any specialized service declared to be duplicative and underutilized on the grounds that rates are to be set so as to cover the costs of "efficient" provision, not low volume provision, of services. Certainly, rate setting should be flexible enough to support the efforts of planning agencies to promote alternatives to acute inpatient care, cooperation in the provision of services, regionalization, etc. An intriguing possibility, just beginning to receive attention, is the concept of relating the amount allowed in hospital rates for depreciation (or growth and development) to future area needs and approved institutional long-range plans. It has been suggested, for example, that hospitals in overbedded areas should not automatically be guaranteed the financial means to replace themselves, while hospitals that are clearly needed should be allowed more than historical depreciation to enable them to accumulate the capital revenues they will need in future years.

BASES OF PAYMENT

Prospective rate-setting systems differ in terms of the basis or unit of payment for which rates are set. This feature is important because the payment unit determines the incentives posed by the system and hence how hospitals are likely to react to it. The alternative bases of payment that might be used are as follows:

1. Apportionment of total budget
2. Apportionment of departmental budgets
3. Capitation
4. Case
5. Day
6. Specific services

Total Budget

The apportionment of total budget method might work in the following way. Hospitals would submit budgets to a rate setting agency or program setting forth and justifying their expected prospective year costs and financial requirements. The agency would assess the reasonableness of each hospital's budget, perhaps by comparing its costs to the costs of similar hospitals, to cost standards, to expected inflation trends, or by a line by line budget review. Hospitals would be asked to defend or modify any parts of their budgets appearing out of line. Agreement on a final budget satisfactory to both parties might be automatic if a budget, as originally submitted or as modified, fell within acceptable parameters, or agreement might be reached through a formal hearings process, an informal negotiations process, or a combination of the two. Once a hospital's budget was agreed upon, each third party would be obligated to pay its share of budgeted costs, regardless (following the basic principle of prospective payment) of the costs actually incurred by the hospital during the prospective year. Apportionment of budgeted costs to different third parties could be based on each third party's share of the hospital's charges, admissions, or patient days, or could be determined by the departmental RCC method (applied to budgeted vs. actual costs). The hospital would be guaranteed its budgeted costs whatever the proportions paid by the different third parties. For example, if a budget of $6,000,000 were agreed upon for a hospital, the hospital would get this amount regardless of what its costs actually turned out to be. If a particular third party were responsible for half the hospital's patients, it would be obligated to pay $3,000,000 (which it might simply forward in monthly $250,000 installments). Quarterly checks could be made to determine each third party's exact share of the $2,000,000 due the hospital for the quarter.

Michigan Blue Cross and Washington's State Hospital Commission are currently experimenting with the apportionment of budget method of prospective payment. Military and Veteran's Administration hospitals and hospitals in a number of Canadian provinces essentially operate on fixed budgets set in advance of each operating year. Obviously, this approach to prospective payment provides an incentive to control both the cost per unit and volume of services provided, since both contribute to the total cost of operating an institution. In actual practice, provision would undoubtedly be made to adjust the budgeted cost figure agreed to for a hospital, if its actual costs or volume diverge substantially from its budgeted costs because of major, uncontrollable, unpredictable occurrences. It merits repeating, however, that automatically adjusting what a hospital is paid based on how it actually operates during the prospective year removes the incentive to control operations.

Departmental Budgets

The apportionment of departmental budgets method of prospective payment is similar, except that cost figures are set for individual departments, and each third party's payment responsibility is determined by the proportion of each department's services going to its patients. The advantage of this approach is the "fine tuning" it makes possible in focusing financial incentives on specific areas of operation. In addition, it allows the elimination of departments over which the administrator has little or no control from prospective rate setting. Or, only the routine daily service and "hotel" cost centers might be included under the assumption that their costs are less influenced by changes in case mix, intensity of service, technology, etc., than the ancillary cost centers. The Connecticut Hospital Association has experimented with a modified version of the departmental budgets method in setting cost targets.

Capitation

The capitation method of prospective payment, as an approach to hospital vs. physician payment, would work best where hospitals are associated with or part of health plans or health maintenance organizations. Each hospital would agree to provide to the enrollees of the plan with which it is associated all needed hospital services in return for a fixed amount per person per year. Although it is conceivable that the capitation approach to payment could be used for hospitals not associated with health plans, this would require that groups of people in areas served by one or more hospitals identify themselves with specific hospitals that would accept responsibility for meeting their hospital needs. It is difficult to see how this would work in metropolitan areas. People do not identify directly with hospitals as they do with physicians, and so it would be difficult to determine which hospital was responsible for which people unless physicians were involved. Nevertheless, in a 1964 experiment conducted by Colorado Blue Cross in Yuma County, Colorado, the Plan made capitation payments to the two hospitals in the County which, in turn, agreed to provide all hospital services needed by Blue Cross subscribers. Yuma County is quite isolated, however, and each hospital's share of Blue Cross's business in the County was well known.

Per Case, Per Diem

Per case, per diem, or per specific services prospective rates are more familiar. The actual determination of per unit rates can be arrived at by dividing approved budgeted costs by expected volume, or by asking hospitals to propose rate structures that will generate just enough revenue to cover approved budgeted costs at expected volumes, or by applying some sort of formula to project historical costs forward into prospective rates or to translate hospital and patient workload characteristics into prospective rates. The only operating per case rate-prospective payment program is an experiment being conducted by Blue Cross of Northeastern Pennsylvania with two hospitals in Wilkes-Barre. However, Phase IV of the Economic Stabilization Program, which of course was never implemented because of the termination of the program, would have employed as its basic cost-control mechanism a limit of 7.5 percent on annual increases in revenue per case. In the prospective rate-setting programs sponsored by Blue Cross plans, choice of a payment unit generally follows the approach to reimbursement that the plan used before. Thus, plans that reimbursed costs tend to set per diem prospective rates, and plans that paid billed charges tend to set specific services rates.

Specific Services

A practical advantage of using specific services as the basis of payment is that services represent a common denominator applicable to all purchasers of hospital services—Blue Cross, commercial insurance, self-pay patients, Medicare, Medicaid, etc. Third parties reimbursing hospitals all-inclusive per diem costs tend to prefer per diem prospective rates. However, it would be inappropriate to charge individual self-pay patients average per diem rates, since some would end up paying for much more service than they actually used and some for less. Therefore, either a dual rate structure would be required to satisfy third parties and individual self-pay patients, or all purchasers would have to agree on specific services as the basis of payment. State commissions, concerned about getting all purchasers to pay the same rates for the same services, seem to favor specific services rates, and several commissions have attempted to get Medicare and Medicaid to waive their cost reimbursement regulations and agree to pay the rates they set. Another advantage of specific service rates is that they permit the costs of similar services to be compared across hospitals. This might encourage patients and physicians to give costs more weight in choosing hospitals. It has also been suggested that third parties might use this information to make co-payment and deductible payments by patients dependent on the costliness of the hospitals they use.

A disadvantage of specific services rates is that hospitals charge for hundreds of services, and a detailed review of the "reasonableness" of each rate is impossible. In practice, prospective rate setting agencies and programs typically review budgeted costs, not rates. Once a hospital's budget is agreed upon, the hospital is asked to propose a rate structure that will generate just enough revenue to cover its approved budget at its expected volume (perhaps adhering to certain guidelines; for example, that rates be set so that each patient service department comes within specified parameters of breaking even). Presumably, the commission would check the hospital's financial reports at the end of the year to determine if the rates proposed by the hospital and approved by the commission did in fact generate only the allowed revenue. Despite this shortcut (i.e., elimination of reviews of hundreds of individual rates), some commissions are beginning to consider requesting that all hospitals under their jurisdiction use a considerably simplified, uniform rate structure.

IMPACT OF PROSPECTIVE RATE SETTING ON HOSPITAL OPERATION

The impact a prospective rate-setting system is likely to have on hospitals depends in large part on the basis of payment used, because the incentives posed by the different payment units differ. The areas of hospital operation that might be affected by prospective reimbursement can be identified *a priori* by considering the factors that determine costs in hospitals. The following is proposed as a complete although general list of these cost-influencing factors.

1. Cases treated
2. Case mix
3. Length of stay
4. Intensity of service
5. Scope of service
6. Amenity level
7. Quality level
8. Efficiency
9. Input prices
10. Investment in the improvement or maintenance of human and physical resources
11. Teaching programs

TABLE 1*

Expected Changes in Hospital Performance Under Alternative Payment Units

Payment Unit	Cases Treated	Length of Stay[1]	Complexity of Case-Mix[2]	Intensity of Service[1]	Scope of Service	Amenity Level	Quality Level	Efficiency	Input Prices	Investment in Resources	Teaching Programs
Total hospital budget	↓	↓	↓	↓	↓	↓	↓	↑	↓	↓	↓
Departmental budgets	↓	↓	↓	↓	↓	↓	↓	↑	↓	↓	↓
Family or person (capitation)	↓	↓	↓	↓	↓	↓	↓	↑	↓	↓	↓
Case or stay	↑	↓	↓	↓	↓	↓	↓	↑	↓	↓	↓
Day	↑	↑	↓	↓	↓	↓	↓	↑	↓	↓	↓
Specific services	↑	↑[3]	↑	↑	↑	↓	↓	↑	↓	↓	↓

[1] It is assumed that intensity of service and length of stay are not substitutes (i.e., hospitals do not have to increase intensity in order to discharge patients sooner). Underlying this assumption is the belief that reductions in lengths of stay would come from the last few days of hospitalization, which are primarily convalescent.

[2] Admissions and case-mix are interrelated in that the case types that would be denied admission if admissions were reduced would be the least complex. Therefore, the case-mix of hospitalized patients that would result would include a higher proportion of more complex case types. At the same time, however, a hospital could attempt to select easier case types whenever possible.

[3] The direction of change in length of stay depends on the occupancy level. If a hospital is operating at high occupancy and has patients waiting for admission, payment on a per service basis should cause it to discharge patients sooner (reducing the average length of stay) in order to substitute patients requiring the more service-intensive first few days of hospitalization. Hospitals operating at low occupancy could both admit more patients and increase the length of stay to increase the quantity of services produced. The direction of change indicated is based on the observation that hospitals have extra or unfilled beds much of the time.

*Reprinted with minor modifications from Dowling, W. L. "Prospective Reimbursement of Hospitals." *Inquiry* 11:3 (Sept. 1974).

It is proposed that hospitals must act through these variables in attempting to keep their costs below their prospective rates. Further, given the payment unit used by a prospective rate-setting system, the changes in these areas of operation that might be expected to occur can be predicted. It should be emphasized, however, that these predictions are based on the assumption that prospective payment is the only constraint or incentive to which hospitals must respond. Clearly, other goals and pressures affect hospitals; therefore, the predictions proposed may not hold in any particular situation.

Table 1 shows the changes in the areas of operation expected to occur under the different payment units. The payment units are ordered from the most aggregate to the most specific. It is important to note that hospital revenue under the first three payment units is not directly related to output, since once the amount to be paid is set for the prospective year, it does not vary with the actual quantity of services provided in that year. Under the other three payment units, which are in effect different measures of output, hospital revenue is directly related to output.

As Table 1 indicates, the total budget, departmental budgets, or capitation bases of payment discourage increases in *cases treated* and *lengths of stay* because these methods of payment do not link the amounts hospitals are paid to the number of patients admitted or days of care provided. Hospitals might attempt to admit more selectively and to discharge patients sooner to alternative facilities or to their homes. Depending on the adequacy of payment for out-of-hospital services, hospitals might develop preadmission testing, outpatient surgery, outpatient diagnostic and treatment services, and home-care programs to prevent or shorten hospitalizations.

In addition to the incentive to reduce admissions and patient days, these bases of payment provide an incentive for hospitals to contain increases in per unit costs by changing the mix of patients treated and by changing the nature of the services provided them. Hospitals might admit fewer complex or serious case types, thereby shifting toward a less costly *case-mix*. Hospitals might discontinue (or delay adding) costly programs and services, thereby reducing the *scope of service* they offer. These actions tend to reinforce each other. Hospitals might also curtail the *amenity level, quality level,* and *intensity of service* they provide. An incentive exists for hospitals to improve *efficiency*, both by increasing input productivity and by shifting toward a less costly input mix. Assuming that hospitals have some buying power, an incentive exists to resist increases in *input prices*. An incentive also exists to reduce *investments in human and physical resources*. Cuts might be made in programs designed to improve employee morale and productivity and in programs designed to prevent deterioration of equipment and physical plant (although such actions would tend to increase costs in the long run). Finally, an incentive exists to curtail *teaching programs*, both because of the direct expenditures involved, and because of the indirect impact of these programs on case-mix, intensity of service, and scope of service.

The overall effect of using any of these bases of payment in a prospective rate-setting system should be to discourage increases in both the quantity and cost per unit of hospital services, so that increases in aggregate costs should be slowed.

In contrast, the overall effect on aggregate costs of using any of the output-related bases of payment—cases, days, or specific services—cannot be predicted, since they simultaneously motivate hospitals to increase output (both to directly increase revenue and to spread fixed costs over more units of output to reduce the average cost per unit); and to contain increases in the cost per unit of output, by containing the amenity level, quality level, intensity, and scope of service provided; by increasing efficiency; and by containing input prices, investments in resources, and teaching programs.

Specifically, payment of a fixed amount per case would motivate hospitals to admit more patients, but, if possible, to admit less complex case types, to shorten stays, and to reduce the intensity and scope of services provided. Payment of a fixed amount per day would motivate hospitals to increase the days of care provided, by increasing ad-

FIGURE 4A. PROSPECTIVE PER CASE, DAY OR SPECIFIC SERVICE RATES

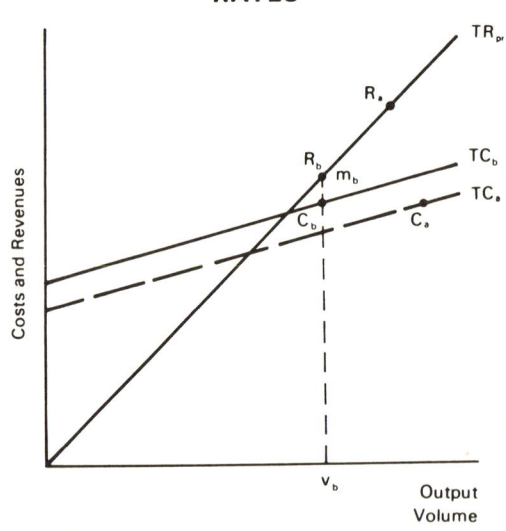

missions and lengths of stay, and to shift from more costly to less costly days by admitting less complex case types and by reducing the intensity and scope of services provided. Payment of fixed amounts for specific services (e.g., nursing care, laboratory tests, surgical procedures, x-rays, etc.) would motivate hospitals to provide more services by increasing admissions and lengths of stay to increase the number of patients requiring services, and by increasing the intensity of service provided. In contrast to the other payment units, hospitals might attempt to admit the more complex case types, since they need the most services.

Figures 4a and 4b contrast the incentives inherent in the output-related and non-output-related bases of payment. Figure 4a illustrates the situation of a hypothetical hospital operating under prospective per case, per day, or per specific service rates. TC_b represents the hospital's approved budgeted costs, TR_{pr} the revenue the hospital's prospective rates will generate at different volumes, m_b the agreed to operating margin, and v_b the expected volume. Since TR_{pr} depends directly on volume, an incentive

FIGURE 4B. PROSPECTIVE TOTAL BUDGET PAYMENT PROGRAM

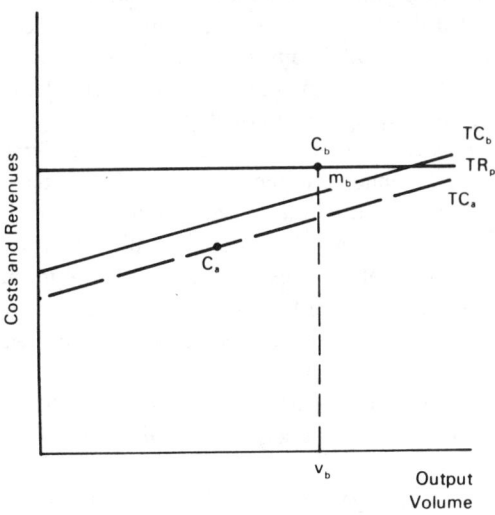

[Graph showing Costs and Revenues on the y-axis and Output Volume on the x-axis. Lines labeled TC_b, TR_{pr}, and TC_a are shown, with points C_b, m_b, C_a marked, and v_b on the x-axis.]

exists to increase volume or at least to keep it from falling below v_b. In addition, an incentive exists to contain costs (as represented by TC_a), whatever the volume. Both actions act to increase the operating margin. Since increases in volume increase costs while cost containment efforts reduce them, it cannot be predicted whether actual total costs C_a will be above or below budgeted total costs C_b. It is quite possible, however, for actual revenue R_a (which is equivalent to patient and third party outlays) to exceed budgeted revenue R_b.

Figure 4b illustrates the situation of a hypothetical hospital operating under a prospective total budget payment program. TC_b represents the hospital's approved budgeted costs and TR_{pr} its guaranteed total revenue, set so as to provide an agreed upon operating margin m_b at the expected volume v_b. Since TR_{pr} does not depend on volume, an incentive exists to reduce volume or keep it from rising above v_b. A cost containment incentive TC_a also exists. Since both actions act to reduce costs, actual total costs C_a should be below budgeted total costs C_b. It is not possible for actual revenue to exceed budgeted revenue, since the approved budget figure is all the hospital will be paid.

All of the output related payment units then provide an incentive for hospitals to increase output, and this might be reinforced by long-run goals of growth and prestige. Of concern, of course, is whether inappropriate use would result. It should be emphasized that no payment unit is without potential negative impacts, and this is a dilemma that must be faced in designing prospective rate-setting systems. It appears that controls over quality and utilization may assume more importance as cost containment incentives are introduced. Another approach would be to aim additional financial incentives directly at certain areas of operation; for example, by directly rewarding hospitals for reducing their average length of stay.

In summary, hospitals can attempt to contain costs in different ways. The actions hospitals are likely to take under prospective rate-setting systems will depend on the basis of payment used. Selection of the payment unit, therefore, depends on how one wishes to change hospital performance. Hospitals could be left free to respond as best fits their situation, or additional controls could be applied to influence their responses. Hospital preferences for the different payment units would depend in part on their expectations about future use. If an increase in use is expected, the output related payment units would be preferred; if a decrease is expected, the budget or capitation payment units would be preferred. The magnitudes of the changes in operations predicted to occur under prospective rate setting depend on several factors:

1. The tightness of the prospective rates. Obviously, if hospitals must take extreme measures to maintain their financial viability, changes would be greater than if the rates were more "reasonable."

2. The firmness of the prospective rates. If rates are adjusted for actual volume or for changes in case-mix, input prices, etc., the impact of prospective rate setting would be moderated.

3. The size of potential rewards or penalties. This depends on the proportion of any difference between actual costs and prospective rates that hospitals are at risk for and on the proportion of their patients covered by prospective payment. Also, if hospitals are able to offset potential losses by increasing charges to self pay patients, the influence of prospective rate setting would be moderated.

4. The present state of hospital performance. Admissions or lengths of stay, for example, might decrease more under the appropriate payments units in hospitals where inappropriate use is occurring than in those where there is little overuse.

5. The disposition of physicians toward cooperating with hospital cost containment efforts. Admissions, case-mix, length of stay, etc., depend largely on decisions made by physicians; and therefore, changes in the medically related areas of operation require their support.

PROSPECTIVE RATE SETTING METHODS

Prospective rate setting is a fairly recent innovation in hospital payment, and as a result, the rate-setting methods currently in use are relatively unsophisticated. Although all methods attempt to establish "fair but tight" rates, the range of factors taken into account in determining rates, the degree of sensitivity to the idiosyncracies of individual institutions, the data required, and the criteria and procedures used differ greatly. In addition, the rate setting method used can affect the incentives placed on hospitals by prospective payment systems. The most commonly used rate setting methods[2] are as follows:

1. Projection of past and/or present year costs forward to become prospective year rates, with projections based upon:
    - peer group cost levels and trends,
    - economic indices,
    - normative standards,
    - or a combination of these bases.
2. Budget review to determine the reasonableness of prospective year costs and rates, with budget reviews based on:
    - comparison of budgeted costs to past year costs,
    - comparison of budgeted costs to peer group costs,
    - comparison of budgeted costs to normative cost standards,
    - or a combination of these bases.

Formulas

Negotiation is generally cited as another method of determining rates, and it is certainly conceivable that decisions about rates could depend solely upon bargaining skill and market power. However, in actual practice, negotiation tends to be the final step used to come to closure after budget reviews or projection techniques have defined a fairly narrow range of acceptable costs or rates. Whereas negotiation may serve as the final step in rate setting, "formulas" often serve as the first step. The term formula has come to mean any automatic, mechanical, rule-like method for defining acceptable parameters around costs or rates or for directly setting rates. Formulas may incorporate peer group cost means or trends, economic inflation indices, coefficients derived from statistically estimated cost functions or points derived from expert panels (both reflecting the scope and sophistication of the programs and services offered by hospitals), or simply arbitrary (or "normative") ceilings or parameters.

Formulas may be used to define how historical costs are to be projected forward into prospective rates, to translate hospital or patient characteristics into acceptable cost or rate parameters, or to define parameters that can be employed in screening budgets to identify costs that appear out of line. Generally, the application of a formula is followed by a detailed review and/or negotiation step, although in a few prospective rate-setting systems, final rates are set directly by formulas, and these rates can only be challenged by a formal appeal. Formula methods of rate setting are certainly less costly to administer than budget reviews or negotiations (although the costs of appeals and court cases may be substantial where formulas are too arbitrary or simplistic). It appears that when formulas are used to isolate questionable situations that are then considered in detail, the advantages of the cost savings inherent in formulas and the fairness and thoroughness inherent in individual reviews can both be achieved. This two-stage process has come to be called the "detailed review by exception" approach to rate setting.

Empirical Standards

Lacking normative standards of "reasonableness," empirical standards are commonly used in the budget review and projection methods of rate setting. Hospitals are grouped according to cost-influencing characteristics like ownership, location, size, scope of services, outpatient programs, teaching programs, etc. Projections or judgments about cost levels or trends can then be based on a comparison of each hospital with its peer group. Although the costs or rates for a particular hospital may appear out of line, only if the hospital is compared to truly similar hospitals can a decision that its costs are actually unreasonable be made with conviction. As a result, the characteristics considered and techniques used in grouping hospitals are critical to the effectiveness and equity of prospective rate setting. The debate between the Social Security Administration and hospital representatives about the adequacy of the grouping scheme used to establish ceilings on reasonable costs in implementing Section 223 of PL 92-603 demonstrates the concern over this matter.

Output Mix, Input Prices

Theoretically, hospitals should be grouped according to two major variables—output mix and input prices. Output mix would be measured by the diagnostic types, complexity, and severity of patients treated by each hospital. Input prices would be measured by the price and salary levels prevailing in each hospital's input market. Capital and teaching costs would be isolated and evaluated separately. Focusing on operating costs then, if output mix and input prices could be measured accurately enough that hospitals treating equally complex case mixes and operating in equally costly input markets could be grouped together, ceilings or projections of costs or rates based on peer group means would be defensible on the grounds that out-of-line costs could be due only to more costly than typical treatment patterns or to inefficient operations. The burden of proof would shift to high-cost hospitals to demonstrate why they could not treat a case mix of the same complexity as cheaply as other hospitals in their peer group. However, the case mix data required to implement such a grouping scheme are not available from most hospitals, and therefore, existing grouping schemes use hospital size, services, and other structural variables. Although these schemes may give groupings of hospitals with fairly comparable cost structures, they do not allow the burden of proof to be shifted to high-cost hospitals as would groupings based on output mix and input prices.

PROJECTION METHODS

Projection methods of rate setting begin with a hospital's costs for the past and/or present year and extrapolate or trend them forward to become prospective year rates using group means or trends, economic indices, normative standards, or a combination of these, as bases for projections. The New York Blue Cross formula for setting prospective rates provides an example:

        Audited base year   +   % increase in estimated
        per diem cost*   current year cost over base
                                     year cost**

    + % increase for projected = Prospective per
       input cost increases***   diem rate for coming year

*Adjusted downward if the hospital's average per diem cost is more than 15% above the weighted average per diem cost for its group.
**Adjusted downward (upward) if the percent increase in the hospital's per diem cost is more than 10% above (below) the percent increase in the weighted average per diem cost for its group.
***Based on a projection of the three-year moving average increase in economic indices reflecting the components of hospital costs.

This formula was used by New York Blue Cross from 1970 through 1975. Although Blue Cross has not changed its basic approach to rate setting since then, two specific changes have been made in the way in which the formula is applied that are extremely significant. First, base year cost ceilings are applied to ancillary and routine service costs separately, and second, for each, the 50th percentile average per diem cost for a hospital's peer group is used as the acceptable cost ceiling. Thus, a hospital's base year average per diem ancillary cost and its average per diem routine cost must both be at or below the 50th percentile figure for its group for formula application purposes. Note that this formula uses both peer group costs and an economic index in projecting prospective rates. The adjustments or ceilings are intended to assure that high-cost hospitals (i.e., hospitals with high base year costs or high base to intermediate year cost increases rates compared to their peers) are not automatically rewarded by high rates, and the economic index is intended to keep hospital cost increases in line with inflation rates in the general economy—an explicit goal of the New York scheme.

The best example of projections based on normative standard come from the ESP program. Phases II and III limited hospital cost and price increases to 6%, and the proposed Phase IV would have limited annual revenue per admission increases to 7.5%. Although clearly somewhat arbitrary, these figures were supposedly based on expert judgment about what was reasonable. The 7.5% figure, for example, represented a composite of (1) an estimated inflation rate of 5.9%, (2) an allowance for increased intensity of 2.5%, and (3) an adjustment or offset for improved productivity of -1.0%.

Problems

Two fundamental problems with projection methods of rate setting are apparent. (1) changes from year to year in each hospital's case mix, intensity, programs and services, etc., are not fully accounted for, and (2) long-run cost containment incentives are poor.

Since the actual costs of each hospital in the past and/or present year serve as the starting point for determining prospective year rates when projection methods are used, differences between hospitals existing initially are presumably taken into account. The problem is with changes over time. Major changes in facilities, teaching programs, or other factors used as classification variables might result in hospitals being regrouped. However, most year-to-year changes, unless very substantial, would not automatically be recognized in this manner. As a result, hospitals caring for a more complex case mix, for example, requiring more intensive and sophisticated services, might be penalized by inappropriately tight rates. So might a hospital adding to or upgrading its programs and services to keep up with advances in medical technology or new community needs.

To deal with these problems, grouping schemes can be refined to take more factors into account. Processes can be established for requesting rate adjustments for approved new facilities and services. A "costliness of case mix" index, as proposed in Phase IV, could be developed to show the cost implications of changes in case mix. A "costliness of services" index could be used in the same way. Diagnostic-specific per case rates might be paid, so that changes in case mix automatically influence the amounts hospitals received. Finally, an appeals process is generally available for hospitals that feel they have been treated unfairly. Nevertheless, projection methods of rate setting tend to be more arbitrary and insensitive to institutional uniquenesses than budget review methods.

When prospective rates are insensitive to changes over time in cost influencing factors like case mix, intensity, programs and services, etc., hospitals may be unfairly under- or over-paid. On the other hand, if changes in these factors are automatically and fully adjusted in hospital rates, the incentives deliberately imposed by prospective rate-setting systems to encourage hospitals to be aware of, concerned about, and to attempt to control costs in all areas of operation are moderated. For example, many believe that prospective rate setting should encourage hospitals not only to improve their operating efficiency, but also:

1. to make definite decisions about what case types to treat and what case types to refer to other hospitals,

2. to attempt to control overuse of ancillary services and overly long lengths of stay,
3. to make cost-effective decisions about adding new programs and services,
4. to avoid duplicating services available in nearby hospitals,
5. to attempt to develop outpatient services as a substitute for inpatient care.

Those who would like to put hospitals at risk for making (or not making) cost-influencing decisions like these are reluctant to see rates adjusted too readily for actual experience during the prospective years, arguing that this eases the pressure on hospitals to act on these matters.

Another problem with projecting historical costs forward into prospective rates is that each hospital's future rates depend on its present cost containment successes. Thus, if a hospital cuts its costs one year, its rates will be lower in future years when the first year's costs become the base or starting point for rate projections. Hospitals are motivated, therefore, to spend right up to their prospective rate each year to avoid putting themselves in a tighter financial position in future years. This problem, perhaps more than anything else, has plagued the design of prospective rate setting systems. It can only be solved if rate projections are based on something other than a hospital's own cost performance. Peer group performance or normative measures of performance are possibilities. It is crucial that this problem be dealt with in the design of prospective rate-setting systems, so that they truly offer positive long-run cost containment incentives, and so that efficient hospitals are rewarded and inefficient hospitals penalized.

BUDGET REVIEW METHODS

The budget review approach to rate setting is clearly more sensitive than projection methods to differences among hospitals in the quantity and types of patients treated, facilities and services, input prices, teaching programs, amenity, quality, productivity, etc. Assuming arbitrary decision rules are not used, budget review is the fairest (in the sense of examining each hospital's situation individually) method of determining the reasonableness of costs in that it permits the affect of each cost influencing factor on each hospital to be taken into account. Hospitals have an opportunity to explain and defend their budgets, and the rate setting agency or program has an opportunity to question items that appear out of line. Budget review gives the agency more of a chance to influence specific hospital activities and plans before decisions about them are implemented.

Cost Examination

In short, a detailed, institution by institution examination of costs and cost-influencing factors characterizes the budget-review method of rate setting. To many, this is the attractive feature of this method; to others, its basic drawback. Meaningful budget reviews require considerable expertise—in accounting, economics, finance, and hospital management—which many rate-setting agencies and programs do not have. Comprehensive and thorough reviews also require comparable and fairly detailed cost and statistical data; a knowledge of the assumptions, modes of operation, and plans that underlie the figures presented; a knowledge of the need for new programs and services proposed; etc. The tendency is for the agency to ask for more and more data and get more and more involved. For example, suppose a hospital's radiology cost per case or per day appears high. This could be due to a case mix requiring extensive and sophisticated radiology procedures, or to the intensity of X-ray services provided to patients generally, productivity, salaries, etc., as the following formula indicates:

$$\frac{\text{Average X-Ray Cost}}{\text{Case}} = \sum \begin{array}{c} \text{Cases}_1 \\ \text{Cases}_2 \end{array} \cdot \begin{array}{c} \frac{\text{Ave X-rays}}{\text{Case}_1} \\ \frac{\text{Ave X-rays}}{\text{Case}_2} \end{array} \cdot \begin{array}{c} \frac{\text{Ave Manhours}}{\text{X-ray}} \\ \frac{\text{Ave Manhours}}{\text{X-ray}} \end{array} \cdot \begin{array}{c} \frac{\text{Ave Salary}}{\text{Manhour}} \\ \frac{\text{Ave Salary}}{\text{Manhour}} \end{array}$$

| | *Case Mix* | *Intensity* | *Productivity* | *Salaries* |

Questions could also be asked about the kinds of radiology procedures commonly done for each case type, the skill mix of the department's personnel, the quantity and types of supplies used, and so on. The point is, of course, that it is difficult to draw the line on "second guessing" hospital management. Few people believe that rate setting agencies can run the hospitals they are supposed to regulate as well as the governing boards and management staffs of these hospitals (typically, the management staffs of a few large hospitals taken together are larger than the entire agency staff), but it is not clear how encroachment on management prerogatives can be prevented.

Case Mix Data Approach

One approach, suggested above, is to concentrate on better case mix data rather than better operating data, so that the "burden of proof" can be shifted to hospitals whose costs appear out of line to demonstrate why they are unable to care for a case mix of comparable complexity as cheaply as their peers. Whether because of intensity, productivity, salaries, skill mix, or supplies, it would be up to the hospital to determine and correct its problems. Another more common approach is the "detailed review by exceptions" process, also discussed above, wherein budgets are screened, perhaps automatically by a computerized process, and only the third or so that appear out of line in terms of certain guidelines, parameters, or standards "flagged" for a detailed review. Thus, an administrator would know that if his budget was kept within reasonable bounds, he would not be second-guessed. This concept could be furthered if the guidelines used for screening were made known in advance. An administrator could budget with these guidelines in mind, knowing that his budget would definitely not be reviewed as long as it fell within the guidelines. Finally, it should be noted that the entire process of reviewing individual hospital budgets may take place within the constraint of a predetermined aggregate state-wide cost increase limit—a "maxi-cap"— as is the case in Rhode Island.

Level of Detail

Related to this is the question of what level of detail to focus on. For example, if a hospital's "bottom line," as represented by, say, its overall cost per case compares favorably with its peers, is further review required? If so, what if its overall routine daily services cost, ancillary services cost, and "hotel" services costs are all in line, is further review required? Should reviews stop at function or program costs, departmental costs, or line item costs? Obviously, a balance between the detail of reviews and the time, effort, data requirements, etc., of carrying them out must be maintained.

Data and Staff Requirements

Two other concerns with regard to budget reviews should be mentioned. First, this approach to rate setting almost inevitably leads rate-setting agencies to want hospitals to convert to a uniform chart of accounts, uniform output and productivity statistics, uniform budgeting, and uniform financial reporting, so that finer and finer comparisons can be made. Second, the budget review approach requires more and better staff than projection methods of rate setting (some estimates are as high as one budget reviewer—knowledgeable about both accounting and hospital management—for every ten hospitals), although staff requirements can be moderated somewhat by the use of screening techniques. Rate-setting agencies frequently find it difficult to get an adequate budget from the state and to attract sufficient numbers of qualified personnel.

YEAR END COMPLIANCE

Compliance Check

It appears that an end-of-year "compliance check" process of some sort will become more common in prospective rate setting systems for three reasons:

1. As noted above, it is literally impossible for a rate-setting agency to individually review and approve all of the rates that characterize a typical hospital's rate structure. Rather, after approving a hospital's budget for the prospective year, an agency may simply ask the hospital to propose a set of rates that in its judgment will generate just enough revenue to cover its approved costs at its expected volume. These rates are rarely reviewed in detail, and so a check may be necessary to assure that the rates are not too high.

2. Also, as noted above, per case, per day, and per specific services prospective payment systems tend to encourage hospitals to increase volume, because this acts to increase their operating margins. Hence, a check may be necessary to assure that unreasonable margins are not made as a result of increases in volume (or by deliberately underestimating volume in the budget).

3. A check may also be necessary in attempting to assure that efficient hospitals are rewarded and inefficient hospitals penalized by the prospective payment system.

Goals

The goals of an end-of-year compliance check can be examined by means of the cost-revenue-volume model. Suppose a prospective rate-setting system has determined as a matter of policy that well-run hospitals should receive a certain margin above operating costs. The rate-setting agency reviews and approves (perhaps after modification) hospital budgets and then essentially accepts the set of specific services rates proposed by each hospital as sufficient to generate just enough revenue to cover its approved costs. Figure 5 illustrates this situation. Approved budgeted cost is represented by TC_b, the revenue the approved rates will generate at different volumes by TR_b, the agreed to operating margin by m_b, and the expected volume by v_b.

Operating Margin

The actual operating margin for the prospective year may exceed the agreed to margin m_b for three reasons:

1. The rates proposed by the hospital and approved by the agency may have been "too high" as represented by TR_a (i.e., they may have generated more revenue than necessary to cover approved costs and provide the agreed to operating margin). This is shown by margin m_{a_1}. Presumably, the hospital should not benefit financially from the fact that its rates were set "too high."

2. The actual volume for the year may have exceeded budgeted volume, resulting in margin m_{a_2}. Presumably, the hospital should not benefit from the fact that its actual volume was higher than its budgeted volume.

3. The actual costs for the year may have been lower than budgeted costs, as reflected by TC_{a_3} resulting in margin m_{a_3}. Assuming that the agency's budget review was rigorous and thorough, the additional operating margin achieved in this situation

FIGURE 5

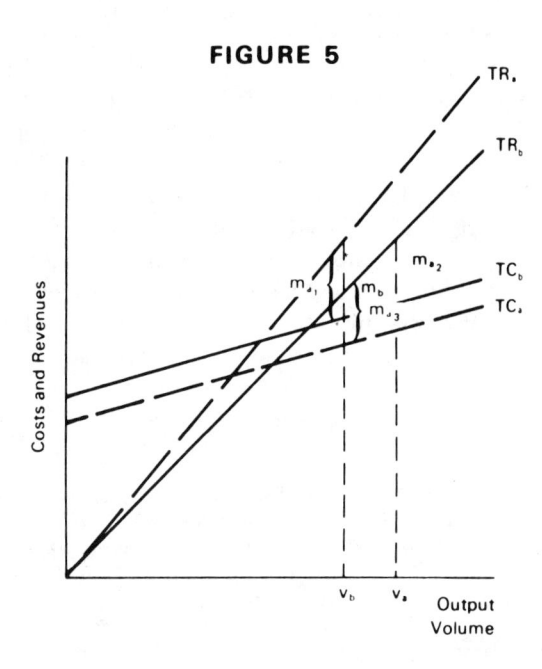

Graph showing Costs and Revenues vs. Output Volume, with lines TR$_a$, TR$_b$, TC$_b$, TC$_a$, and points m_{a_1}, m_b, m_{a_2}, m_{a_3} at volumes V_b and V_a.

can be attributed to improved operating efficiency, and presumably the hospital should benefit from its cost-containment success. In short, it appears that rate setting agencies will begin to develop methods for determining the nature of the surpluses (or losses) that hospitals experience under prospective payment in an attempt to control the system and to make sure that only deserving hospitals are rewarded by it.

POTENTIAL

As this discussion of the dilemmas and problems inherent in translating the concept of prospective rate setting into practice should make clear, prospective payment is not a simple panacea for the cost inflation problem confronting the nation's hospitals. It is not a fully developed, tested, and proven strategy, and much refinement of data, methods, and techniques will be necessary before fair but tight rates can be set with assurance. Moreover, even with refinement, few believe that rate setting, in isolation from controls over facilities, services, and utilization and mechanisms for encouraging consumers and physicians to use hospitals more prudently, can impact significantly on the cost problem.

Despite the problems, however, prospective rate setting appears to have considerable potential. Living under a fixed budget or rate is just fundamentally different from operating under the conventional methods of reimbursement. Prospective rate-setting causes costs to be given more weight in decisions about current operations or future programs. It should lead to better budgeting, planning, cost finding, and cost control. It should make cash flow and revenue more predictable. It may provide a basis for straightening out differences in payment among the different third parties. Perhaps most important, it gives administrators and financial managers a clear mandate to attack the cost problem in their institutions. The critical question is whether the cost containment potential of prospective rate setting can be exploited with enough sensitivity that the quality and financial viability of the hospital system is maintained.

SUGGESTED READING

Bauer, K. "Hospital Rate Setting—This Way to Salvation?" In: *Hospital Cost Containment,* Zubkoff, M. and Raskin, I. (eds.), Milbank Fund, Washington, D.C., 1976.

Bauer, K. and Densen, P. *Some Issues in the Incentive Reimbursement Approach to Cost Containment: An Overview,* Health Care Policy Discussion Paper No. 7, Harvard Center for Community Health and Medical Care, Harvard University, 1973.

Dowling, W.L. "Prospective Reimbursement of Hospitals," *Inquiry* 6:163 (September 1974).

Feldstein, P. "An Analysis of Reimbursement Plans." In: *Reimbursement Incentives for Hospital and Medical Care,* SSA Research Report No. 26 Government Printing Office, Washington, D.C., 1968.

Goldstrom, G. *Prospective Payment to Hospitals: Methods of Rate Determination,* Occasional Papers in Hospital and Health Administration 2, Graduate Program in Hospital Administration, University of California, Berkeley, 1973.

Hardwick, C., Meyers, S., and Woodruff, L. *Incentive Reimbursement: Prospects, Proposals, Plans, and Programs,* Research Series No. 6, Blue Cross of Western Pennsylvania, 1969.

Ludicina, S. *Prospective Reimbursement for Hospitals: A Guide for Policymakers,* Community Service Society of New York, New York, October 1976.

Pauly, M. "Efficiency, Incentives, and Reimbursement for Health Care," *Inquiry* 7:14 (March 1970).

Sattler, F.L. (ed.) *Hospital Prospective Payment—Issues and Experiences,* Interstudy, Minneapolis, Minnesota, June 1976.

Sigmond, R. "The Notion of Hospital Incentives," *Hospital Progress* 50:63 (January 1969); and *Prospective Reimbursement Studies, Experiments, and Demonstrations.* Social Security Administration, U.S. Department of Health, Education, and Welfare, Report to the Congress of the United States, August 1974.

Detailed descriptions of specific prospective rate setting systems can be found in:

Arthur D. Little—

The Prospective Reimbursement Program of Connecticut Blue Cross, Office of Research and Statistics, Social Security Administration, 1974.

The Prospective Reimbursement Programs in the State of Colorado, Office of Research and Statistics, Social Security Administration, 1974.

The Prospective Reimbursement Program of Blue Cross of Northeast Pennsylvania. Office of Research and Statistics, Social Security Administration, 1974.

The Prospective Hospital Rate Review Program for Blue Cross of Wisconsin Payments to Hospitals. Office of Research and Statistics, Social Security Administration, 1974.

The Prospective Reimbursement Program of Blue Cross of Northeast Ohio, Office of Research and Statistics, Social Security Administration, 1974.

Bauer, Katharine G.—

The Combined Budget Review and Formula Approach to Prospective Reimbursement by the Blue Cross of Western Pennsylvania. Harvard Center for Community Health and Medical Care, April, 1974.

Bauer, Katharine G. and Clark, Arva R.—

The New Jersey Budget Review Program. Harvard Center for Community Health and Medical Care, March, 1974.

The Indiana Controlled Charges System. Harvard Center for Community Health and Medical Care, March, 1974.

Budget Reviews and Prospective Rate Setting for Rhode Island Hospitals. Harvard Center for Community Health and Medical Care, February, 1974.

New York: The Formula Approach to Prospective Reimbursement. Harvard Center for Community Health and Medical Care, March 1974.

FOOTNOTES

[1] Although the concepts and issues surrounding prospective rate setting appear applicable to all institutional providers, in actual practice almost all of the operating systems focus on hospitals. Hence, reference is made hereafter to "hospitals" rather than to "providers."

[2] Two additional methods of rate setting have been suggested but not tried: *Determination of reasonable costs of specific services:* The National Advisory Committee on Health Manpower recommended that payment of hospitals be based on: ... a small number of well-defined services or treatments. Those chosen should be well enough defined so that there would be reasonable assurance of meeting the criterion of equal payment for equal services, e.g., certain laboratory or radiology procedures, or the treatment of specified orthopedic or surgical cases. Careful studies would be made to determine the reasonable cost of providing each service. Evaluation would be made of the quality of each service in the participating hospitals. For each one, all hospitals in a locality would receive an equal base payment plus an increment that varied with the standard of service. See: National Advisory Commission on Health Manpower. *Report,* Vol. 1 (Washington, D.C.: GPO, 1967) p. 59; *Bidding:* The bidding method of rate setting might operate as follows: Hospitals should submit bids reflecting their expected costs of producing specific services (for which specifications would be developed), or their expected costs per day. For each service the average of the bids would be accepted as the reasonable cost. If a hospital's actual cost per unit of

service was below its bid, it would be paid its actual cost plus a varying percent of the differences between its actual cost and its bid, the percent depending on how far the hospital's bid was below the average of all bids (to encourage hospitals to make low bids). Hospitals with actual costs above their bid or above the average of the bids would suffer losses. See: Hinderer, H., "Reimbursement: Past, Present, and Future," *Public Control and Hospital Operations,* Graduate Program in Hospital Administration, University of Chicago, 1972, pp. 4-9.

# 37.
Institutional Providers and the Professional Standards Review Organization

KURT DARR

Kurt Darr, J.D., Sc.D., is Professor of Health Care Administration and Assistant Dean - School of Government and Business Administration - The George Washington University.

> ... [I]t is the purpose of this part to assure, through the application of suitable procedures of professional standards review, that the services for which payment may be made under the Social Security Act will conform to appropriate standards for the provision of health care ...
> —*from Declaration of Purpose, Part B, Title XI, Public Law 92-603.*

INTRODUCTION

H.R. 1, the Social Security Amendments of 1972, which passed the United States Congress on October 30, 1972, became Public Law 92-603. This omnibus bill included among its wide variety of amendments one that would shake the health care industry and have profound consequences on the delivery of health care services. This amendment added Part B to Title XI of the Social Security Act of 1935. Section 1151, *et. seq.*, contains provisions for professional standards review, known as PSROs. The purpose of professional standards review is to promote effective, efficient, and economical delivery of health care services of proper quality for any payment of federal monies under Titles 5, 18, and 19 of the Social Security Act, maternal and child health, Medicare, and Medicaid, respectively.*

Former Senator Wallace F. Bennett (R-Utah) is known as the father of PSRO legislation. The ranking minority member of the Senate Finance Committee, he originally sought passage of a bill in 1970; but a PSRO amendment, though approved by the Senate, was never considered by conference committee because it

---

*Relationships between a PSRO and the Title 5, 18, and 19 programs vary because of different state and federal levels of responsibility, i.e., PSRO quality of care review under Title 5 is advisory only, reimbursement decisions are the state agency's; Title 18 is exclusively federal and fiscal intermediaries are specifically directed to pay or withhold payment; and state Medicaid agencies determine coverage decisions, while the PSRO determines medical necessity.

This article was written for this book.

was too late in the legislative session. This proposal contained substantive parts of a peer review program suggested by the American Medical Association.[1] Early in 1972, Senator Bennett introduced another amendment for professional standards review. His statement in the *Congressional Record* leaves no question that he intended PSROs to be controlled by physicians and be educational rather than punitive.[2] But debate about the functions, and the benefit of PSROs continues.

Some proponents of the legislation have stated that a primary purpose is to improve quality of health care services delivered to federal beneficiaries. Others have argued that quality is secondary and that the primary intent of professional standards review is to reduce, or at least limit increases in the cost of providing these services. The evidence points to reduce and limit; both the preamble and the statement of duties and functions of the PSRO make repeated reference to efficiency, effectiveness, medical necessity, and care which can be provided on an outpatient basis—or more economically in an inpatient health care facility of a different type. The law makes only one reference to the quality of these services.

There are problems in the health care field which support both positions. The costs of Medicare and Medicaid have risen sharply, and evidence suggests that quality of care is not what it should be.

PROVISIONS

The legislation directed the Secretary of Health, Education, and Welfare to designate areas wherein professional standards review organizations can be established. The secretary has designated 203 areas. Within each area there is to be a group of local doctors of medicine or osteopathy organized into a voluntary nonprofit PSRO.** The program presumes that physicians (defined by the law as doctors of medicine and doctors of osteopathy) are best qualified to evaluate the quality of medical services, and that the most appropriate means is through a peer review mechanism. Equally important is the determination by these practitioners of the content of care and level of services utilized by the patient. Such requirements begin to address questions of efficiency, effectiveness, and appropriateness.

In any states having three or more PSROs, statewide professional standards review councils must be established. The legislation requires that membership include PSRO representatives, physicians, and public representatives. The councils must also have advisory groups composed of representatives of nonphysician health care practitioners and health care facilities, including hospitals.

The secretary is also directed to establish a National Professional Standards Review Council to: advise the secretary in administration of the law; provide for development and distribution among councils and PSROs of information and data to assist in

---

**PSRO membership must be distinguished from its governing authority. The governing authority is responsible for overall PSRO policy and management. Composed primarily of physicians, it may nonetheless include persons other than physicians and a number do.

carrying out their duties and functions; review operations of statewide councils and local review organizations; advise the secretary on PSRO effectiveness, and make recommendations for improvement. The council is exclusively composed of physicians, eleven in number. The majority must be selected from nominees of national organizations representing practicing physicians. Other members of the council shall include physicians who are recommended by consumers and other health care interests. The limitation on practitioners other than physicians is obvious. The council has only advisory power, but in this respect it has substantial legislatively mandated responsibilities.

The law also provides for review of payment disputes between the PSRO and providers. It specifically identifies section 205 of the Social Security Act as that containing the administrative review process.

Attempts to improve efficiency in the use of health care services and review quality of care are not new for federal government. A plan for utilization review (UR) was a necessary part of hospital participation in Medicare under the original legislation passed in 1965 (P.L. 89-97). The UR plan was required to provide:

1. for the review, on a sample or other basis, of admissions to the institution, the duration of stays therein, and the professional services (including drugs and biologicals) furnished, (a) with respect to the medical necessity of the services, and (b) for the purpose of promoting the most efficient use of available health facilities and services.[3]

The Medicare legislation suggested a variety of general approaches for UR. One, commonly used by hospitals, had a staff committee of the institution review medical care provided for federal beneficiaries. But, in practice UR was performed in only a perfunctory manner. The review provision was never adequately enforced, however, and Congress apparently preferred passage of specific professional standards review legislation to applying existing law.

In the late 1960s, preceding passage of the PSRO legislation, considerable information and insights on medical care appraisal had been developed by the Experimental Medical Care Review Organizations (EMCRO) Program.[4] EMCROs were supported by the National Center for Health Services Research, part of HEW's Health Resources Administration, and were directed to develop methods for assessing objectively the content of office and hospital medical practice.

INHOUSE REVIEW

Under the PSRO legislation, a hospital has the option of developing its own review plan and system, or submitting data on federal patients for review by the area professional standards review organization. It is likely that most larger hospitals will choose inhouse review, or be asked to do it by the PSRO. An important reason to implement inhouse review is that hospital control will seem desirable to many governing authorities and medical staffs—despite the requirement for approval and PSRO scrutiny of the program. This advantage diminishes if, as is likely, PSRO review becomes increasingly stringent and burdensome. Smaller hospitals may join in a cooperative inhouse review effort; otherwise they might be unable to afford to meet program criteria and the PSRO would perform the review.

Because of the large number of federal discharges, approximately 15 million in 1978, there are likely to be substantial problems in processing the tremendous volume of data generated for PSROs. In addition, the need for a uniform hospital data set and format is obvious.

It is distinctly advantageous for the fledging PSRO network that hospitals conduct inhouse review. Inhouse review will substantially ease the initial burden of data systems and personnel which would otherwise have to be provided by the PSRO. The PSRO would have an opportunity to develop its own capability. Should external review predominate, implementation of the program would be further delayed. Indeed, some financially hard-pressed PSROs are requesting that hospitals do in house review

If a hospital chooses external review other problems arise. Most hospitalized patients are not federal beneficiaries. To be accredited by the Joint Commission on Accreditation of Hospitals the care of representative numbers of all hospital patients must be reviewed. Also, other third party payors, e.g., Blue Cross and commercial insurance carriers, are beginning to demand the same kind of review mandated by PSRO legislation. The law permits contracts with PSROs for review of these private patients. These increased emphases make it impossible for hospitals to ignore evaluation of care for nonfederal beneficiary patients. However, the impracticality and expense of dual systems makes it necessary that there be one approach, whether internal or external.

PSRO ACTIVITIES

PSRO legislation requires three independent activities; concurrent review, medical care evaluation studies, and profile analysis. Concurrent review ascertains medical necessity and appropriateness of admission* and continued stay. Medical care evaluation (MCE) studies are short-term retrospective studies analyzing the results of medical care and the medical management practices within the facility. Profile analysis is designed to provide retrospective displays of trends for both physicians and hospitals, and, therefore, care provided for the patients. Concurrent review may be delegated to the hospital; MCE is a shared activity; and profile analysis is exclusively PSRO.

The legislation states that PSRO membership must be composed of a "substantial" number of physicians and osteopaths practicing within the designated PSRO area. This provision is based on the presumption that effective peer review requires broad physician commitment and participation. "Substantial" has been interpreted by the Secretary of HEW to mean 25 percent, and guidelines have put the minimum number at 300 and the maximum at 2,500.

---

*Each PSRO is authorized to assess the medical necessity and appropriateness, prior to admission, of any health care service which is to be provided on an elective basis.

Individual PSROs must develop criteria and norms of care and treatment from practice patterns in their geographic region. These will be compared with standards (desired levels of compliance with criteria or norms). Nonphysician reviewers will identify exceptions for review by physician members of the PSRO. The legislation gives the PSRO authority to make final determinations of medical necessity and appropriateness for purposes of payment. A major problem is developing norms by diagnosis specific enough to be meaningful, and acceptable to physicians.

IMPLEMENTATION AND PROBLEMS

Implementation of PSRO legislation has been slower than expected. It is anticipated that by early 1978 (six years after enactment) approximately one-half of the areas designated by the secretary will have conditional PSROs, reviewing approximately five million hospital discharges. During this conditional period (which may not exceed two years and can be terminated by 90 days notice by either the secretary or the PSRO) the PSRO must implement review programs for care rendered to hospital inpatients and also that provided in long-term care facilities. If satisfied that the PSRO can adequately perform the basic functions and activities required for both types of facilities under the law, the secretary denotes the PSRO as "fully designated," and removes its conditional status. If requested and approved, PSROs have legislative authority to review ambulatory care services. The latter activity is not likely to occur for several years.

Several problems with professional standards review have caused substantial controversy in the health care field and consequently have delayed implementation. Initially, many physicians were hostile. They viewed PSROs as inappropriate federal intervention into the private practice of medicine. A number of physician groups, primarily county and state medical associations, went on record as officially opposed to establishing PSROs. There were modest efforts by organized medicine in Congress to have the legislation repealed; however, repeal is no longer considered viable. Since its adoption, the opposition by physicians has softened somewhat, and there are evidences of increasing cooperation.

A second problem has been the provision of federal funds to assist in establishing conditional PSROs. Congressional support for proposed funding levels has been less than enthusiastic. The retirement of Senator Wallace Bennett, who was a staunch advocate of PSROs, may have had some impact on congressional funding levels. Nonetheless, available funding (Fiscal 1978—$147 million)* is sufficient to sustain program development, albeit at a slower pace.

The PSRO mandate is very broad, and this has resulted in administrative controversies and unclear jurisdictional lines. The agencies and bureaus involved in develop-

---

*Of this amount, $72 million is available for PSRO development and nonhospital review activities (funded from general revenues), and $75 million is available to perform hospital review activities (funded from Medicare Trust Funds).

ing PSROs have been subject to a number of reorganizations. These difficulties resulted in delays of the regulations implementing the legislation and initial designation of areas.

There are other potential administrative problems. PSROs are characterized as autonomous organizational units, yet they are required to comply with federal policies, procedures, regulations, and pressures from other components in the health care system. The extent to which PSROs will be able to maintain autonomy is questionable.

It should be noted there are a number of areas of activity within hospitals for which PSROs are not responsible. PSROs do not determine whether charges are reasonable. They are not necessarily responsible for hospitalized patients other than federal beneficiaries. If a hospital does not develop an internal review system, the PSRO can only review the care provided for patients who are federal beneficiaries under titles 5, 18, and 19. PSROs do not determine internal management efficiency except as it relates to the patterns of utilization and the internal review which a hospital may develop.

The Health Standards and Quality Bureau in DHEW does not determine national health goals, priorities, or appropriate levels of care, nor the measurement of the quality of that care. The PSRO legislation does not establish a national health insurance system; however, one cannot ignore the importance of PSROs if a national health insurance program were enacted.

ISSUES AND QUESTIONS

The establishment of PSROs has raised a number of issues and questions. Reputedly, PSROs were established to insure that quality medical care is being received by certain patients. To date, the Health Standards and Quality Bureau has provided little guidance to assist PSROs and institutions in identifying what quality care is and how it may be measured. When one considers there will be 203 PSROs, all authorized to develop criteria, norms, and standards* defining the care for each diagnosis, it would appear to be very difficult to insure comparability on a national basis, especially for medical problems which have significant regional variations in frequency and treatment patterns. However, there is some information about the long-term intent at the federal level. HEW has contracted with the American Medical Association to assist in developing national criteria for judging hospital care.

A basic underlying assumption of the PSRO legislation is that medical practitioners will respond to information about the quality of their practices—the educational com-

---

*HEW has proposed the following definitions: *criteria*—predetermined elements of health care, developed by health professionals relying on professional expertise, prior experience, and the professional literature, with which aspects of the quality, medical necessity, and appropriateness of a health care service may be compared; *norms*—numerical or statistical measures of usual observed performance of health care services; *standards*—professionally developed expressions of the range of acceptable variation from a norm or criterion.

ponent. This is not an unreasonable assumption. But no relationship between medical education and the quality of a practitioner's performance has been established,[5] and there is evidence to the contrary. The Commission on Professional and Hospital Activities at Ann Arbor, Michigan, has been providing physicians in hospitals with feedback about their practices for more than twenty years. Its director, Dr. Vergil Slee, recently concluded that in the vast majority of situations physicians do know what should be done.[6] For their own reasons they choose a different course of action. This suggests substantial questions about the value of education in modifying behavior and increases the prospects for punitive measures through government intervention.

Questions of cost-benefit ratios in PSRO development have never been addressed. Except for some medical care foundations, there are too few pre-PSRO data available in PSRO areas. Therefore, truly meaningful studies of the impact of PSROs may be impossible. Included under this rubric is the situation where physicians have under-utilized health care services in treating a patient.

An important part of the rationale for PSROs were allegations of a chronic problem with over-utilization of medical care services. Nowhere has the question of under-utilization been addressed. Assuming that each PSRO will develop a systematic set of utilization guidelines and medical practice criteria, it seems reasonable to conclude that providers who had previously been under-utilizing certain types of services would be prompted, if not compelled, to include them in all medical regimens. These patients will have increased utilization and consequently increased costs. It may be argued that requiring certain content in medical practice will enhance the quality of care; however, such regimentation ignores the not insignificant portion of medical practice which is still an art and not yet a science.

Preliminary evidence from some hospitals shows that initially presence of PSRO review has led to increased length of stay. This may be a result of PSRO norms permitting longer stay than that allowed by the hospital's existing utilization review program. It does, however, provide some indication about the problem of under-utilization.

Bureaucracies are often inflexible and unresponsive to change. Although PSROs presently must develop criteria, norms, and standards based on local medical practice patterns, this is likely to be an interim arrangement. The trend in courts of law is that physicians sued for malpractice are held to a national standard—the locality rule is disappearing. A similar situation may develop for PSROs. This will mean that innovations and changes in medical practice will have to undergo a bureaucratic as well as a professional test of acceptability.

The establishment of PSROs is based on the continued dominance of allopathic medicine in the United States. This theory of medical practice holds that where the body's functioning deviates, a counteracting force is applied. It presumes a general similarity among patients with the same diagnosis and a general similarity in treating disease, and therefore minimizes individual differences in patients.[7] The ability of PSROs to assess quality (appropriateness) of care by analyzing patterns of practice will be diminished to the extent to which medicine learns about individuals. Behavior patterns, genetic makeup, stress, life style, psychological components of illness, and responses to environmental stimuli are only now beginning to be understood as important. An increase in number and importance of nonquantifiable factors or a large number of records which require individual analysis will make PSRO review prohibitively expensive. PSROs may encourage cookbook medicine which will reduce the responsiveness of medical practitioners to individual patients—a diminution in the quality of care—when the statistics will show that the quality of care based on other criteria has increased. Truly, a paradox.

CONCLUSION

A mechanism such as the Professional Standards Review Organization was an inevitable result of large scale federal involvement in the financing of health services. Congress has a responsibility to scrutinize how public monies are used. The trend will be toward even more regulation as efforts are made to fine-tune the process. Little serious consideration will be given to lessening the federal role in the field, thereby eliminating one need for regulation. It may well be necessary for PSROs to assume a punitive posture if education is not effective in modifying physician behavior. Even more highly unpredictable is whether physician dominance of PSROs will continue, especially if the regulatory purpose, as opposed to the educational, becomes predominant. As with so many federal programs, the extent to which PSROs successfully meet legislative and regulatory objectives may never be clear.

BIBLIOGRAPHY

Bennett, Wallace. "Professional Standards Review Organization." *Jounal of the Kentucky Medical Association* 71(February 1973): 96-100.

Bonner, Paul, and Decker, Barry, eds. *PSRO: Organization for Regional Peer Review.* Cambridge, Mass.: Ballinger Publishing Co., 1973.

Flashner, Bruce; Reed, Shirley; Coburn, Robert; and Fine, Philip. "PSROs." *Journal of the American Medical Association* 223(1973): 1473-84.

Slee, Vergil. "PSRO and the Hospital's Quality Control." *Annals of Internal Medicine* 81(July 1974): 97-105.

Tucker, Jeanne, and Rogers, Jane. "New Federal Regulations, PSRO, JCAH and Criteria Development." *Medical Record News* 46(February 1975): 24-37.

U.S., Congress, House. *Compilation of the Social Security Laws,* Vol. 1, 93d Cong., 1st sess. Washington, D.C.: Government Printing Office, 1973.

U.S., Department of Health, Education, and Welfare, Health Services and Mental Health Administration, National Center for Health Services Research and Development. *Experimental Medical Care Review Organization (EMCRO) Programs.* Washington, D.C.: Government Printing Office, 1973.

U.S., Department of Health, Education, and Welfare, Health Care Financing Administration, Health Standards and Quality Bureau. *PSRO Factbook.* Washington, D.C.: Government Printing Office, 1977.

U.S., Department of Health, Education, and Welfare. *PSRO Program Manual.* Washington, D.C.: Government Printing Office, 1974.

Welch, Claude. "PSROs–Problems and Prospects." *New England Journal of Medicine* 289(9 August 1973): 291-95.

FOOTNOTES

[1] Initially the American Medical Association (AMA) had opposed the concept of a formal utilization review committee or plan.[a]

In 1965 Representative King and Senator Anderson introduced H.R.1/S.1 (a new variation of their proposal), which expanded the concept of a utilization review committee and defined it more specifically. The AMA at this time gave limited acceptance by supporting Blue Cross administration of utilization committees (which would monitor and evaluate the effectiveness of review).[b]

Representative Mills introduced H.R. 6675 (incorporating the King-Anderson approach and two other proposals), and stipulated medicare utilization review requirements similar to those in H.R. 1. The AMA, though still opposed to utilization review, recommended provisions guaranteeing immunity from civil liability for members of review committees.[c] The bill passed (Senator Bennett voted against) and was signed into law on 30 July 1965, Public Law 89-97.

Later in the 89th Congress, the Senate Finance Committee showed continued interest in Medicare/Medicaid. Some congressmen introduced bills to limit the two programs; most other proposals sought to greatly expand coverage and benefits. Senator Frank Moss introduced S. 3436 to extend state plan requirements under Medicaid; some of those requirements related to utilization review and would have extended functions of the National Medical Review Committee to include Medicaid as well as Medicare.

Representative Mills introduced H.R. 5710 in the 90th Congress, which would have increased the membership of the National Medical Review Committee and would have eliminated initial physician certification requirements for inpatient hospital services. (The AMA opposed certification and recommended deletion of recertification provisions.[d]) Senator Moss reintroduced his proposal, S. 1661, and added requirements for recordkeeping by persons and institutions. Representative Mills introduced H.R. 12080 (a new version of H.R. 5710), which would have eliminated the National Medical Review Committee (it had not been formed yet) and transferred its functions to the Health Insurance Benefits Advisory Council, established in P.L. 89-97. The Moss amendment (recordkeeping) was incorporated and H.R. 12080 became law on 2 January 1968, Public Law 90-238. (Senator Bennett voted against.)

In the 91st Congress with the cost spiral upward, the Senate Finance Committee ordered a staff study. There was a significant gap between estimated utilization of benefits and actual utilization of benefits. The committee staff believed utilization review procedures were at fault.[e,f] The administration submitted a new proposal, the Health Cost Effectiveness Amendments. This bill gave the government increased authority to withhold payment, and in this connection the Secretary of HEW would create a national program of medical review and evaluation, and appoint one or more review teams in each state. The AMA did not object to utilization review per se at this juncture, but cited the tremendous burden on the review committee. (Also note that testimony here by Blue Cross was a precursor to the "area" approach, and that the AFL-CIO recommended a combination of the "local" concept with the use of norms. These components of PSROs were later to be synthesized into a comprehensive whole.)[g]

The Senate Finance Committee responded to its staff report almost immediately by holding more hearings. Chairman Long said: "This medicare program is completely out of hand...." After a few days of hearings, the investigation was delegated to a five-member Subcommittee on Medicare and Medicaid. Senator Anderson, the father of Medicare, and Senator Bennett, the father of PSROs, were members.

At this point the AMA abandoned its "hold-the-line" position. "We feel that peer review is necessary and we have a program of peer review which we plan to submit at a later date."[h] This AMA program would be the concept which Senator Bennett would use significantly in drafting his PSRO legislation.

Thus, by mid-1970 all necessary elements for a drastic revision of Medicare and Medicaid utilization review procedures were established. That is, sufficient analysis, study, and discussion of the problems involved had transpired to warrant the institution of a major revision. The medical profession had conceded that alterations were necessary. A medium for change would soon be provided through a traditional all-inclusive revision bill by Representative Mills. And, Senator Bennett was sufficiently acquainted with the problem to create a solution.

- a. U.S., Congress, House, Committee on Ways and Means, *Hearings on H.R. 4222/S. 509,* 87th Cong., 1st sess., 1961, vols. 145-146, pp. 1321-22 (vol. 146 begins on page 12950); and U.S., Congress, House, Committee on Ways and Means, *Hearings on H.R. 3920/S. 880* (based on Anderson S. 3565), 88th Cong., 1st and 2d sess., 1963, vols. 125-126, pp. 663-64 (vol. 126 begins on page 603).
- b. U.S., Congress, House, Committee on Ways and Means, *Hearings on H.R. 1/S. 1,* 89th Cong., 1st sess., 1965, vol. 139, p. 287.
- c. U.S., Congress, Senate, Committee on Finance, *Hearings on H.R. 6675,* 89th Cong., 1st sess., 1965, vol. 198, p. 615, and Appendix 1, Hearing 4.
- d. U.S., Congress, House, Committee on Ways and Means, *Hearings on H.R. 5710,* 90th Cong., 1st sess., 1967, vols. 140-141, p. 1660 (vol. 141 begins on page 1197).
- e. U.S., Congress, Senate, Committee on Finance, *Hearings on Medicare and Medicaid,* 91st Cong., 1st sess., 1969, vol. 282, pp. 47-48.
- f. U.S., Congress, Senate, Committee on Finance Staff, *Medicare and Medicaid—Problems, Issues, and Alternatives,* 91st Cong., 2d sess., 1970.
- g. U.S., Congress, House, Committee on Ways and Means, *Hearings,* 91st Cong., 1st sess., 1969, vols. 183-184, AMA, p. 1425; Blue Cross, p. 1706-09; AFL-CIO, p. 1789 (vol. 184 begins on page 1413).
- h. U.S., Congress, Senate, Committee on Finance, *Hearings on Medicare and Medicaid,* 91st Cong., 2d sess., 1970, vol. 283, p. 649.

[2] U.S., Congress, Senate, *Congressional Record,* vol. 118, no. 152, pp. S16111-12.

[3] P.L. 89-97, Section 1861 (k).

[4] U.S., Department of Health, Education, and Welfare, Health Services and Mental Health Administration. National Center for Health Services Research and Development, *Experimental Medical Care Review Organizations.* (Washington, D.C.: Government Printing Office, 1973), p. v.

[5] Richard Greene, *Assuring Quality in Medical Care: The State of the Art* (Cambridge, Mass.: Ballinger Publishing Co., 1976), p. 139.

[6] Vergil N. Slee, "PSRO and the Hospital's Quality Control," *Annals of Internal Medicine,* 81 (July 1974), p. 103.

[7] Brian Inglis, *Fringe Medicine* (London: Faber and Faber, 1964), p. 15.

Health Care Policy Issues

This section addresses broad policy issues such as regulation and national health insurance. Selection 38, "THE CRISIS IN THE HEALTH CARE SYSTEM: A CONTRARY OPINION" by S. David Pomrinse, describes the many factors and problems of health care delivery. Policy questions such as system reorganization, paying and organizing physician providers, and education and use of medical personnel are addressed. David B. Starkweather describes in Selection 39 the potential impact of hospital regulation in "WHAT CAN BE LEARNED FROM REGULATION OF OTHER INDUSTRIES?" The analogies and comparisons drawn are useful in understanding the benefits and problems. In discussing the implications of regulation for the hospital field, the writer reaches some rather startling conclusions. In Selection 40, "POLICY CONSIDERATIONS IN NATIONAL HEALTH INSURANCE," Kurt Darr identifies and discusses the issues inherent in any national health insurance program. He describes the major previous congressional attempts to enact NHI. The article is especially concerned with questions of how to achieve equity for all consumers of health care service under such a program. The final Selection, "HEALTH AND PUBLIC POLICY" by Herman M. Somers, describes a number of health care policies developed by federal government and their positive and negative aspects. It concludes with a discussion of the relationships between health policies and goals, health care services, and health.

38.

The Crisis in the Health Care System: A Contrary Opinion

S. DAVID POMRINSE

S. David Pomrinse, M.D., is Executive Vice President, Mount Sinai Hospital, and Edmond A. Guggenheim Professor of Administrative Medicine, The Mount Sinai School of Medicine.

When I was thinking about a title for this paper, I considered a number of possibilities. One thought recurred with great regularity, and I shall use it both as a subtitle and a continuing theme: "It ain't simple." Any discussion of health care in the United States must address itself to the intrinsic complexities involved or it will be caught in the trap (or should I say clap-trap) of over-simplification which one finds in most of what is written on this subject. The erroneous conclusions drawn from such over-simplification end up being included in many of the proposed solutions. I do not trust easy anwers to complicated problems. If I leave you with nothing else, I hope you will at least be challenged to question glib, superficial solutions to the problems of a group of perhaps the most subtly interacting systems in our society. For we are dealing not with a single health care system, nor with the pejoratively titled "non-system," but with many systems. If we truly had a non-system 3 million health workers would be unable to treat 200 million Americans with any effectiveness, death and morbidity rates would have skyrocketed and our institutions would not function at all.

Let me list some of the systems we do have. Among others, we have systems for private practice, for institutional care, for manpower development, for governmental service, for research, for special target population groups, for financing, for regulation, for the maintenance of professional values, for the protection of workers' rights, for the promotion of quality, etc. The surprising thing is not that the interplay among these systems doesn't work perfectly, but that the group of systems works as well as it does. I have yet to learn how perfection can be measured, and I have certainly not learned how it can be attained in all parameters at once, since one of the basic concepts of systems analysis is that of trade-offs: substituting all or part of one goal in

---

Reprinted by permission from *Hospital Administration* (currently *Hospital and Health Services Administration*): *Quarterly Journal of the American College of Hospital Administrators,* Chicago, Vol. 19 (Winter 1974), pp. 10-29. Copyright 1974 by the American College of Hospital Administrators. All rights reserved.

favor of more complete attainment of another. We simply cannot have all the many health services instantly available to everybody, provided by expert practitioners at minimal cost.

A RULE TO APPLY

The title of this paper is "A Contrary Opinion." The term is used in the same sense that it is in stock-market forecasting where the presumption is that when everybody is thinking the same way, the smart trader acts in the opposite way. If everybody's buying, sell! At the moment, in the health field, everybody's buying "crisis," "inefficiency," "HMO," and "national health insurance." Contrary opinion would question whether there is a crisis, how efficient we are, what's good about fee-for-service and what's good about our present insurance arrangements. Obviously, I'm not suggesting that all is well and that we must not change a thing. My basic point is that we may be much better off as a nation by keeping what is good and adjusting those parts of the systems that appear to need it without destroying the fundamental ability of the system to function. Every physician is taught the fundamental rule of pharmacology: *primum non nocere*—above all, do no harm. Let's apply that rule to health care system planning.

Having introduced a medical concept, let's examine the problem the way a physician approaches his patient. First, he takes a history. Our patient, the health care system, appeared to be vigorous, growing in a healthy fashion, and well-loved (we mustn't forget his mental health) as long as his image was dominated by the friendly general practitioner who charged fees according to the patient's ability to pay, and by the relatively small voluntary hospital with a warm and involved community relationship, willing and able to support its modest deficits by fund-raising efforts. However, lest we forget, almost 40 years ago, in the midst of these halcyon days, the Committee on the Costs of Medical Care recommended many of the same organizational and financing changes which are widely touted today. This Committee may have been exceedingly far-sighted or they may have been guilty of over-prescribing.

But the picture I have painted of the family doctor and the protective hospital was slowly but inexorably changed by the accelerating pace of technology. The most able physicians were not satisfied passing out sugar pills and sugar-coated philosophy when more accurate methods of diagnosis and more effective modes of treatment became available. So the leaders of medicine became specialists and trained young doctors in their own image, and gradually a series of professional and academic rewards developed which, in turn, led to a financial reward system favoring the specialist over the generalist. The specialist, of course, needs more sophisticated equipment, and more and better prepared nurses and technicians, and he demanded that the hospital supply them. You are all familiar with what this has done to hospital costs, and since larger hospitals are better able to meet the needs of specialists and super-specialists it has led to increased hospital size. The need for around-the-clock medical coverage and the desire to train more young physicians led to an enormous growth in the size of house staffs, another large component of cost.

INCREASE OF EFFECTIVE DEMAND

But what of more recent history? The nation decided that as a matter of public policy, health care was to be considered a right, and arranged for financial support for the aged and the poor through Medicare and Medicaid since these two groups were least able to pay for their own care. What happened? As the economists say, effective demand increased; the supply of doctors, nurses and beds was fixed, so, as could have been predicted, the price went up. The concept of donated services by volunteer physicians disappeared. Because of open-ended cost reimbursement, hospital employees through their unions were able to demand and get sharply increased salaries. Hospitals were able to and did increase their programs and services in response to professional as well as community demands, thus adding to cost escalation. Predictably, governments reacted by reducing eligibility for their programs and restricting payment both to physicians and institutions. In other words, having whetted the appetite of the consumer for service, governments said: "Oh yes, health care is a right, but we didn't realize it would be so expensive so it must be the providers' fault." Unfortunately, the law of supply and demand has not been repealed and if demand is significantly increased and supply held constant, prices will rise and all the control techniques can do is slow the rise, not stop it.

So much for our patient's history. The next step in the physician's problem-solving approach is to do a physical examination and to look at each of the patient's visible organs to see what he can find.

Cost inflation in hospitals is constantly identified as a particularly troubled part of the total health care system. We know that *per diem* costs have been rising at more than twice the rate of the total Consumer Price Index. The conclusion is then drawn that it must be because we are inefficient.

USE OF STRIKE THREAT

Salaries and fringe benefits constitute about 75 percent of total hospital costs and the rate of increase in salary levels has been far greater than that of the average worker. Unskilled hospital workers, with the effective assistance of their unions, have moved from being among the lowest paid service workers in this region to being the highest paid. And this increase has perforce rippled up through the skilled, technical, and professional employees. A key reason for the inordinate rate of increase has been the use of the strike threat, a perfectly acceptable mechanism in industry where decisions can be made on purely economic grounds, but totally inappropriate in a hospital where the decision to take a strike is a decision to permit some patients to die. Interestingly enough, the cost of local city government has also been increasing at a rate similar to that of hospitals and for much the same reason: the city cannot tolerate a strike either.

The other reason for hospital inflation is a change in the mix of services. Ten years ago Mount Sinai had no intensive care units, no coronary care unit and essentially no cardiac surgery program. Each of these is vastly more expensive than the cost of an average patient day. Yet they are included in total hospital service costs, so the average cost of all patient days goes up. American industry has a historical increase in productivity of 3 percent per year. In hospitals, productivity is measured by considering how many man-hours it takes to produce a patient day or a clinic visit. This productivity figure has declined about 3 percent per year, reflecting these newer, more expensive services. Incidentally, the demands of governmental agencies for higher standards of patient care and more complex reporting systems have added significantly to the reduction in productivity.

Let's look at inefficiency—inefficient compared to what? Some months ago, we put together our costs for operating the Mount Sinai Hotel, including everything we would have to spend if all we took care of were healthy people. Our total expense, including room service from a selective menu three times a day, was about half what a guest would be charged in one of the better commercial-level hotels in New York. Yes, the hotel pays taxes and shows a profit, but still we must be doing something right! This doesn't mean we can't be more efficient, but the potential for major savings is small. Interestingly enough, our hotel costs were only 20 percent of our total costs. In other words, 80 cents out of every dollar pays for patient care, professionally related costs which are much less amenable to comparison with the commercial world, and are generated and controlled more by the doctor than by the hospital manager.

HIGH RATE OF INFLATION

Inflation of hospital costs is not just an American phenomenon. Average hospital costs in England, Sweden, and Canada have been inflating at a slightly greater rate than ours and yet each of those countries has one form or another of governmental control of hospitals. The politicians like to say that if we don't control costs, they'll take us over. I say fine; if you do, the rate of inflation will quicken and God help the quality of care. It won't even be safe. The only two areas of the economy inflating at a higher rate than hospital costs are construction and the cost of local government, and for many of the same reasons.

This brings us to the physician. He initiates use of the hospital by having the patient admitted, he orders all those tests and procedures (X-ray use is increasing over 10 percent a year compounded), and he determines when to discharge the patient. In hospitals, we surround him with all sorts of bureaucratic controls which are being extended to his office practice in the hope of reducing expenditures. Payments to physicians constitute about 22 percent of the health care dollar and about one-third of that goes to pay his overhead. This net 15 percent of all health care expenditures, which is the doctor's income, is sufficient to develop an annual average income of just over $40,000 per year for America's practitioners, putting them in one of the highest income brackets in this country. By comparison with other countries, we treat our doctors well. Yet the potential for saving money by limiting his income is small—some percentage of the 15 percent. On the other hand, if he is motivated to use fewer hospital days, fewer nursing home beds, less expensive drugs, etc., the potential is enormous.

A REORGANIZATION SYSTEM

How about reorganization of doctors into group practice? According to *Medical Economics*, the average physician in a group practice nets a bit more than his solo practice colleague. He is also a bit more productive, but there's no magic in group practice, unless the financing mechanism and the incentive system are changed also. We presently reward doctors for over-utilizing—the more visits, the more hospital days, the more surgical procedures, the higher the individual doctor's income. One of the prime reasons for this reverse incentive system is, I believe, the split between Blue Cross and Blue Shield. The payments the doctor receives bear little relationship to the hospital bill and indeed most physicians have no idea of the size of the patient's hospital bill and, consequently, little reason to be concerned about it.

Possibly the most important organ of our medical care system is money. The importance of money is not its gross amount, but the way it flows and the actions this flow causes. It is impossible to argue that there is not enough money going into medical care in this country when we spend 7.4 percent of our Gross National Product and other industrialized countries spend around 5 percent. If we were spending less than 5 percent, mine would be one of the loudest voices calling for more total dollars. But there's enough money in the pot, So how about its flow?

What happened when the flow to hospitals was in the form of open-ended cost reimbursement is a matter of record. With no external reason to say no, salary levels soared, physicians' requests for staff were honored, new programs were started and hospitals reached out to their communities. Recent changes in reimbursement levels and techniques have put an abrupt halt to this approach.

The doctor has almost always been paid on a fee-for-service basis. This is both good and bad. It's good because it makes him clearly responsible to his patient. It's bad because it tends to encourage over-utilization. How about the alternatives to fee-for-service? There are really only two. The first is salary. If a doctor knows he will not profit from unnecessary care, he is less likely to provide it. The problem with salaried physicians is that they tend not to work as hard, as a carefully done study by Maloney of UCLA has shown. Unfortunately, doctors are not immune to the civil service mentality so that we must be concerned also with productivity. Consider what would happen if America's doctors who now work a 60-hour week were all to become salaried and work a 40-hour week; we'd need 50 percent more doctors!

A MONTHLY PAYMENT FEE

The other alternative method to pay doctors is by having them share in the net proceeds of partnership income. If the partners charge on a fee-for-service basis, no special economies are likely to result. However, if the group collects prepayment on a monthly basis from subscribers, it is to its advantage to reduce expenditures, particularly if the members share in any reduction of hospital use. Certainly the experience of the Kaiser plan must be noted where significantly fewer hospital days per thousand members are used than in the general population. Dr. Herbert Klarman has shown that when appropriate statistical corrections are made, the saving in hospital days is about 20 percent. One cannot help but wonder, however, how much under-treatment occurs in the Kaiser system, and whether adequate consideration is given to the 15 percent of care which their members buy in the fee-for-service market, even though they've already paid for total care under the prepayment mechanism. In summary, no technique for paying doctors is perfect since each method tends to encourage either over-utilization or under-utilization and the latter may be hazardous to health. Fortunately, the great bulk of physicians are basically honest and make their decisions on professional grounds. But as a former practitioner I can testify that economic considerations cannot help but sway marginal decisions on individual patients, and if we can structure payment mechanisms to encourage appropriate utilization of all health services, we will have made a most valuable contribution to the American health system.

Is there evidence that, properly organized and controlled, private practicing physicians will reduce hospital use and, therefore, cost? Let's look at GHI's experience. They provide fee-for-service medicine at a fixed fee schedule. About half of New York's doctors agree to accept the payment and make no additional charge. Payment for lab and X-ray is made. GHI competes with HIP and Blue Shield to cover New York City employees. They perform careful and effective claims review. Recently, New York City published data which showed that GHI subscribers used only 1 percent more hospital care than HIP and there was, of course, free choice of doctor and no prepaid group practice. Interestingly enough, Blue Shield subscribers used 35 percent more hospital care than HIP—an indication that to make fee-for-service work takes administrative know-how and good controls, but it can work and compete with prepaid group practice.

Another bit of evidence against swallowing the HMO concept whole: the Social Security Administration has published data showing that Medicare patients cared for by prepaid group practice in New York cost 11 percent more per person than those cared for in private practice.

One could examine many other organs of our system, but let us consider just one more: health manpower. I've concentrated on the doctor, but he represents less than 10 percent of all health workers. Largely in response to the growth of technology, we have seen an almost bewildering growth in varieties of personnel working in health, and, consequently, an increasing difficulty in relating them to each other in any rational way. Each group develops a self-protective definition of its functions and defies all others to trespass on its turf. So we have great rigidity in job function which leads to as many as 34 different types of people walking into a patient's hospital room to provide some part of his care. No wonder the patient gets confused and no wonder costs rise. Each group institutionalizes its job definition with credentials and laws and strives for professional status. In New York State, only a physician or a certified X-ray technician may take a chest film—a job that can be taught in a day or two. Yet to be certified as an X-ray technician, one needs two years of training. Nurses are trying to define a job function that has less and less to do with the physician's concept of what the patient needs; so a new group of people called physician's associates are being trained and will receive credentials in New York State. Right now the most careful hair-splitting of roles for physicians, nurses, and physician's associates is underway. I can see two things happening; initially costs will rise since these new people will have to get paid. Later, if the associates work out as anticipated, we will have fewer nurses. In a sense the nurses will define themselves out of a job since their newer job expectations, no matter how desirable, are not critical to patient care. They may find they've won a battle and lost a war as we learn how to provide care at lower cost using a combination of physician associates and better-trained aides.

PUBLIC ACCEPTANCE OF BASIC SERVICES

As the cost control pressures increase, consumers will have to accept only the more basic services and eliminate the more global efforts to consider total psychosocial and family needs, if they are not relevant to the medical problem at hand. In other words, if the patient sprained his ankle, we'll not be concerned if no member of the health team gets worried about whether his child is doing well in school. In a sense, some health personnel have gone looking for new business instead of just dealing expeditiously with what's at hand. We shall increasingly treat what the patient wants treated and not what the health professional thinks might be good for him, whether or not the extra service has any meaningful value to the patient. This is not to decry preventive medicine, but rather to expect that there will be enough public health education so that patients come to expect effective preventive services and don't consider them "unneccessary." This can work, as the experience with Pap smears has demonstrated.

In performing his work-up, following a physical examination, the physician turns next to the laboratory to gather objective data. Sometimes he over-utilizes the lab; I will try not to be guilty of that wasteful approach in continuing my diagnostic exploration.

Finding data accurate for comparison purposes among various health systems is not simple since the purposes for which the data are collected and, therefore, the format of how they are collected, vary so much. Hospital Administrative Services (HAS) has helped to begin the standardization of operating data, but still has a way to go. Utilization rates for a non-prepaid population can be obtained from special studies based on sampling. But our biggest problem is with output measurements—what did the care accomplish? Until we know definitively what we have done, we can't know how efficiently we've done it. Perhaps the greatest need in this entire field is to concentrate on disability rates, morbidity rates, and mortality rates, rather than on inputs such as personnel and dollars.

MORE MEDICAL SERVICE?

Where outputs have been measured, the organization of care has been directly affected: it was the demonstration of a reduced mortality rate from coronary occlusion in coronary care units which led to the very rapid establishment of these units in almost all hospitals. Unfortunately, crude rates are less than useful. America's relatively high infant mortality rate is used to damn our health care system without considering the effects of the greater social pathology in the ghettoes of this country related to bad housing, and inadequate income for which medical care hardly appears to be the best method of therapy. Contrary opinion would question whether more medical service is a better investment than more food for pregnant women; or whether prepaid group practice would have more of an effect than a rat control program, better elementary education, more jobs or better housing.

Now, as a final diagnostic method, let's put the X-ray on hospital management itself and see whether my earlier comments regarding inefficiency can be supported. Voluntary hospital administrators are constantly accused of poor management because of the excessive rate of inflation, and urged to be businesslike. We're told that Kaiser is very efficient. I concur that as a system it is efficient because it provides only half as many hospital beds per thousand as is provided for the rest of the population in its areas. But as hospital managers, they do not do better than their colleagues. Moreover, do the vaunted techniques of business management actually work at Kaiser hospitals? With the help of statistical consultants, data from 17 Kaiser hospitals on *per diem* cost and length of stay from the guide issue of *Hospitals* were compared with comparable hospitals in the same geographic regions. In summary, there was *no* statistically significant difference either in *per diem* cost or in length of stay between the Kaiser hospitals and those serving the general community.

COMMERCIAL HOSPITAL CHAINS

How about the commercial chains of hospitals? There is no doubt that they can run a hospital at less cost than the voluntary hospitals in the same areas. But they can only do it by eliminating programs which lose money such as education, or clinics, or by providing fewer hours of care per patient per day, assuming that pay scales are comparable. There's no magic involved: if you have as many hours of care multiplied by the same hourly rate, the personnel cost must be equal; personnel costs make up 75 percent of total hospital costs. Therefore, if you want to operate more cheaply you drop high-cost programs and do only bread and butter care; you decide which programs you will operate only on the basis of the bottom line financial result and ignore the community needs for the service.

Voluntary hospitals have always taken the other approach: see what needs to be done and then figure out how to finance it. In the long run, some hospitals will have to perform the necessary but money-losing functions, and the voluntary hospitals had better be kept viable so that they are around to pick up what the commercials reject.

One more point. The essence of good business management is an ability to make sensible long-range plans which lend themselves to necessary short-range modifications. How is one to plan when in the last four years we have had four different reimbursement schemes, some favoring one approach to cost management and some another. (The decision as to whether to lease or buy equipment is one example of this confusion.) Reimbursement controls are in the hands of the same state agency which is responsible for controlling Medicaid expenditures: can the judge be totally unbiased? At labor contract negotiation time, decisions on wages must be made if an unnecessary strike is to be avoided. Yet decisions on payment rates to cover the extra costs must come from three different agencies in normal times and four different agencies this year. At the critical hour, management doesn't know how much money it has. In capital planning we are controlled by an agency which is supposed to guide the hospitals into efficient use of community resources and rational organization of care facilities. Yet this very agency changes its basic policies almost cavalierly and ignores sizable capital expenditures made by individual hospitals in precise accord with its earlier position. I challenge any business executive to maximize efficiency when controlled by multiple, inefficient, poorly coordinated regulatory agencies.

DIAGNOSIS AND TREATMENT

We've completed the data gathering from and about our patient. Now let us proceed to diagnosis and treatment. We shall not use outdated methods of reporting our findings; we shall use the coming method called the "problem-oriented record" which takes each of the major identified problems, tries to establish a cause, recommends a treatment and follows it to cure. Obviously, today we will not be able to report on progress towards cure of any of the proposed solutions since it is not very likely that the patient will take his medicine!

Problem one: Excessive and improper demand. Fueled by money made available with little direct personal involvement, medical care is sought for trivia, for social reasons (clinics are good places to meet your friends), as a substitute for welfare services, for status purposes, and as a relief for psychological pressures. Just think of all the hours of doctor time which would be available if the uncomplicated common cold was barred from the doctor's office—he can't do anything for it anyway. Suppose everyone with a tension headache learned to talk it out with his spouse or his boss. What if lonely old people were really encouraged to visit day centers? These three moves alone would make a sizeable dent in the volume of visits patients make to doctors, reduce cost sharply, and make it possible for doctors to have the time to spend with patients for whom they could do some good. If nothing else, clearing medical care flow would reduce physician boredom and would thus aid greatly in improving patient-physician relationships.

A major public health education campaign is recommended to try to get people to use doctors appropriately for prevention and early treatment but not for functions which non-physicians can perform better than physicians. But such a campaign needs to work and that means mobilizing the entertainment television programs, the comic books and similar behavior-modifying media, not the stultified approaches typical of professional health educators.

Problem two: Manpower. Conventional wisdom argues that since it's difficult to get a doctor to do things he doesn't want to do, practice in a ghetto, make home calls or be available the moment a patient wants him—there must be a shortage of physicians. Contrary opinion points out that demand is elastic and will expand to fit the available resources of physicians and dollars. Thus, the more doctors trained and the more money made available by government, the more demand there will be. The result is more money put into health services, not less.

A SUFFICIENCY OF SURGEONS

There is little doubt that we have a sufficiency of many types of physicians such as surgeons, along with a shortage of specialists such as radiologists and, particularly, of generalists. To control the supply of the various specialists we need approval of training programs geared to the national need, not the educational interests of chiefs of services and their staffs. Let's stop creating so many surgeons and the rate of questionable surgical procedures will drop. It's just that simple. And this is the first time I've said anything in this field is simple.

The generalist question is more complex. Anyone trained for six to eight years after high school plus two years of family practice residency has a pretty impressive image of himself. Since he studied all those years to gain his union card as a family physician he must be pretty good and able to handle much of the illness he sees. He's taught to be a doctor, a curer. While he's also taught to refer, it's a challenge to his intellect and to his ego to go just a bit further than might be wise. He's taught to make a diagnosis and accept responsibility, and he will. Now what really should he be doing? Since over 80 percent of the conditions which bring people to doctors are self-curing, he must recognize them and treat symptomatically. Perhaps 8 to 10 percent are really too complicated for the generalist and should be referred, but, he may be tempted to handle them himself. So we prepare full-fledged doctors who should intervene therapeutically and make it count in only 10 to 12 percent of the cases they see. What a waste. Think of the boredom facing a man with this much education who functions largely as a referral point. Remember these are highly intelligent people whom we're asking to function basically as technicians. In my opinion, which in all modesty is contrary to that of the United States Congress, most medical educators and leading professional societies, we don't need any more primary care generalist physicians. We need more primary care technicians who can do the sorting function and refer the 20 percent which require specific intervention to the appropriate specialists. The primary care technician is another name for the physician's associate. Having no more than four years of higher education, belonging to a group whose intelligence levels are a notch below that of the physician, presenting no self-image as a scientist and not trained to be the last word on anything, he is far less likely to exceed his proper bounds. If he's paid a salary rather than fees, he has no reason to do so. Will he make mistakes? Of course, but they will be a different quality than that of the generalist physician. He will get scared faster and get help sooner. I believe we should structure a primary care system based on technicians, closely related to those physicians who know them, who can supervise and control them and who will be legally responsible for them.

Within hospitals, I see a cadre of personnel trained as just described who will provide most of the ongoing care under the general orders of a physician. They will do many of the repetitive functions and, in smaller hospitals, will come to replace the foreign-trained house staffs. I see these people, many of them former nurses whose orientation has been changed, becoming the ward generalists. They will either provide or supervise all the care along with a cadre of aides. They will function as pharmacist aides and give medication, take an ECG, draw blood for the laboratory, write histories, do physicals, make observations of patient behavior, do procedures or help with them. Perhaps I've described a Renaissance person and am expecting too much. I don't think so. Such a person working with a small group of patients (six or eight) and doing everything for them would sharply reduce the over-all numbers of personnel needed in a hospital. It would stop the conflict of people from different departments competing for the patient in order to carry out separate functions and give the patient the security of a continuing relationship with one person. Can all this be taught in two to four years following high school? Of course it can. How many doctors have office assistants who do most of these functions and retain for themselves only the critical part of the procedures? How many public health nurses have functioned in patient's homes in this way and kept quiet about it because they're afraid of being accused of practicing medicine? Will it be done? That depends on whether the nurses associations decide to act like the dinosaur and not adapt to a changing world or seize the opportunity of redefining their role in a way that would be fulfilling for the nurses and useful for the nation.

USING THE NURSE

In my contrary opinion, we need control of the numbers and types of specialists and the rapid development of large numbers of primary care technicians who function both in the hospital and out. The reservoir available, with little additional training, to fill this role is the nurse. Longer range, educational programs should be pointed directly at this newer job definition. Money redirected from creating new medical schools would more than suffice to support this education.

Problem three: Access. This refers to the difficulties people have in getting medical care when they think they need it. But this cannot be discussed without looking at organization. Medicine has been called a cottage industry. Some industries should continue to have a large number of small units rather than become totally centralized. On the other hand, doctors do not need to work entirely alone. To my mind, the small multi-specialty group practice of six to ten doctors in association with at least an equal number of primary care technicians is about right. The size permits coverage in the different specialties yet doesn't get so big that it becomes bureaucratic. The group needs and can afford X-ray and lab service, social work, and a business manager. I would like to see these group practice units scattered throughout our cities and rural areas. And, if financing is available, they will be. Doctors don't practice in ghettoes because they can't make a living. Given some form of insurance covering the poor who pay at rates similar to that collected from the middle-class, doctors will move into ghettoes. They started to do this in New York when Medicaid was liberal and moved out again when it was cut back.

GROWTH OF PRIVATE PRACTICE GROUPS

In my opinion, it will be a rare doctor who chooses to work alone in the future, particularly since in a group he would have a pool of primary care technicians to draw on and would not have to be their personnel officer as well as their supervisor. More doctors are joining groups because it's easier on the doctors as well as being better for the patients. And the really rapid growth is not in prepaid groups but in fee-for-service, private practice groups.

Given large numbers of such groups with an on-call roster of physicians and primary care technicians, patients will be able to see someone whom they know is a member of the group and in whom they have confidence. Wouldn't this be better than the commercial home-call services using moonlighting residents which are now springing up in all our cities?

But let me be perfectly clear. I don't mean that such groups should be mandated, but that they will evolve because they tend to be the most satisfactory form of practice arrangement for both patients and for doctors. Government should not use its funds to push doctors into such groups, but rather it should subsidize groups to locate in economically unviable geographic areas if the general method of payment for services is inadequate.

Problem four: Quality. Needless to say, no organizational pattern will be worthwhile if the quality of the service is not at an acceptable level. The conventional jargon says excellence for all. Nonsense, all service cannot be excellent since some physicians are going to be better than others, better being defined in any way you wish. However, all service should be at levels defined from time to time by national bodies as attainable by the majority of practitioners.

Then it must be monitored. One of the most promising methods for such monitoring of care outside the hospital is the medical foundation which uses a claims review technique. My only concern is that the foundations will become so enamored of financial controls that they will forget to watch quality.

For in-hospital care, the organized medical staff now functions in this regard. It is not necessary to create a whole new organizational pattern, but rather to define accepted, objective standards for what is meant by adequate care. How high should the post-operative infection rate be before corrective action is required? What death rate from acute myocardial infarction is considered acceptable? These are value questions having immediate impact on the behavior of doctors, as well as on the cost of care. Until we are prepared to face up to them, discussions of quality have little meaning.

APPROACHES TO FINANCING

Problem five: Money. There are many ramifications of this problem. *The first* is the source of the money to pay for care. As far as I'm concerned this is a political, rather than an economic or operational, question. There's only one source of money, and that's the production stream of the national economy. Whether medical care is paid directly by labor and management as a fringe benefit or whether taxes are paid and the government purchases the care is not as basic as how the care is provided. There's no question that some method of spreading the risk of illness is necessary. The number of organizations who handle the funds is related to administrative cost and should be decided on the basis of how it can be done most economically.

Second. What part of the bill most bothers people? For the young it is the grossly inadequate coverage provided by Blue Cross for obstetrical care; for the middle-aged, the threat of being wiped out by a major illness; and for the poor, the cost of any medical service. We have tried, it seems to me, to do too much for too many with single forms of coverage and, consequently, have not done enough for some and, perhaps, too much for others. We need insurance (or payment) programs aimed at the major economical and medical threats. The alternative is to provide comprehensive coverage for all, medical and dental services to all, recognizing how this would increase effective demand even more, and would raise costs to levels which our political and business leadership would find unacceptable.

Third. How can we give physicians incentives to reduce the costs of hospital care, as well as ambulatory drugs, laboratories, and X-rays? Our present Blue Cross/Blue Shield policies reward the doctor for over-utilization. I have two suggestions. One is to pay the under-utilizing physician at a higher fee schedule than the average and to pay the over-utilizing physician at a lower rate. He'll get the message quickly. The other idea is to award the physician a total amount, and let him pay the hospital bill, keeping the remainder for himself. Watch his length of stay and his unnecessary ordering of lab and X-ray drop! A working, rather than a theoretical model of cost control via physician activity is the medical foundation. By reviewing individual doctor's claims it can spot apparent excessive utilization, and by peer pressure it can help to reduce it. In some foundations there is a total pot of money, and each service is paid for at a percentage of the sum. Don't think there isn't careful scrutiny of claims and firm pressure on the high utilizers.

LOOKING AT HOSPITAL COSTS

Fourth. How about hospital costs? Let's consider *per diem* costs first. They are made up basically of salary rates and levels of care or complexity of service. Until society finds a way to control salary rates in hospitals, costs will rise. And until society says, and means it, that it will settle for less than the best, the levels of care will rise and will increase costs. But let us consider community-wide hospital costs. Here the answer is clearer and simpler. If you want to reduce the cost of hospitalization, reduce the number of beds. This means strong regional planning and a willingness to accept long waiting lists. But if fewer beds are operating, the cost of hospital operation drops. The quickest and surest way to reduce hospital costs is to close one-fourth of the present operating beds in a city, starting with the poorest physical plants. Many communities now have three beds for each 1,000 potential users versus the national four per 1,000. The pain in reorganizing medical staffs and trustee relationships will be great. But until it's done, I will not believe that we want to do something about the high cost of hospital care.

Fifth. What about alternatives to hospitalization? Ambulatory care, home care, extended care facilities, and nursing homes are cheaper units of care, but they all add up as additional services which must be paid for. New services mean new costs. They may reduce the pressure for expansion of hospitals, but they won't save money.

Sixth. We need a national consensus on what we're willing to accept as a level of care. We can't have everything for everybody and expect it to be cheap. We can make the system run better, but we have to translate our value systems into quantifiable terms: How low should the infant mortality be? What percentage of cervix cancer patients should live? How much money are we prepared to spend? These questions are inseparable and must be faced for our solutions to be rational.

A NATIONAL HEALTH INSURANCE SCHEME

Given all of the above, a source of funds, incentives for physicians, identification of special needs of different groups, a reduction of hospital beds and operational targets, we can devise a national health insurance scheme that will work. I don't mean it must be operated by the government; we could legislate mandatory coverage for the working, with payment by government for the indigent. This pragmatic, cautious approach of gradually adjusting components of the total system, while being sensitive to how each change affects the rest of the system, is contrary to the usual one of testing political waters and seeing what will fly. My approach may not garner votes, but it's more likely to work.

I've tried in this paper to cast light, rather than to quote dogma. I've tried to make you see that much of conventional wisdom in the medical care field is based on false assumptions and inadequate data. I've suggested an approach which might correct the present problems and ease the present concerns. But my major concern is that given the complex systems we have in this field, we should try new things carefully and with thorough documentation and study. Let us not force four million health workers and 200 million potential patients into operational modes which may not work. My proposed solutions to individual problems in the total system do not vitiate the basic proposal that we are dealing with extreme complexity. Each change will produce unknown results on other parts of the total system. Without change, we will finally have revolution. With careful change, we can have evolution.

I believe that in a pluralistic society there should be many approaches to health care organization and, given honestly free choice, the best overall system will evolve. It may or may not resemble what I've been describing, but I think these approaches should be tried.

We need diversity in this country. We have thrived so far because of it. We need experimentation. We need to make mistakes and to learn from them. We cannot afford to stop the present medical machinery while we attempt to create something perfect. No human endeavor is perfect, some are less imperfect than others. America now has a superb system of care by expert specialists. It needs to improve its primary care system and its financing mechanisms. Let's adjust our machine to strengthen its weak points and get on with the job of caring for the sick.

A quotation from Isaiah is very apt: "Where there is no vision, the people perish."

What Can Be Learned from Regulation of Other Industries?

DAVID B. STARKWEATHER

David B. Starkweather, Dr. P.H., is Associate Professor of Public Health and head of a group of graduate curricula in Administrative Sciences - The University of California, Berkeley.

There is no question that hospitals *can* be regulated by public utility commissions. This method of controlling hospital affairs, probably at the state level, represents a sudden and dramatic trend in the evolution of events which most certainly are propelling hospitals toward new forms of social control. Whether or not it is justified, public disdain over rising, uncontrolled, and unexplained costs makes commission regulation appear as an attractive and appropriate legislative response.

The singular focus on hospitals is, at least, partially unfair. Given the inseparability of hospital patient care and the practice of medicine, physicians should also be included in any new controls. Further, given the interdependencies between hospitals and health insurance, government reimbursement, the marketing of drugs, the development of medical equipment and the training of virtually all health manpower, the question can legitimately be asked: can regulation of hospitals *alone* achieve the desired social objectives? Nonetheless, as a practical matter, hospitals are the only element in the health system that have the capacity to respond to new forms of regulation (i.e., they can uniformly gather and report operating data, they possess the concentrations of resources which provide the basis of decision making by utility commissions, and they are linked to other elements of the health care industry in a way that makes them attractive conduits for more generalized scrutiny).

It can be argued that hospitals are already regulated to the hilt. Yet, in terms of widely accepted features of commission-type regulation, existing hospital controls are incomplete. These features include the *adequacy of service* which is partially fulfilled by licensure, the *control of market entry* which is represented in some states by hospital franchising laws and the *rate control* which is represented indirectly in some re-

---

Reprinted by permission from *Hospital Administration* (currently *Hospital and Health Services Administration*): Quarterly Journal of the American College of Hospital Administrators, Chicago, Vol. 17 (Spring 1972), pp. 65-72. Copyright 1972 by the American College of Hospital Administrators. All rights reserved.

spects by *indirect* controls of health insurance rates and reimbursement provisos.

Features of typical utility regulation which do not currently hold for hospitals are *uniformly adequate service to* a defined geographic area, *control of market entry regarding services* as compared to beds, *control of abandonment of service* and *direct rate setting*. Thus from the viewpoint of "classical" utility regulation, there remains much with which hospital managements can and must deal: factors affecting the very essence of institutional survival.

IMPLICATIONS OF REGULATED HOSPITALS

There is wide variation in evidence, conclusion and opinion regarding the worth of utility commission regulation as an instrument of public good. Most studies have been undertaken by economists, and they reveal little concerning management implications. Further, there is a dearth of literature which compares and contrasts regulation across various industries. In short, there are few available generalizations which seem suitable for direct application to the management of hospitals as regulated enterprises.

Still, the notion remains compelling that whatever might be extracted from a comparative review of the evolution of regulation in other industries should certainly be used by hospitals as a background for thought and action. Based on such a comparative review, this paper attempts to summarize a few things which appear to be true concerning commission regulation in other industries and couples these with hospital management implications.[1]

The format of presentation is an unusual one: it assumes a highly tentative stage of generalization, based on the fact that analysis in this realm is, by its very nature, of low articulation. Some "syntheses" are stated which represent gleanings from cross-industry inquiry, followed by "implications" which represent useful topics for consideration by hospital managements.

Synthesis:

The distribution of control among firms in an industry is altered by regulation, that is, there is industry restructuring. If regulation is for the purpose of preserving a degree of competition (e.g., trucking), the firms which might not otherwise survive in the free marketplace will be protected. If regulation is for the purpose of controlling a "natural monopoly" (e.g., power), there is a long run tendency towards concentration of firms.

Implication: Hospital and medical care by their very nature are inclined more to the second characterization than the first; the consumer is in no position to make informed choices among competing products. Thus, assuming regulation, the structure of the hospital industry will move towards federations, consortia, mergers, and other forms of institutional concentration. Initiative in these realms rests with hospital administrators.

Synthesis:

Regulation of industries which are "naturally monopolistic" includes the obligation to serve markets which may be unprofitable in their own right. (e.g., long-run passenger runs on railroads).

Implication: Hospitals in a regulated industry may not ignore underserved areas. Hospital concentrations that are permitted or encouraged, and may be justified on efficiency grounds, will also be required to provide at least an adequate level of uniform service to an entire assigned jurisdiction. They may not abandon that service once it is established. This will call for the development of satellite ambulatory care operations, primary care centers backed by specialty-oriented facilities and the careful integration of many health care activities in an area on a multi-location, multi-facility, and multi-function basis. This is a management challenge of the first magnitude.

Synthesis:

Utility regulation is a function of state government, except in cases where interstate commerce is a significant aspect of an industry's activity.

Some examples are the state regulation of insurance, federal regulation of communication, and both state and federal regulation of power production and distribution.

Implication: Since the interstate aspects of hospital care are not apparent, state government is the obvious source of regulatory legislation. This introduces the crucial question of whether hospitals should fall under the supervision of generic, multi-industry, public utility commissions, or whether separate commissions should be created specifically for hospitals. Since hospitals are manifestly different than most other regulated industries, it is in hospitals' best interests to urge the creation of separate commissions. This will take place only if there is effective cooperative activity by hospitals in the political arena.

Synthesis:

Most regulated industries are capital-intensive with regulation based in major part on "rate base" considerations (i.e., the determination of assets which are necessary in order to provide service and upon which return be earned fairly).[2] This simplifies the process of financial review and rate making although it leaves room for dispute over what constitutes a reasonable rate of return. States vary considerably on both the calculation and level of rate-base and rate of return.

Implication: Hospitals are labor intensive enterprises and are both for-profit and nonprofit in corporate form. This substantially complicates the job of rate setting, since the significant capital rate base characterizing most regulated industries is relatively unimportant in the hospital industry. The question of return on non-commercial capital is a complicated matter of public policy which cannot be answered simply for both profit-making and charitable hospitals. New bases of rate setting will need to be established, probably using the "financial requirements" approach,[3] which reduces dependence on rate base and rate of return considerations. Methods of dealing fairly and simply with operating expense considerations will have to be devised in order to avoid severe problems associated with enormously complex tariff schedules.

Only hospital managements have sufficient knowledge to deal with these matters. In the absence of positive initiative, "solutions" will be imposed which have been drawn from other regulated industries and are fundamentally incompatible with the economics of effective hospital service.

Synthesis:

One factor clearly defined by commission regulation is jurisdiction of service. Once this geographic area is spelled out, reasonable demands from within the area must be met, and service may not be abandoned without clear justification. Conversely, a regulated firm may not be forced to go beyond its area of service, although various financial inducements may make it worthwhile to do so, as in the case of rural electrification.

Implication: The definition of service area has plagued hospital and health services planners in most communities, not only because of complicated patient referral patterns but because most hospitals have overlapping service areas. Access by all people in a defined jurisdiction to a uniform basic level of health care is as much a concomitant of utility status for hospitals as it is a "human right." Hospital managements could shape decision-making by utility commissions if boundary and jurisdictional matters were settled through voluntary collaboration.

Synthesis:

The process of regulation forces industry-wide agreement on the definition of services, measurement of performance and appropriate levels of quality. In fact, many regulated industries find it to their advantage to operate at relatively high-quality levels.

Implication: An acceptable definition of hospital output is difficult to derive, partly because of the inseparability of hospital and medical care, and partly because of the obscure relationship between hospital output and health status. Nonetheless, hospitals can and should actively seek new measurements which are output-related rather than activity-related, incorporate the influence of medical practice on hospital operations, and recognize genuine differences between hospitals. It is in the hospitals' best interests to do so. There is probably no potential more damaging to hospitals than new controls applied on the basis of inappropriate indicators.

Synthesis:

While regulation is often coupled with heavy "external subsidies" from government (e.g., early development of railroads, subsidies to airlines for mail), elements of "internal subsidization" usually remain: the exercise of government power to compel some members of the public who purchase goods or services to support services to other areas which the free market would serve only at reduced levels, or not at all.[4]

Implication: Regulation of hospitals will undoubtedly be infused with both government financing and legitimized "robin-hooding." The mix of these financing mechanisms is an important public policy issue upon which different elements of the health industry have widely varying and strongly held views. It is in the best interests of both hospitals and the public to prepare careful documentation of the amount of subsidy and the identity of recipients and payors and to place such information in the public record in order to bring the issues to light. This calls for careful, and in many instances new, forms of hospital financial analysis—a management responsibility.

IMPLICATIONS FOR HOSPITAL MANAGEMENT

The foregoing is a small sample of the many aspects of utility regulation which must become common knowledge to hospital management if regulation by commission comes to pass. In fact, regulation is often sought by leading firms in an industry, which seek protection from marginal and unethical operators. Thus, the active pursuit of regulation by hospitals may be in their enlightened self-interest. Whether or not this is true, many of the foregoing statements of management implication have by their intrinsic merit value, *regardless* of possible commission regulation. The value of utility regulation of hospitals will long be debated, and the arguments will be intense. Yet, the several actions suggested here and inspired by the "threat" of regulation are in themselves *pro bono publico.*

FURTHER READINGS SUGGESTED BY THE AUTHOR

(Compiled in part by the Cooperative Information Center for Hospital Management Studies of the University of Michigan.)

Berstein, M. H. *Regulating Business by Independent Commission.* Princeton, N.J.: Princeton University Press, 1965. (paperback.)

Brigham, J. A. "Questions about Public Utility Status and Prepayment and Insurance Plans," *Hospital Progress,* Vol. 51, July, 1970, p. 6.

"Cohen Hints at Public Utility Status for Hospitals," *Hospital Progress,* Vol. 48, 1967. p. 480.

Edleman, J. "Public Utility Regulation," *Hospitals,* Vol. 44, November 1, 1970. p. 120+.

Edwards, S. A. "Are Hospitals Public Utilities?" *Hospitals,* Vol. 39, January 16, 1965. p. 51+.

"Hospital of Future Seen as Public Utility or Self-Help 'Cafeteria,' " *Modern Hospitals,* Vol. 108, April, 1967. pp. 26-27.

Levey, S. "Hospital and Public Utility–Are They Related?" *Hospital Topics,* Vol. 41, March, 1963. pp. 36-39.

McWilliams, W. V. and Bamberger, E. C., Jr. "Rising Hospital Costs and Public Concern–Two Plans for Action: Make Hospitals Public Utilities; Let the Critics Help Make the Decisions," *Hospitals,* Vol. 34, October 1, 1960. pp. 44-48.

Morrissey, F. P. "The Dilemma of Hospitals–Is Public Utility Status the Answer?" *Hospital Administration,* Vol. 16, No. 4, Fall, 1971. p. 10+.

Mott, A. T. and others. "Should Hospitals Seek Public Utility Status?" *Modern Hospital,* Vol. 108, June, 1967 (N., p. 36). p. 93.

Phillips, C. F., Jr. *The Economics of Regulation.* Homewood, Ill.: Irwin, 1965.

Posner, R. A. "Taxation by Regulation." *Bell Journal of Economics and Management Science,* Vol. 2, Spring, 1971, p. 22+.

Priest, A. J. A. "Possible Adoption of Public Utility Concepts in the Health Care Field," *Law and Contemporary Problems, Part II,* Vol. 35, Autumn, 1970. p. 839+.

Somers, Anne R. *Hospital Regulations: The Dilemma of Public Policy.* Princeton, N.J.: Princeton University Press, 1969.

Somers, Anne R. "These are the Questions about Regulation: What Kind? How Much? By Whom? Why?" *Modern Hospital,* Vol. 113, No. 3, September, 1969, pp. 137-141.

"State Regulation of Hospitals: Span of Control: From Hands Off to Handcuffs," *Modern Hospital,* Vol. 115, No. 6, December, 1970. pp. 62-75.

Stigler, A. J. "The Theory of Economic Regulation," *Bell Journal of Economics and Management Science,* Vol. 2, Spring, 1971. p. 3+.

"Storm in New York City as City Suggests Public Utility Status for All Hospitals," *Modern Hospital,* Vol. 109, October, 1967. p. 46+.

FOOTNOTES

[1] The industries compared are railroad, air, power, banking and communication.

[2] For brief descriptions of the process of establishing utility rates, see F. P. Morrissey, "The Dilemma of Hospitals–Is Public Utility Status the Answer?" *Hospital Administration,* Vol. 16, No. 4, Fall, 1971, pp. 14-16, and A. J. A. Priest, "Possible Adoption of Public Utility Concepts in the Health Care Field," *Law and Contemporary Problems, Part II,* Vol. 35, Autumn, 1970, pp. 845-847.

[3] Priest, pp. 845-847.

[4] For full discussion of the concept of internal subsidization, see R. A. Posner, "Taxation by Regulation," *Bell Journal of Economics and Management Science,* Vol. 2, Spring, 1971, pp. 28-34.

40.
Policy Considerations in National Health Insurance

KURT DARR

Kurt Darr, J.D., Sc.D., Professor of Health Care Administration and Assistant Dean - School of Government and Business Administration - The George Washington University. Washington, D.C.

BACKGROUND

National health insurance (NHI) is not a new issue, either for the United States or other nations. A health insurance program was first used in industrialized western Europe in 1883 by Chancellor von Bismarck for certain working class Germans. In 1911 national health insurance was passed in England, and 37 years later the National Health Service was established, and included state ownership and control of the health care system. Other European countries had significant governmental involvement in this same period, but only those in eastern Europe since World War II have complete state ownership of facilities, and employment of medical personnel.

At the turn of the century, an apparent greater social awareness stimulated attempts to pass social legislation.[1] In the United States, it was the era of state workman's compensation legislation. In addition, during World War I, there were efforts in some state legislatures to enact health insurance legislation. These attempts diminished after opposition by organized medicine and the prosperity of the 1920s. President Franklin D. Roosevelt refused to ask for inclusion of health insurance in the Social Security Act of 1935. There is evidence he feared his entire economic security package would fail politically if health insurance were added.[2]

EARLY BILLS AND FEDERAL INVOLVEMENT

National health insurance legislation was introduced in Congress in the late 30s and early 40s. Most notable was the Wagner-Murray-Dingell bill. A similar version of this proposal was introduced in almost every Congress during the 1940s. The 1947 version, entitled "The National Health Insurance and Public Health Act of 1947," proposed to amend the Social Security Act of 1935. It provided for federal preemption of virtually the entire health care system. Title 2 outlined prepaid personal health

---

This article was written for this book.

services. Benefits included: medical, dental, home nursing, and hospital services, as well as auxiliary benefits such as eyeglasses, and X-rays. A patient could choose any doctor who participated in the program. Individuals not automatically insured, including the poor, could be covered through premiums paid for them by public agencies. Participation by health services professionals was through a voluntary agreement with the state administrative agency. Payment was determined (1) according to a fee schedule, (2) on a per capita basis, (3) salary basis, or any combination of these, if approved by the federal unit.

Title 2 also provided that administrative responsibility for local health services be decentralized to the greatest possible extent, and that states could assume complete responsibility if they submitted a plan approved by the National Health Insurance Board. The National Health Insurance Board was to be composed of five members, three appointed by the president and approved by the Senate, and the other two were the surgeon general and the commissioner of social security. A National Advisory Medical Policy Council would advise the Insurance Board. United States preoccupation with World War II undoubtedly contributed to the lack of serious consideration of NHI, but now, for the reformers, the time was opportune.

The 1947 bill was very comprehensive. However, its predecessor, the 1943 Wagner-Murray-Dingell bill, was even more comprehensive and envisioned a system of national health insurance controlled through a federal bureaucracy.

In 1949, the 1947 bill was reintroduced in the 81st Congress, and achieved national prominence when the putative reformers faced strong opposition. In following months the American public witnessed significant discussion on health and medical problems and the question of government involvement. This debate degenerated into vitriolic and irrational attacks by both parties, and by 1950 it disappeared from the national political scene.

Though the United States found itself in the middle of the 20th century as the only major western industrialized country without some form of national health insurance, the federal government had not been inactive in the health care field. Billions of federal dollars had been spent to support the delivery of health care services. In areas such as biomedical research it had achieved an almost exclusive role. In training and educating health care manpower, and in constructing, and remodeling health care facilities, it had certainly achieved the role of partner with the states and private groups. In addition, Congress saw fit to provide substantial medical care programs to various special groups including military personnel, veterans, and the Indian population.[3]

Increasingly during the late 1950s and early 1960s the emphasis shifted. Congress began to pay for actual health care rather than to provide the resources to assist in its delivery. Rather than seek passage of national health insurance, advocates of the Wagner-Murray-Dingell bill took a new tack and sought coverage for a limited group, i.e., old age and survivors hospitalization insurance. This was the first evidence of legislation to provide—on the basis of entitlement rather than charity—certain forms of health coverage for any person eligible for old age and survivors insurance under the

Social Security Act. Primarily, it was designed to provide hospital coverage. Administered where possible through state agencies, it would establish a trust fund to handle the financing. That 1952 legislative proposal was the first effort to provide old age insurance which was finally enacted in the Social Security Amendments of 1965 (Medicare).

Before the passage of Medicare in 1965, however, an interim and almost unnoticed legislative event occurred. In 1960, the Kerr-Mills bill became law. The "Medical Assistance Act" financed health care services to the needy elderly. Today, this would be Medicaid for the over-65 population. However, it was received unenthusiastically and fewer than half of the states passed the enabling legislation permitting them to receive matching federal funds.

In the 60s, too, public statements began to refer to health care as a "right."[4] Health planning legislation provides one example of this philosophy's emergence. The Comprehensive Health Planning and Public Health Services Amendments of 1966 which amended section 314 of the Public Health Service Act states that "fulfillment of our national purpose depends on promoting and assuring the highest level of health attainable for every person," and that federal financial assistance would be used to "assure comprehensive health services of high quality for every person." Previously, society had charged government with guaranteeing only liberty rights. The implications of any effort to guarantee a right to health care are obvious. This can only be carried out by great public expenditures and, necessarily therefore, with federal involvement in previously non-federal sectors of the economy.

POLITICIZING HEALTH CARE

Enactment of Medicare and Medicaid in 1965 was a dramatic step toward involvement of federal government in the health care field. In many ways, this was hardly unexpected or unprecedented; hospital care for the over-65 population had been a political issue since the early 1950s. Ironically, massive government involvement in financing health care not only for the elderly, but for the needy, hastened the politicization of health care problems on a much broader and substantially more conceptual basis. There is evidence that a significant reason for health care inflation has been the tremendous increase in federal expenditures.[5] Regulators and legislators are seeking means to control costs. This has further brought the health care system into the political arena. Recent major legislation has been directed at controlling costs of programs already enacted or costs in the health care field more generally; e.g., P.L. 92-603, the Social Security Act Amendments of 1972; and P.L. 93-641, the National Health Planning and Resources Development Act of 1974. These are only first steps in control efforts and are likely to become increasingly common. The problem of rising costs is not unique to the United States. Countries such as Sweden and England with health care systems more highly regulated than ours have experienced similar problems in controlling costs.[6]

Politicization has had a number of clear benefits, e.g., identification of problems in the delivery, financing, and organization of health care services. Issues have been joined, and in many cases there has been meaningful debate. Leaders and thinkers in a number of fields have increasingly sought and proposed means to solve these problems. Concomitantly, this politicization is not without problems, however; some NHI proposals evidence little understanding and even some misunderstanding of the health care system. Perhaps political gain is a primary motivation. Furthermore, tampering with the health care system may cause unintended harmful results, e.g., Medicare and Medicaid, and their impact on inflation in health care costs.

After an absence of twenty years, Congress in the late 1960s once again began to consider national health insurance proposals. These proposals had a wide range of philosophical bases and suggested federal involvement in a variety of ways. Most included a continuation of the traditional federal-state cooperation characteristic of federal intervention in the health care field. A new element is the presence of proposals advocated by provider and financing groups as well as reformers. Specifically, the American Medical Association, the American Hospital Association, the Health Insurance Association of America, and AFL-CIO have participated in drafting bills and advocating their passage. For the AFL-CIO, activity is not unusual since organized labor has been a rather consistent and firm advocate of health care legislation. The fact that provider groups are actively supporting federal involvement in the health care field indicates the extent to which issues and problems in health care have become politicized.*

At least among the political and other power elite who are now active in developing national health insurance legislation, there seems to be little disagreement about the need for some federal role in health insurance. The American people generally, however, are much less sure. Responses in a 1971 nationwide household survey of health care use and expenditures show substantial equivocation.[7] While 76 percent answered "yes" when asked: "Is there a health care 'crisis' today?" only 18 percent favored extending Medicare to the entire population. Questions about the impact of a government health insurance program found: Would NHI—

Do a better job than private health insurance?	51% agree
Provide all people with access to high-quality care?	60% agree
Result in too much government regulation of health care?	54% agree
Mean a longer wait to see the doctor?	60% agree

The responses indicate a reasonably sophisticated understanding of the issues. The uncertainty of constituents is clearly reflected by the lack of congressional action on national health insurance.

---

*There is a public affairs theory for industry which is, "If there is going to be a law or regulation, why not help write it." This may explain proposals by AMA and AHA.

ALTERNATIVES

National health insurance is defined by Tomkins as:

> Any federally initiated financing mechanism for the consumer purchase of health care services which (1) is nationwide in scope; (2) covers general health and medical care (rather than being limited to specific diseases, occupational hazards, etc.); and (3) is extended non-categorically to the total population (though not precluding distinctions among subpopulations for different treatment within the general plan structure).[8]

Coverage is usually mandatory, most often through payroll deductions. NHI does not necessarily preclude substantial involvement from the private sector, e.g., Blue Cross.

Of bills introduced during the 1970s, the narrowest proposals provide for some form of catastrophic health insurance coverage. Funding is on an insurance basis through employee and employer contributions.

The broadest proposals include those which would have a substantial impact on other areas of the present system, e.g., organization. However, they stop short of federal ownership of facilities and employment of medical personnel. They are universal (all persons are included) and comprehensive (all medical problems are treated). They provide for reorganization, cost and quality controls, and greatly expanded regulation of all types of providers. Funding comes from a combination of general revenue and specific taxes and premiums—the latter much like social security. Major proposals of the 95th Congress, 1977, are outlined in the accompanying table.

Writers in the health care field have identified a number of issues which should be addressed in considering national health insurance. Accessibility, acceptability, organization, quality of care, and accountability (including cost control) are most commonly mentioned. Present proposals deal with these problems in a variety of ways, if at all. With the possible exceptions of reorganization and accountability, solving them is primarily a function of the financing level which federal government is willing to provide. Some provisions for reorganization are based on financial incentives and/or disincentives; others include outright controls. As costs continue to rise and the frustration of policy-makers grows, controls become more likely. To a lesser extent, accountability is also a function of the willingness of government to spend the funds necessary to determine levels of responsiveness, use of resources, and the performance of providers. Although adequate funding will not solve all these problems, it is a necessary precursor to reasonable efforts.

SOCIAL GOALS AND FINANCING

There is a significant complication when analyzing and understanding some NHI proposals. Those suggesting a substantial federal government role tend to include goals which are not specifically related to health care. Granted that in many cases it is difficult to distinguish where social goals end and health goals begin—many health problems have social components. However, some proposed program elements are clearly on the periphery of alleviating illness and solving problems of health care delivery. These include using the financing of NHI to redistribute wealth or using the law to change practice patterns to those that comply more closely with what some experts think is desirable, e.g., group practice. Perhaps, though, large scale intervention invariably has social consequences and dislocation.

Whatever the level of federal expenditures, there are issues concerning the sources of these monies. No proposal to date has suggested that funding be provided solely by general revenues. Assuming that our federal income tax structure is redistributive, substantial financing of a national health insurance program from general revenues would have social consequences beyond health care.

If the funding mechanism is primarily social insurance (payroll taxes and/or premiums), i.e., each person pays relatively the same sum for similar services or benefits, then questions of regressive taxation will emerge. It is probable that in the near future any national health insurance program will be substantially funded through a social insurance, as opposed to a general revenue mechanism. There are several reasons for this. This approach is known to the population (social security taxes and Blue Cross premiums) and the people are likely to consider it an equitable means of funding. Secondly, it would avoid more direct competition between health care expenditures and expenditures for other purposes such as defense and education, i.e., the program would have its own specific funding. Thirdly, it might encourage more attention to budgets and the amount of money available. Finally, it may put a clear budget ceiling on national health insurance expenditures and therefore potentially have a significant impact on cost control.

Such a budget ceiling would have negative features as well. Health care as a matter of legislative entitlement means that theoretically, all persons are eligible for the same care. Assuming budget limits, this would reduce services to the lowest common denominator. This is probably undesirable; however, it is an inevitable part of attempts to achieve equity within budgetary limitations.

EQUITY

There are other issues which go beyond the types and levels of financing and cost of any nationally focused program with substantial federal involvement. The most dominant is equity—or who gets what. Such questions are politically very sensitive. This may explain why even in countries where universal and comprehensive national health programs have been in existence for some time, issues of equity have not been publicly addressed. In Great Britain and Sweden there is evidence that problems of equitable distribution of health care resources exist. In Great Britain, for example, there is wide variation in utilization of health services by socio-economic classes. And in Sweden there is apparently a greater potential demand for kidney dialysis units than treatments actually being given. In the past, economics played a substantial role, i.e., those persons who could not afford the treatment did not receive it. This had the

Basic Content of Major National Health Insurance Bills
95th Congress - 1977

Title and Bill Number	Congressional Sponsors	Organizations Supporting	Coverage	Financing	Government Involvement
National Health Care Act H.R. 5 S.5 (94th Congress: H.R. 5990 S. 1438)	Rep. Omar Burleson (D-TX) Sen. Thomas J. McIntyre (D-NH)	Health Insurance Association of America	Voluntary for all U.S. citizens. Identifies minimum coverage requirements for voluntary plans to qualify: 100% of specified examinations, X-rays and laboratory tests, drugs, and 80% of specified hospital, surgical, professional, and ambulatory health care; also, basic dental, maternal, child, family planning, and mental health care.	Purchase of private insurance: (1) employer-employee arranged premiums, or (2) individual policy holder pays full premium, or (3) state plan enrollee premium contribution for poor and near poor. Medicaid would cover additional services. Some deductibles. Business income tax deductions for qualifying plans; unlimited personal income tax deduction for qualifying health plan.	Private insurance carriers would administer their own policies which must be approved by state insurance departments. Each state must establish health insurance pool for reinsurance and other purposes. Secretary DHEW authorized to review rate level of institutional reimbursement.
National Health Insurance Act H.R. 16 (94th Congress: H.R. 94)	Rep. John Dingell (D-MI)		Almost all employees and self-employed covered; all persons eligible for social security benefits covered. Broad medical benefits, but specific control of benefits package is at state level. Standard benefits: 60 days general hospital (30 days psychiatric, TB) inpatient care; outpatient care; physicians, dentists, podiatrists, and optometrists services; check-ups; home health; physical therapy, X-ray, and other ancillary services.	Establishment of personal health service account; account would receive 3% of total earnings (as defined under present social security law). Dental, home health, and certain other services financed by additional 1% payment. Another 1% of earnings to be appropriated in first year of enactment to establish reserve. Bill authorizes additional expenditures from general revenues to meet needs.	Major operating responsibilities at state and local levels. Each state to develop health plan to be submitted for approval to national health insurance board. Federal government will contract with state for administration of program.

450

The Health Security Act H.R. 21 S. 3 (94th Congress: same numbers)	Rep. James C. Corman (D-CA) Sen. Edward M. Kennedy (D-MA)	Committee for National Health Insurance; AFL-CIO; major unions and consumer groups	All U.S. residents. Unlimited for most services, including inpatient and outpatient services. Most physician and health professional services covered. Certain limitations on mental health and skilled nursing home care services. Dental care coverage phased in. Optometrist and podiatrist services covered. No coinsurance or deductibles.	Financed by combination of: 50% payroll taxes (employees—1%, employers—3.5%, unearned income—2.5%); and 50% general federal revenues. Medicare repealed; Medicaid retained to cover additional services. No private health insurance organizations to be used.	To be administered by DHEW through 5 member health security board which develops regulations and guidelines. National advisory council established to advise on policy and provide program evaluation. Establishes commission on quality of health care to monitor providers.
Health Care Insurance Act H.R. 760	Rep. Charles E. Bennett (D-FL)		Voluntary coverage of eligible beneficiaries (married persons under 65) and dependents, through issuance of health insurance certificates. To be qualified, voluntary plan must provide: (1) basic coverage for all expenses incurred for institutional care, emergency and outpatient services, medical care, dental and oral surgery, and ambulance services; and (2) catastrophic expense coverage.	Eligible beneficiary receives health insurance certificate of entitlement. Value assigned certificate is sum of: (1) yearly allowable premiums for qualified health insurance multiplied by applicable percentage (from 100% for persons with $0.0 income tax liability to 10% for persons with tax of $891 or more); and (2) 100% of allowable premiums paid for yearly catastrophic expense coverage. Deductibles and coinsurance on institutional care.	Establishes health insurance advisory board to develop federal standards for use by state insurance departments to identify qualified plans and carriers. Board shall develop programs for monitoring quality care, effective utilization of resources, etc.

Comprehensive Health Care Insurance Act H.R. 1818 S. 218	Rep. Tim Lee Carter (R-KY) Sen. Clifford P. Hansen (R-WY)	American Medical Association	Requires all employers to offer employees and their families qualified health insurance program. Coverage shall be optional with the employees. Qualified plan has broad hospital, medical, and other health care services. Excludes: personal comfort items; eyeglasses, hearing aids, and orthopedic shoes; and private rooms. Sets limits of aggregate expenditures for catastrophic illness expenses for individuals. Sets requirements which must be met by qualified health care insurance plans. Employers contribute to cost of coverage at least 65% of premium; employee contributes remainder. For low-income employees a program of certificates of entitlement or income tax credit formulas is developed. Establishes federal health insurance redemption fund. Authorizes appropriations to fund to pay full premium for those with low income and to pay decreasing amounts to those with higher incomes. Permits income tax credits for premiums paid for qualified insurance plans. Carriers offering qualified health care insurance policies must participate in assigned risk pool established by appropriate state agency. Federal health insurance advisory board: develops regulations to implement act; establishes minimum standards for qualified policies to be enforced by states; plans, reviews, and develops programs to maintain quality of care; and review effectiveness of programs.
Catastrophic Health Insurance and Medical Assistance Reform Act H.R. 4684	Rep. Edward J. Patten (D-NJ)	Insurance industry	Catastrophic health insurance for all legal U.S. residents: (1) federally administered public plan for unemployed, welfare recipients, aged, and persons not opting for private coverage, or (2) private catastrophic insurance plan for employers. Medical assistance plan to be financed from general revenues and state funds. Catastrophic insurance plan to be financed through 1% payroll tax on empoyers, no employee contribution. Approved employer plans Administered through Social Security Administration. Secretary DHEW required to establish separate organizational unit within HEW under an assistant secretary for health insurance adminis-

452

(Bill contains major elements of a bill with the same name introduced in the 94th Congress by Senators Russell Long and Abraham Ribicoff and Rep. Joe Waggoner.)

ployers and self-employed, on voluntary basis. Covers inpatient hospital services past 60 days and inpatient hospital benefits exceeding $2,000 per family per year. Benefits: catastrophic plan—similar to Parts A and B of Medicare, except no upper limit on hospital days or home health visits, some mental health services covered; medical assistance plan—broad coverage of hospital and medical services necessary prior to catastrophic, plus catastrophic coverage.

(those with at least same minimum benefits) may be used instead; employers eligible for income tax credit for costs.

tration who has policy and administrative responsibility for act.

Cost estimates for these bills were not available at the time of publication.

Other nonsimilar bills include: Rep. Robert J. Lagomarsino's (R-CA) National Voluntary Medical and Hospital Insurance Act (H.R. 957), Rep. Robert A. Roe's (D-NJ) National Catastrophic Illness Protection Act of 1977 (H.R. 2150), and Rep. Ronald Dellums' (D-CA) Health Service Act (H.R. 6894). The first two stress voluntary action and would require few changes in the present delivery system, e.g., utilizing private insurers to cover catastrophic costs. At the opposite end of a governmental involvement continuum, the latter would create health regions and districts to provide all health services to all persons. Dellums' bill goes much further than Kennedy-Corman in reorganizing the existing health services system.

As of April 1978 Rep. Al Ullman's (D-OR) National Health Care Services Reorganization and Financing Act (H.R. 1 in the 94th Congress) has not been introduced. Its reintroduction is contingent on the Carter administration's activities in NHI.

effect of providing a filter or automatic demand-limitation. At the very least, national health insurance would suggest that all persons can receive the level of treatment their problem requires. Thus, it becomes politically unfeasible to identify the existence of these shortages, at least publicly. The informed observer should therefore treat with skepticism the statements that a particular plan is universal and comprehensive. These are, at best, goals to be attempted, rather than easily accomplished fact.

In a country like the United States, with its heterogeneity in population density, geographic expanse, racial composition, and social attitudes towards health, it is unrealistic to believe that we can be very successful in achieving equity. Certain portions of the population will almost certainly receive less health care than others. These patterns will probably develop by neglect or as an unintended consequence of a policy decision rather than purposeful action.

It may well be necessary or even desirable that varying technological levels exist for different groups or persons. However, assuming the likelihood of budgetary limitations, it is quite probable that even where the technology can be provided there will be difficulty in selecting those who are to receive the treatment. This problem is exacerbated by the high cost of most new medical technologies. Somehow available treatments or procedures must be rationed, but these questions have yet to be squarely addressed, even in those countries where they have been identified. The questions "by whom?" and "with what criteria?" pose difficult ethical problems for a society whose health care leaders are only now beginning to identify thoroughly the issues and seek enlightened but humane answers.

CONCLUSION

Politicians and reformers have showered us with rhetoric, but there seems to be significant reluctance on the part of the American people to direct their representatives to involve the federal government massively in the health care field. Health care professionals might well ask if they are not primarily talking to each other and a few national political leaders. National health insurance is clearly not a priority among the population. It should also be remembered that Medicare, despite its slow emergence and substantial supporting evidence of the problems, came perilously close to not passing the Congress. This was true even in the presence of a strong Democratic party Medicare plank, an overwhelming Democratic majority in Congress, and an advocate president. The national health insurance issue must be viewed in this context.

The dramatic rise in costs of health care has sounded a note of caution heard by Congress and public alike. It is reasonably certain that unless means to control costs can be found, there will be continued reluctance to pass national health insurance legislation, despite the need to improve access and solve other problems in the health care field.

BIBLIOGRAPHY

Anderson, Odin W. *The Uneasy Equilibrium: Private and Public Financing of Health Services in the United States, 1875-1965.* New Haven: College and University Press, 1968.

Chapman, Carleton, and Talmadge, John. "The Evolution of the Right to Health Concept in the United States." *The Pharos,* January 1971, pp. 30-51.

Davis, Karen. "The Case for National Health Insurance." *Trustee* 29 (March 1976): 21-23.

——————. *National Health Insurance: Benefits, Costs, and Consequences.* Washington, D.C.: The Brookings Institution, 1975.

Falk, I.S. "National Health Insurance: A Review of Politics and Proposals." *Law and Contemporary Problems* 35(Autumn 1970): 669-96.

Fuchs, Victor. *Who Shall Live?* New York: Basic Books, 1974.

Gehrig, Leo, and Lesparre, Michael. "National Health Insurance: Forecasting the Political Climate." *Hospitals* 50(1 March 1976): 45-48.

Mitchell, Bridger, and Schwartz, William. "The Financing of National Health Insurance." *Science* 192(14 May 1976): 621-29.

——————. "Strategies for Financing National Health Insurance: Who Wins and Who Loses." *New England Journal of Medicine* 295(14 October 1976): 866-71.

Newhouse, J.P.; Phelps, C.E.; and Schwartz, W.B. "Policy Options and the Impact of National Health Insurance." *New England Journal of Medicine* 290(13 June 1974): 1345-59.

O'Connor, Robin. "National Health Insurance: The Time Has Come to Wait Some More." *Hospitals* 50(1 March 1976): 55-60.

Tomkins, Richard M. "Evaluating National Health Insurance Legislation: A Summary Review." *Hospital Administration* 19(Summer 1974): 74-84.

FOOTNOTES

[1] Odin W. Anderson, *The Uneasy Equilibrium: Private and Public Financing of Health Services in the United States, 1875-1965* (New Haven: College and University Press, 1968), pp. 52-90.

[2] Edwin E. Witte, *The Development of the Social Security Act* (Madison, Wisconsin: University of Wisconsin Press, 1962).

[3] Anderson, *Equilibrium,* pp. 104-9.

[4] Ibid., p. 131.

[5] Victor R. Fuchs, *Who Shall Live?* (New York: Basic Books, 1974), p. 94.

[6] Odin W. Anderson, "All Health Care Systems Struggle Against Rising Costs," *Hospitals* 50 (1 October 1976): 97.

[7] Ronald Anderson; Odin W. Anderson; and Joanna Kravits, "The Public's View of the Crisis in Medical Care: An Impetus for Changing Delivery Systems," *Economic and Business Bulletin* 24(Fall 1971).

[8] Richard M. Tomkins, "Evaluating National Health Insurance Legislation: Summary Review," *Hospital Administration* 19(Summer 1974): 74-84.

41.

Health and Public Policy

HERMAN M. SOMERS

Herman M. Somers, Ph.D., is Professor of Politics and Public Affairs - The Woodrow Wilson School of Public and International Affairs - Princeton University

Complaints are frequent that the United States lacks a national health policy. What that allegation means is rarely made clear. Policy means different things to different people. But, if by policy one means legislative and governmental administrative actions, it is conspicuous that this nation has been spawning health policies at a proliferating and bewildering rate ever since World War II. Keeping up with the multiplicity of policies has become a formidable challenge, and few succeed.

In this fiscal year (1975) the nation is spending for health and medical care about $116 billion,[1] in 1950, we spent $12-billion. That is almost a 10-fold increase. On a per capita basis we have moved from about $78 to an estimated $530 per person. Even in constant dollars—removing the influence of inflation—the increases are impressive. The public portion of these expenditures has accelerated at a far more rapid pace than the total. Government, at all levels, spent well over $41 billion for health care in 1974, compared to $3 billion in 1950. During the 10-year period, 1965 to 1974, government increased its payments by 333 percent. Public expenditures moved from 25 percent of the total in 1950 to 40 percent in 1974.[2]

This, I submit, in itself represents a policy—and an important one. Government has now committed itself to massive expenditures for health care. It has allotted progressively larger portions of the government budget and induced steadily higher proportions of our total wealth—gross national product—to this field. This has been accompanied by governmental involvement in the full spectrum of health activities.

Access

The largest and most obvious outlet for these expenditures has been the attempt to enlarge access to health care through such programs as Medicare and Medicaid. Precise data are not available, but indications are that utilization of health services has been substantially increased, probably more than doubled per capita since 1950.

Reprinted by permission from *Inquiry*, Vol. 12 (June 1975), pp. 87-96. Copyright 1975 by *Inquiry*, The Blue Cross Association. All rights reserved.

In recent years the poor on average have become as active utilizers of services as the rest of the population, although, of course, they need much more—and other serious historical inequities remain. In fact, to a large extent it has been the improvement in the circumstances of the relatively deprived that has helped sensitize us to the many gross inequities that remain.

There have been unhappy and unplanned "side effects" of these new expenditures such as an acceleration of an already serious inflation of prices and costs, and various abuses and corruption, particularly in nursing homes.

Research and Construction

For some time now, government has been paying for more than 90 percent of all serious biomedical research in this country. This is an important policy. There are many who are convinced that by far the most important improvements we can look forward to in health care are likely to result from the products of the research centers rather than direct expenditures for health services.

But, here, too, there are many protests about undesirable "side effects." It is alleged that an unduly large proportion of physicians have been diverted from delivery of health care to research, and that the large research grants flowing from government to medical schools have distorted the teaching functions of the schools.

Government has also steadily increased its financial support for construction of medical facilities: hospitals, clinics, etc. Last year more than a third of all construction costs for both private and public facilities was paid for by government.

Medical Manpower

A few years ago the nation decided on an all-out drive to increase the supply of medical manpower in all categories. Federal support for health profession education reached its legislative apogée with the passage of the Comprehensive Health Manpower Training Act of 1971. Massive support has been furnished to encourage increased enrollments and development of new schools.

Between 1968 and 1974, 20 new medical schools were created, bringing the total to 114, or 25 percent more schools than in 1951. The number of students increased even more rapidly. In 1974 we graduated 84 percent more M.D.s than in 1951, and 42 percent more than in 1968. The accelerating trend is perhaps best indicated by pointing out that the first-year class in medical schools in 1973-1974 was 14,124, and this was 25 percent more than that year's graduating class.[3] As a result of such movement, the physician/population ratio rose to a record high in 1974, and now compares favorably with any other Western society.

This policy also is subject to mounting attacks. There are increasing fears that we may have gone too far and that we are moving toward a costly surplus of physicians. (The province of Ontario has recently undertaken to limit the admission of additional physicians in order to contain costs; the government calculates that every additional physician generates at least $150,000 of additional medical costs annually.) It is also questioned whether medical schools have been encouraged to operate on too extravagant a scale. There are increasing allegations that the training the schools are offering with the new money is, in fact, not being directed toward meeting the health needs that were the justification for the additional financial support. The schools are being blamed for an excessive movement to specialization, so that even though we increase the supply of physicians there is a decline in the number available for primary care.

There are increasing protests that at the same time that we have been rapidly expanding our own supply of physicians we have been encouraging an even more rapid entry of foreign medical graduates, whose training for delivery of health services is widely questioned. In 1972, 46 percent of all new licentiates were FMGs.[4] In each of the last four years for which data are available (1970-1973), the number of FMGs admitted to the United States exceeded the total number graduated that year from U.S. medical schools. The wide use of undereducated physicians, often unlicensed, who have either not taken or have failed a licensing examination, and who have never passed a proficiency examination, was recently labeled a "medical underground" in one of our leading medical journals.[5]

The federal government has tried to cope with the problem of geographic imbalance by subsidizing clinical facilities in rural and underserved areas and by creation of the National Health Service Corps, which subsidizes young physicians who agree to serve for a limited period in underserved areas. Its history is yet too brief to evaluate results.

Structure and Organization

Government has even undertaken to reform the organization and structure of the delivery system. Almost 30 years ago, the Congress passed the Hospital Survey and Construction Act, commonly known as Hill-Burton. The preamble of that act has often been described as one of the most advanced statements of public policy ever made in this country for the development of regionalized medical care. The legislation, many times renewed over the following years, did stimulate and help finance thousands of new and modernized hospital beds, particularly in rural areas.

Now the complaint is that the country is substantially over-bedded and that this is a major factor in the inflation of costs. Many people are calling for an absolute moratorium on all construction and expansion of hospital capacity. Moreover, no visible progress has been made toward regionalization or rationalization of services or health care institutions. Clearly, a public policy pronouncement, however earnest its intent, is not to be confused with pragmatic achievement.

With a similar goal, the Congress passed the Regional Medical Program legislation in 1965 (P.L. 89-239). Some very useful individual and special projects mark the history of RMP, but its underlying goal of regionalization completely eluded the program, which is now entering its final days.

In 1966, Congress passed the Comprehensive Health Planning Act (P.L. 89-749), subsidizing the operation of health planning agencies in every state and in smaller geographic areas throughout the country. The functions of such agencies were only vaguely defined, but systemization of health care delivery was a primary policy intent. CHP is now being phased out in favor of a new legislative effort, the National Health Planning and Resources Development Act of 1974 (P.L. 93-641). But we are no closer to systemization now than we were in 1966, and fragmentation remains the most conspicuous hallmark of the delivery structure.

Both the legislation of 1966 and the new 1974 law contain ringing declarations of public policy in their preambles. The 1966 Act declared that access to adequate health care was a right of every citizen; and the 1974 Act opens with the statement, "The achievement of equal access to quality health care at a reasonable cost is a priority of the Federal Government." A priority is, I presume, intended to be a policy, but it would not be fair to expect the 1974 law alone to bring us very much closer to the goal than did the 1966 legislation.

HMOs

Five years ago, in 1970, the Department of Health, Education and Welfare, then under Elliot Richardson, proclaimed with considerable fanfare that the promotion and support of health maintenance organizations was to be the "centerpiece" of the Administration's health care strategy, because HMOs represented a more efficient way of organizing and delivering health services. HEW announced its intention of spotting the country with enough HMOs to be available to 90 percent of the population by 1980.[6]

HEW promptly undertook to furnish financial support for the policy, even in advance of congressional action. In 1973, Congress finally enacted the Health Maintenance Organization Act, authorizing $375-million to assist in the financing of HMOs. It also undertook to stimulate HMOs by passing a mandatory requirement that all employers of 25 or more employees covered by the Fair Labor Standards Act must, in their employee health insurance plan, offer an HMO option to each employee, wherever one exists. It also authorized the by-passing of any restrictive state laws against HMOs.

Despite all this, the movement toward HMOs has been disappointingly slow. Best estimates are that HMOs are now serving about six to seven million people, less than 4 percent of the population.[7] It has again been made clear that even laws, public policy, and public monies do not rapidly alter patterns of behavior of consumers or providers, and that human institutions have a stubborn tenacity for survival.

Experience and Perspective

This list is, of course, only a sampling of some of the better known federal activities of recent years and omits mention of a significant multitude of state actions. Yet I have found that in our impatience for more progress and new action, we often tend to overlook or understate the extraordinary volume and variety of past and present governmental efforts—currently costing about $43-billion a year and sweeping upward. The amount of experience we have accumulated with governmental activity in health care is now prodigious; it should be instructive. Yet the historical experience seems in the main to go unappraised, almost unnoticed, as I believe examination of current literature and contemporary policy debate will confirm. It is commendable and necessary to look ahead, but it is also prudent to look back periodically. It may add enlightenment to our vision of the future.

The lessons of our experience are numerous and widely suggestive. However, I will confine myself to two areas: the first concerns the politics of health, and the second has to do with the effect of medical care on health, a matter that has become of profound concern to me.

POLITICS AND POLICY

When people complain about a lack of national policy, they obviously cannot mean quite that, as it is too apparent that policies are legion. They are really saying that they are displeased with the policies; or, more frequently, they complain that the various policies lack coherence, that they are frequently contradictory, often fragmentary, tentative and halting.

This is, of course, very true. I do find puzzling, however, the apparent notion that this in some way differentiates the health field from other areas of public concern. That phenomenon characterizes foreign policy, economic policy, labor policy, welfare policy, and all others of importance. With some variations in particulars, related to each field, the reasons are essentially the same. The policies emerge from essentially the same political process.

In a country of continental dimensions, large issues cut across a multitude of diverse and conflicting interests, and the stakes are often high. We are sometimes told government is not responsive. Yet the problems people point at usually are direct consequences of the fact that governmental machinery, both legislative and administrative, dances to many tunes because it *is* responsive. It is, as it must be, responsive to diverse constituencies pursuing different goals. It marches to discordant beats of varied drummers, each of whom has a large enough drum to be heard and respected—each of whom has some power base among the multitude of power centers in our society, rarely powerful enough to get its own way but influential enough to be able to stop the opposition from getting its way.

The normal pattern is either to accept stalemate or to get some kind of action through a process of bargaining, compromise, and accommodation. This may come about in a settlement that gives two or three proponents of divergent policies their own partial victories on condition they permit the others to have their victories simultaneously. Or, the bargaining may lead to elimination or softening of particular provisions that are completely offensive to one or more large interests too strong to be overcome, resulting in a program that is acceptable to the majority of interests, although not fully satisfactory to any of them. Not surprisingly, such legislation will tend to be general, ambiguous, even conflicting, and subject to many different interpretations and actions at the administrative level.

Similar pressures impinge upon and influence the administrative policy process. As a result we frequently hear demands for reorganization or "coordination" of the administrative structure. There is almost always a good case to be made for reorganization—if only to avoid bureaucratic arteriosclerosis—but no amount of reorganization is likely to produce full agreement on goals, or how best to achieve them, or end the fragmentation among health interests. Policies, administrative and legislative, will reflect these realities.

This, of course, tends to sound messy and unsatisfactory, especially if, in our mind's eye, we envision the alternative as being a clear and coherent expression of policy that we support. It may not seem quite so unsatisfactory, and the messiness more tolerable, if we consider the possibility that the clear and coherent policy could be one that we would utterly deplore. A winner-take-all game is only attractive to the winner.

In any case, where controversy is many-faceted and deeply felt, the only way to a unified and consistent national policy is through authoritarianism. Those who would function effectively in a democratic society learn to live with inconsistencies and compromises and try to make progress incrementally within a bargaining process. It may rankle, but as Woodrow Wilson wrote a long time ago, "It is a strenuous thing this living the life of a free people." I often think of the appropriateness of George Shultz's observation when he became the first director of the Office of Management and Budget a few years ago, "Those who can't stand ambiguity can't be creative here."

Some Special Factors

There are, additionally, some special complicating factors in the case of health care. Among these are, *first*, that despite the great degree of public financing, health care remains predominantly a private sector industry. The creation and administration of public policy for a widely dispersed and varied set of enterprises dominated by the private sector involves numerous delicate legal and bureaucratic complexities. Things often have to be done by indirection and devising of roundabout procedures.

Second, there are historical and practical problems of intergovernmental relations. Historically and, many believe, constitutionally the states are the regulators of health care. They alone, for example, license practitioners and institutions and set standards. By its inherent character as a personal and individualized service, health care is provided at the local level. The problems of reconciling into a national policy the interests and functions of all levels of government that must be involved are both sensitive and formidable.

Third, health care is full of unresolved issues about which our factual knowledge is sparse and uncertain. For example, we have been debating the question of quality of care for a long time and most people accept the idea that some sort of policy is needed to assure a reasonable standard of quality. But the concept of quality is as elusive as it is important. There is little agreement on its definition, or on criteria, or upon how one goes about effectuating quality controls.

The problem is illustrated by the Professional Standards Review Organizations (PSRO) legislation passed by Congress two years ago (P.L. 92-603). The purpose was the monitoring and promotion of quality of care as well as cost containment. Necessarily, the law states mainly high level objectives; it could not and does not attempt to spell out what quality is. It leaves that to the administrators and the hundreds of local PSRO organizations, most yet to be established, to determine. We are all aware of the struggles, the compromises, and the evasions now in progress in the attempt to find acceptable standards and procedures. The American Medical Association has, in another context, taken court action against the government, claiming that it does not have the power to mandate peer review. And a great many physicians honestly fear that the process could actually prove a set-back to quality. Yet, it is clear that protection of quality does require professional peer review, within a context of public accountability, and all one can do is to explore within such parameters.

Another example is the delivery system. For a great many years we have been hearing eloquent demands that the delivery system needs to be reformed. By now most people appear to agree that reform is desirable, if not necessary. But what kind of reform? What specifically are the next steps? Here the consensus collapses. There appear to be as many different notions of how best to reorder delivery as there are advocates of reform. And, as in the case of quality, none can definitively demonstrate that he is right or that his reform would really be an improvement. The policy process becomes ensnared in situations where no witnesses can offer persuasive positive facts.

There is thus a certain inevitability about the vagueness, the complexity, and the unresolved issues that characterize our most recent assault on the problem of systemization, the National Health Planning and Resources Development Act of 1974, which was signed into law on January 4, 1975. This law is also facing a court test by the AMA. The Act, among other things, replaces Hill-Burton, Comprehensive Health Planning, and the Regional Medical Program, and moves on to a somewhat different track. The mood is frankly experimental and exploratory. It is hoped that the uncertainties and conflicts will be worked out in the process of administrative action, and that at least some framework for regulation may be available by the time national health insurance arrives on the scene.

There is little doubt that we will be in for more frustrations and aggravation. But I would plead for tolerance and restraint. When we cannot be sure of the right road, cautious probing may be the only sensible behavior. Certainly it is better than endless debate and no action.

A final point is perhaps only a corollary—it is a reminder of the limits of human and institutional capacities. Not everything we would like to see done can be done. Not everything that can be done lies within the competence of the federal government. Whenever we discover an inefficiency or an inequity or a malfunctioning that seems to need correcting, we almost instinctively say, why does not the federal government change all that?

If there is anything that should have become visible in the last decade or more it is that there are severe limits on what large bureaucracies can do well, or do at all. Our politicians are responsive—perhaps too much so. If strong enough demands are made they will respond, even when they know the proposed solution may not work. So, if we are tired of failures, we need to be more selective in what we demand of government. We have to develop a greater consciousness of the technical and administrative problems that accompany grand scale proposals. We have to ask: desirable or not, can this program be carried out by government? And, are governmental monopolies any healthier for society than private monopolies? It is one thing to enunciate lofty goals, but quite another to know how to implement them.

National Health Insurance

These political observations seem to have immediate pertinence to at least one major current issue of concern to everybody interested in health care—the debate over national health insurance. For several years now, people have been led to expect that a comprehensive national plan would be passed in that year, and many are still saying, "this year for sure." The fact is that no bill of any description has even been reported out by any committee in either House. People have apparently been misled by the fact that every important interest group—from the AMA to the AFL-CIO to the Health Insurance Association of America and the Administration—has sponsored some sort of NHI proposal, and a majority of congressmen, as well as the public, appear to be in favor of a national plan.

This is misleading because the proposals of the various groups differ sharply on the essentials: how the program will be financed; who will administer it; the scope of the program; and the like. Thus far, most of the leading contestants have not been willing to participate in the normal political process; they have refused to bend or bargain. The result has been a drawn-out stalemate. If postures do not change this will continue because no proposed plan can now, or in the foreseeable future, command anything resembling a majority. Some of the purists allege with pride that they are "standing on principle" when they refuse to compromise. But the nation has been paying a heavy price for their "purity." If the parties had been amenable to compromise, the country could already have been started on the road to comprehensive national health insurance. It would have been a modest and incomplete start, but one that could be added to and adjusted incrementally over the ensuing years. This continues to be true. If the chief contending forces are willing to accept something much smaller than their proposals contemplate, we could have legislation in this session of the Congress. Otherwise, stalemate is sure to continue.

Health Care and Jobs

One last point about the politics of health. The enormous growth of the health care economy has made it a leading source of employment and an important economic prop for many communities. There are now 4.5 million persons employed in the industry, not counting the large number engaged in the manufacture of pharmaceuticals and in the health insurance business. It is one of the largest employers in the nation. Thus, debates over proposals for particular health care expenditures or programs often, in reality, relate more to economic protectionism for providers of all stripes, employees, industries, and communities than they do to health—although the public rhetoric is of course aimed at health. An increasing number of strong vested interests have developed, as is inevitable in a $100-billion industry with so much at stake—and this means more pockets of resistance to change irrespective of basic ideological orientation.

When it was proposed to close some public health hospitals, the real issue became not whether those hospitals were still serving a useful purpose, but the economic blow it would represent to the communities in which they were located. When a new neighborhood health center is under discussion, the central issue is often the employment opportunities it will offer to local people. When a hospital reorganization or merger is contemplated, the position of employee unions will be determined by its effect upon jobs, and the position of the medical staffs by the effects on their practices.

I am not one to take the problem of employment and unemployment lightly, especially in times like the present. But it is always useful to recognize what the real issue is and to understand that many alleged health care decisions are being taken on grounds that have little or nothing to do with health as such, and that most of the pressures influencing health care policy are actually generated from within the health care industry itself.

HEALTH SERVICES AND HEALTH

I now turn to a second broad lesson of recent history. In the waves of enthusiasm for opening up previously barricaded access to medical care, we may have lost our sense of proportion. When people speak of national health policy it usually turns out that they are really talking about health care policy—or, more specifically, medical care. This can be dangerously misleading, for the two are not the same. Our goal presumably is, or should be, health. Medical care is not an end in itself, but one of the instrumentalities toward achievement of health. The utility of medical care as a purveyor of better health can easily become overvalued in relation to the many other factors determining health, and extreme overemphasis on medical care can threaten both the quality of medical services themselves as well as the public health.

The spectacular increases in health care expenditures and in utilization of medical services in recent years has not been accompanied by improvement in the health of Americans, as measured by any available indices of health status. After half a century of steady and marked improvement, the crude death rate for the United States ceased to improve during the 1960s and into the 1970s. It has remained virtually stable for well over a decade, fluctuating between 9.3 and 9.7 per thousand. The age-adjusted death rate was 7.6 in 1960 and 7.3 in 1969; for males it was 9.5 in both 1960 and 1969.[8]

When the data are broken down by age and sex it appears that the overall stability obscures particulars that are far more disturbing. The general stability resulted primarily from the changing age composition of the population. During the 1960s, there was a decline in the infant population (under one year), which has a death rate far above the general or crude rate. On the other hand, the population in the low-risk age groups, between five and 44, increased.[9] This tends to give the overall rate a more favorable skewing.

There has been improvement in infant mortality and length of life for females, and in the control of some remaining infectious diseases such as measles. But these gains have been offset by increases in lung cancer, emphysema, cirrhosis of the liver, motor vehicle accidents, suicide, homicide, and diabetes mellitus.

During the 1960s, death rates rose in every five-year age group from 15 years through 44 years. Significant improvement was registered only for the very young (under five years of age) and the old, particularly those 75 and over.[10]

Death rates of young and middle-aged American males are rising sharply. Mortality for white men, aged 15-24, rose 22 percent. For nonwhites, the rise was a shocking 42 percent. Mortality increases, smaller but still significant, apply to all white males under 45 and to all nonwhites under 75. The leading factors in the upturn for young men, 15-24 years, were motor vehicle accidents, suicide, and homicide.

For those between the ages of 25 and 44, the leading culprits were the automobile, homicide, lung cancer, suicide, and cirrhosis of the liver. For men between 45 and 64, there were substantial increases in the death rate due to lung cancer, emphysema, diseases of the heart and circulatory system, bronchitis, and cirrhosis. There were also substantial increases in the death rates for white women at ages 15-24 and 35-44 years, and for women of other races at ages 15-24 years.

While the overall death rates remain stable, it appears that the most productive years of life for American men are being foreshortened. Disablement and morbidity are not as well reported as deaths. But it can be readily inferred that increased death rates are accompanied by similar or larger morbidity and disability changes from the same causes.

Mortality Rates and Medical Care

It should be noted that the mortality data show a preponderant incidence of preventable causes, but generally not of the kind that lend themselves to medical "cure." They reflect primarily the consequences of life-style and personal behavior and portray circumstances wherein conventional medical intervention is usually too late. The availability of medical care is clearly not the major problem.

The rapidly increasing differential in male-female life expectancy is also revealing. In 1920, the average female baby could expect to live only one year longer than the average male baby; in 1972 the differential was 7.7 years and growing,[11] which explains the rapid increase of widows in our population. In 1910, there were 106 males for every 100 females in the United States; in 1972, only 95. Especially interesting is the fact that sex differentials have become more important than racial differentials in life expectancy. The average black female baby can now expect to live about a year longer than the average white male baby; three years longer in California. Certainly the genetic make-up of males and females has not been altered in recent years. Nor is there a difference in access to health care among males and females. The explanation appears to lie primarily in different life-styles, not in the amount of medical care.

Another revealing statistical phenomenon is that the traditional relationship between life expectancy and per capita income has vanished, except among the very poor.[12] Although high income groups have better access to modern medical care, their health is no better than among middle and lower-middle classes. In fact, evidence indicates that higher incomes often seem to do more harm than good for health. Again, the explanation appears to lie in life-style of the affluent rather than medical care.

Diminishing and Disappearing Returns

Nobody questions that availability of a certain amount of medical care is of great importance and that therapeutic medicine has made significant contributions to improvement in health status. But scholars are increasingly recognizing that additional increments of medical services can eventually lead to diminishing returns. The marginal value of added care is eventually reduced to a point where it does not repay the investment. More important, it is possible for the marginal value to reach zero or even become negative. Duncan Neuhauser, of the Harvard School of Public Health, has suggested the possibility that we may have reached or passed that point in the United States.[13]

There is increasing evidence of the diminishing relative importance of traditional therapy in all advanced societies, and the problem is receiving increased attention of scholars in many countries. Among the growing number of authorities who have been calling into doubt the value of proliferating service expenditures or the burgeoning of increasingly elaborate techniques are A. L. Cochrane, Thomas McKeown, and Brian Abel-Smith in England; A. D. Frazier in Canada; Anne R. Somers and Victor Fuchs in the United States.

The available evidence suggests to me that we have reached a stage where we must examine with care, and some skepticism, any proposal to throw more money and resources into the health care machine, although there is no question that the machine could absorb infinite amounts. As Enoch Powell, the former Minister of Health in Great Britain, reported about a decade ago, "There is virtually no limit to the amount of medical care an individual is capable of absorbing."[14] The caution I urge is not primarily for purposes of trying to save money but because of a concern for health.

First, we must keep in mind that we live in a world of limited resources, and thus every expenditure represents a choice among alternatives. If we feed the health care machine additional resources that do not add to positive health, we are depriving ourselves of the opportunity to use such resources in other pursuits where we know the marginal gains can be great: better food, improved housing, a cleaner environment, etc. Second, we may be nurturing a comfortable illusion that better health is simply for sale, and deflecting people from behavior that can prove more fruitful to health.

Dr. René Dubos, one of the world's most respected health authorities, told us several years ago that "Therapeutic medicine is probably now entering a phase of medically diminishing returns."[15] It now seems that the greatest potential for improving the health of the American people is probably not to be found in increasing the number of physicians or hospital beds, but rather in what people can be taught and motivated to do for themselves, in influencing personal behavior and attitudes.

This is hardly a new thought. Writing almost 35 years ago, Dr. Henry Sigerist, the great medical historian, said, "The state can protect society very effectively against a great many dangers, but the cultivation of health, which requires a definite mode of living, remains, to a large extent, an individual matter."[16] But individual activity and behavior can be promoted, aided, and encouraged by the state in many ways. We have not acted on such knowledge. Discipline is more demanding than shopping for health. Moreover, there is no significant interest group, no professional constituency, no lobby, for health itself—only for health services that can be purchased. Thus, we may be in danger of inflating ourselves into an over-medicated society and increasingly exposing ourselves to iatrogenic illness.

Make no mistake, I am not advocating a retreat into the past or an abandonment of medical services. There is much to be done in health care itself. I strongly favor and advocate comprehensive national health insurance, I was pressing for prepaid group practice many years before it became a popular cause, and I feel it essential that we have a more equitable deployment and distribution of the resources we devote to health care. What I am pleading for here is some sense of balance in resource allocation, that we invest a reasonable proportion of future dollars, and a larger part of present dollars, in positive health promotion, including prevention (by which I do *not* mean primarily more and earlier visits to the doctor), health education, and health motivation. Nobody can guarantee results in health, whatever road we take. But it does seem reasonably clear that the prospective pay-off for investment in health promotion represents a far better bet for society than still more investment in an already prodigious health care economy. "In order to build its own future, each generation must learn both to utilize its past and to escape it."[17]

REFERENCES AND NOTES

[1] Department of Health, Education and Welfare. *Estimated Health Expenditures Under Selected National Health Insurance Bills—A Report to Congress,* July 1974 (processed), p. 3.

[2] Worthington, N. L. "National Health Expenditures, 1929-74," *Social Security Bulletin,* February 1975, p. 5.

[3] *Journal of the American Medical Association,* November 19, 1973, pp. 910, 918. Estimates, 1973-74, from Association of American Medical Colleges.

[4] Association of American Medical Colleges, Task Force on Foreign Medical Graduates. *Graduates of Foreign Medical Schools in the United States: A Challenge to Medical Education* (Washing-

ton, D.C.: AAMC, March 22, 1974) Table 1. Also, Department of Health, Education and Welfare. *The Foreign Medical Graduate and Physician Manpower in the U.S.* DHEW Publication No. (HRA) 74-30; (Washington, D.C.: DHEW, 1974).

[5] Weiss, R. J., *et al.* "The Effect of Importing Physicians—Return to a Pre-Flexnerian Standard," *New England Journal of Medicine* 290:1453–1457 (June 27, 1974); and Weiss, *et al.*, "Foreign Medical Graduates and the Underground," *New England Journal of Medicine* 290:1408-1413 (June 20, 1974). Also see: Dublin, T. D. "Foreign Physicians: Their Impact on U.S. Health Care," *Science* 187:407-414 (August 2, 1974).

[6] Department of Health, Education and Welfare, Office of the Secretary. *Towards a Comprehensive Health Policy for the 1970s—A White Paper* (Washington, D.C.: DHEW, May 1971) p. 37.

[7] Department of Health Education and Welfare, Health Services Administration, Bureau of Community Health Services. *Community Health Service* (Washington, D.C.: DHEW, April 1974).

[8] *Statistical Abstract of the United States,* 1974, p. 60; Department of Health, Education and Welfare, National Center for Health Statistics. *Mortality Trends: Age, Color, and Sex, United States, 1950-69,* Series 20, No. 15 (1973) p. 14.

[9] *Ibid.,* p. 3 ff.

[10] These and data in the next three paragraphs are from *ibid;* Department of Health, Education and Welfare, National Center for Health Statistics. *Mortality Trends for Leading Causes of Death: U.S., 1950-69* Series 20, No. 16 (1974); and *Leading Components of Upturn in Mortality of Men: U.S. 1952-67* (1971).

[11] Department of Health, Education and Welfare, National Center for Health Statistics. *Vital Statistics of the United States, 1972: Vol. 11* Section 5, Life Tables, DHEW Publication No. (HRA) 75-1147, p. 5-15.

[12] Fuchs, Victor R. *Who Shall Live?* (New York: Basic Books, Inc., 1975) p. 31 ff.

[13] Neuhauser, Duncan. "The Future of Proprietaries in American Health Services," in: Havighurst, C. C. (ed.) *Regulating Health Facilities Construction* (Washington, D.C.: American Enterprise Institute for Public Policy Research, 1974) pp. 233-237.

[14] Powell, J. Enoch. *Medicine and Politics* (London: Pitman Medical Publishing Co., 1966) ch. 4.

[15] Dubos, René. *Man, Medicine, and Environment* (New York: New American Library, 1968) p. 119.

[16] Sigerist, Henry. *Medicine and Human Welfare* (New Haven: Yale University Press, 1941) p. 103.

[17] Davis, Michael M. *Medical Care for Tomorrow* (New York: Harper and Brothers, 1955) p. 434.

SUBJECT INDEX

Accountability,
 administrator, 112, 133-134
 .governing authority, 86, 97, 100-101
 medical staff, 10, 13, 86, 133
 of hospitals, 338-339, 360
Accrediting Commission on Education for Health Services Administration, 11
Administrator,
 accountability, 112-113, 133-134
 and unionism, 212-214, 242-245
 as decision-maker, 285-289, 309
 as manager, 46-47
 as professional, 113-114
 authority, 25-26, 28, 347
 challenges of, 41, 123, 164, 174-175
 functions, 11-12, 60-61, 112-113
 responsibility, 7, 26, 111-112
 to governing authority, 78-79, 118-119
 to medical staff, 119-120, 125, 133-134
 see also, Triad
American College of Surgeons, 6
American Hospital Association, 87, 206, 248, 345, 447
American Medical Association, 106, 447, 462
American Nurses Association, 206, 223-224, 250-251
Arbitration, *see* Unionization
Authority,
 hierarchy, 29, 58
 hospital, 21-22
 multiple lines, 23, 25-26

Bargaining units, 210, 223-224, *see also,* Unionization
Behavior,
 and leadership, 185
 approach to management, 108-109
 organizational, 22
 see also, Motivation, Needs
Blue Cross, 337, 339, 386-387, 392, 414
Board of trustees,
 see, Governing authority
 see also, Triad
Break-even analysis, 381-383
Budgets, 277, 390-391
Bureaucracy, 26, 56, 59

Capital budgeting, 320-329
Chief executive officer, *see* Administrator
Collective bargaining, *see* Unionization
Consumers, 81, 97, 99, 112, 339, 368
Constitution, 331-333
Control,
 and physicians, 13, 349
 over hospitals, 339, 360, 439
 need, 23-24
 process, 277
 techniques, 277
Coordination, 21, 23-24, 26, 34-38, 41, 43, 108, 111, 138
Cost-benefit analysis, 320-329

Decision-making,
 and administrator, 117
 and governance, 45
 defined, 274
 group, 193-194
 participatory, 30
 process, 275-276, 286-289
 resource allocation, 111, 273-274, 288-291, 295, 308-309
 types of, 274-275
 see also, Quantitative techniques
Delegation,
 and governing authority, 86
 attitudes, 200-201
 benefits, 157
 defined, 157-158
 description, 25
 process, 122, 201-202
 risks, 158, 199-200
Division of labor, 20-21, 24, 34, 58

Educational programs, 11
Environment
 and planning, 365-370, 376
 and systems, 54
 and unionization, 205-206
 as restrictor, 1, 273-274, 336-337
 health care, I iv-vi
 impact, 64
 to administration, 110
Effectiveness/Efficiency, 23, 28, 68, 132,

469

470   Index

147, 339, 350, 360, 378-379, 386, 412, 424, 426

Flexner report, 5

Governing authority,
  accountability, 85-86, 101, 133-134
  and mergers, 66-67
  authority, 25-26
  characteristics, 75, 99
  composition, 88-89, 97, 125-126
  consumer representatives, 99-100
  physician involvement, 91-96
  responsibility, 76-77, 84-85, 351-354
  roles, 10-11, 20, 98
  structure, 100
  to administrator, 78-79, 118-119
  to medical staff, 79-81, 119-120
  to public, 81-82
  see also, Triad
Governance,
  perspective on, 84-89
  problems of, 43-45
  see also, Triad
Government involvement,
  and construction, 458-459
  financing, 339
  history, 7, 331-336
  pressure, 10
Grievance procedure, 232-233, 246, 269-272.
  see also, Unionization

Health administration,
  as a profession, 12, 106, 113-114
  as a system, 57-60, 105
  definition, 109-110, 114
  education programs, 11
  specialty field, 105
  see also, Administrator
Health care,
  as a right, 331, 338, 346, 356-358
  crisis, I i, 331, 447
  costs, 91, 425, 435-456
  industry, I i-vi, 106-108
  non-crisis, 423-447
  politicizing, 336, 446
Health Maintenance Organizations, 273, 339, 424, 428, 459
Health policy, 460-462, see also, Policy, Societal attitudes

Hierarchy, 12, 29, 34, 43, 167, see also, Organization
Hill-Burton, 458, 462
Hippocrates, 2
Hospital,
  admissions, I iii
  and change, 336-337
  and politics, 336
  and production, 21, 47-49
  anomaly, 43
  as a matrix, 37-40
  as a social system, 60, 164-168, 358-359
  as a system, I iv-vi, 57-58
  authoritarian, 21-22
  characteristics of, 21, 27-28, 345
  complexity, I iv-v, 1-2, 13, 20-21, 93, 132
  constraints on, 336-338
  coordination, 34-36
  corporate structure, 7-9, 64-72, 87-88, 347, 430-431
  consolidation, 6-7
  data, I iv, 6-7
  definition, 19
  history, 2-7
  investor-owned, 70-72, 430-431
  objectives, 19, 60, 171, 177, 354
  organization chart, 8-9
  regulation, 337, 438-442
  role in delivery, I i, 5-6, 354-361
  structure, 38, 46-48
  types of, I iii-iv
  see also, Joint venture, Organization
Hospitalization insurance, see National Health Insurance
Informal organization, 162-163, 166-167, see also, Organization, Management
Input-output, I iv-viii, 97, 109-110, 147, 277, 290, 311, 396-398, 430
Insurance, see National Health Insurance
Involvement,
  employee, 195
  physician, 91-95

Job satisfaction, 149-150, 156-157, 170-171, see also, Motivation, Needs
Joint Commission on Accreditation of Hospitals, 6, 65, 91, 141, 274, 337, 363, 414
Joint ventures,
  conditions, 64-65
  failure, 67
  objectives, 65-66, 339

Labor legislation,
  Non-profit Hospital Amendments to the Taft-Hartley Act, 206, 208-210, 221, 249-250
  Norris-LaGuardia Act, 205
  Taft-Hartley Act, 205, 207-208, 221, 226-227, 234-235
  Wagner Act, 205, 207, 221
  see also, Unionization
Labor organization, 250-251
Labor relations, see Unionization
Leadership,
  and change, 194
  and medical staff, 131
  and motivation, 150
  definition, 150
  decision-authority, 151
  effectiveness, 186-188
  leader, 194-195
  participative, 156-157, 194-197
  supervision, 151-152
  styles, 177-182, 184
Licensure,
  medical staff, 12
  providers, 338
Line-staff, 25
Linear programming, 308-314

Maximization, 286-288, 310-312
Management by objectives, 196
Medical care,
  evolution, 2-4, 333-334
  scientific, 5
Medical education, 4-5, 457-458
Medical staff,
  accountability, 10, 13, 34
  and PSRO, 412-413
  authority, 25-26
  conflict, 138-139, 349
  effectiveness, 141-143
  leadership, 131
  organization, 36-37, 94, 126-129, 132, 137-143
  management, 132-133
  role, 12-13
  to governing authority, 79-81
  to administrator, 119-120, 125, 133-134
  see also, Triad
Medicare-Medicaid, 271, 334-336, 346, 387-389, 392-393, 413, 425, 446-447, 456

Morale, see Motivation, Needs
Motivation, 147-150, 156, 169-171, 177, 193, 211, see also, Job satisfaction, Needs
Management,
  and administrator, 46
  and medical staff, 132-133
  and systems theory, 54
  approaches, 107-109
  need for, 44, 132
  participative, 156-157, 193-197, 212
  styles of, 30-33, 46
  theories of, 34, 57-59, 108, 184-185
  theory X, Y, 154-155
  see also, Hospital administration, Leadership, Organization

National Health Insurance,
  alternatives, 448
  and crisis, 424
  and Medicare, 334-336
  and politics, 446-447, 463
  coverage, 436-437, 450-453
  defined, 448
  equity, 449-454
  financing, 338
  goals, 448-449
  history of, 444-446
  legislation, 450-453
National Labor Relations Board, 210, 222-224, 252, 260, 230-231, see also, Taft-Hartley Act
Needs, 51, 147-149, 162, 165-166, 211-212, see also, Job satisfaction, Motivation
Negotiation, 207-208, 226-232, see also, Unionization
Nightingale, Florence, 5, 11, 169
Nurse,
  and delegation, 199-203
  and leadership, 184
  and motivation, 169-175
  and unionization, 224, 249-255
  as professional, 249, 433
  as supervisor, 174, 184, 199
  authority, 25
  participant, 118, 433-434
  responsibility, 26
Nursing,
  evolution, 5
  specialization, 20

Occupational roles, 20

Operations research,
  linear programming, 316-319
  history, 278
  queuing, 316-319
  techniques, 294-300
  see also, Quantitative techniques
Organization,
  attitude, 165
  authoritarian, 21
  change, 167
  classical theory, 29-31, 57-58, 60, 108
  hospital as, 25
  mergers, 64-73
  other forms, 38-39, 45, 59
  traditional, 46-49
  see also, Hospital, Informal organization

Participative management, *see* Leadership, Management
Patient care, 19, 21, 27, 126-128, 171, 177, 193
Patient care team, 37, 40
Personnel,
  physicians, 25, 93, 131, 141, 457-458
  types of, 20, 24
  see also, Medical staff, Nurse
Physician, *see* Medical staff
Planning,
  agencies, 86-87, 107, 339
  and environment, 365-370
  and reimbursement, 388-389
  benefits, 376
  committees, 363-376
  Comprehensive Health Planning Act, 1966, 335, 458-459
  medical staff, 130
  PL 93-641, 86-87, 273, 446, 459, 462
  premises, 365
  process, 276-277, 350
Policy,
  and NHI, 444-448
  and politics, 460-461
  implementors, 12, 97
  makers, 77, 85, 97, 110
  social, 45, 273
Professionalism, 21-22, 24-25, 33-34, 50-51, 106, 250
Prospective reimbursement,
  bases of payment, 390-393
  definition, 377
  elements of, 378
  implications of, 379-381
  impact of, 393-398
  incentives, 273, 384-386
  purpose, 339, 378-379
  rate setting, 398-407
  see also, Reimbursement
PSRO's,
  activities, 414-415
  and care, 339
  as constraint, 142, 273, 462
  issues, 416-418
  legislation, 411-412
  organization, 412-413

Quality assurance, 338-339
Quality of care,
  and governing authority, 11
  constraints, 339
  control, 434
Quantitative techniques,
  applications, 276-278
  types of, 277-278, 292-293, 297-300, 308-314, 316-329
  see also, Decision-making
Queuing theory, 289-299, 316-319

Recognition, 207, 208, 221-222, *see also,* Unionization
Regulation,
  and hospitals, 438-442
  as a utility, 337
  limitations, 110, 337, 338
Reimbursement,
  and control, 431
  retrospective, 377, 383, 425-427
  types of, 107-108
  see also, Prospective reimbursement, National Health Insurance
Rights,
  distributive, 331-332, 338
  natural, 331-332
  see also, Health care

Scientific medicine, 4-5, 44
Simulation, 278
Societal attitudes,
  and health care, 132, 331, 425, 436
  and hospitals, 5-6, 356-357, 361
  and NHI, 338, 444-447
  and unionization, 213
  as a patient, 172, 193-194

Solicitation, 238, 260-266, *see also,* Unionization
Specialization, *see* Division of labor
Status, 12, 167
Supervision, *see* Leadership
Systems,
 and health administration, 105-111
 characteristics, 55
 concept, I iv-vi
 definition, 53-54
 subsystems, 62-63, 274, 423

Taft-Hartley Act,
 effect of, 207-208
 provisions, 207, 240-241
 unfair labor practices, 207, 224-226, 249-251
 1974 hospital amendments, 208-210, 226-227, 249-250
 see also, Unionization
Third party payers, 45, 92, 107, 110, 339, 377
Triad, 7, 25-26, 43-45, 97, *see also,* Administrator, Governing authority, Medical staff

Unionization,
 and administrator, 212-214, 242-245
 and needs, 148
 and strikes, 213, 247-248
 arbitration, 233-234
 bargaining units, 223
 causes of, 211-212, 245-247, 232-233
 government involvement, 206-211
 grievance procedure, 232-233, 246, 269-272
 history of, 205-206
 issues, 238-239
 negotiation, 221-222
 organizers, 261-262
 solicitation, 260-267
 unfair labor practices, 207, 224-226, 249-251
 see also, Labor legislation, Taft-Hartley
Utilities, 337-338. 438-442
Utilization review, 94, 339

COLLEGE LIBRARY
SUFFOLK UNIVERSITY
BOSTON, MASS. 02114